MITR

Manual for Immunohematology and Transfusion Residents

Dr. Abhishekh B

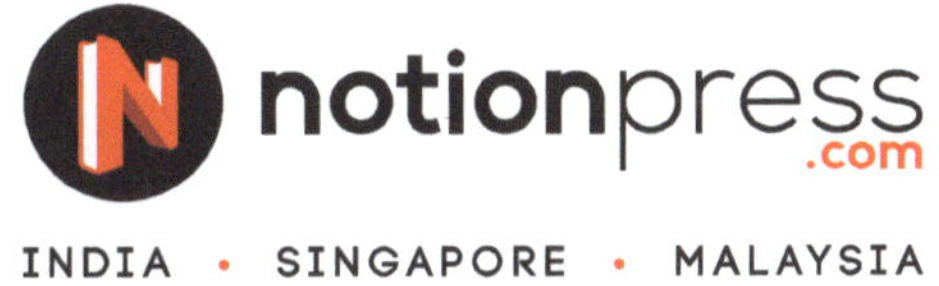

notionpress
.com

INDIA · SINGAPORE · MALAYSIA

ISBN 979-8-88849-371-7

CONTENTS

Section I
Introduction to Transfusion Medicine Residency

Section II
General Skills

Section III
Specific Divisions of Transfusion Medicine

Section IV
Applied Transfusion Medicine and allied specialities

Section V
Management of blood Transfusion Services

Section VI
Concluding Residency

FOREWORD

I feel elated and honoured to be allowed to write the foreword for the first edition of the *Manual for Immunohematology and Transfusion Residents* written by Dr. B. Abhishekh, Additional Professor of the Department of Transfusion Medicine, JIPMER, Puducherry. Dr. Abhishekh is my esteemed colleague in JIPMER, and I have known him since 2014, when he joined the department as a dynamic Assistant Professor. His enthusiasm and concern for transfusion practices, patient care and, most of all, the training of the residents are unmatched. 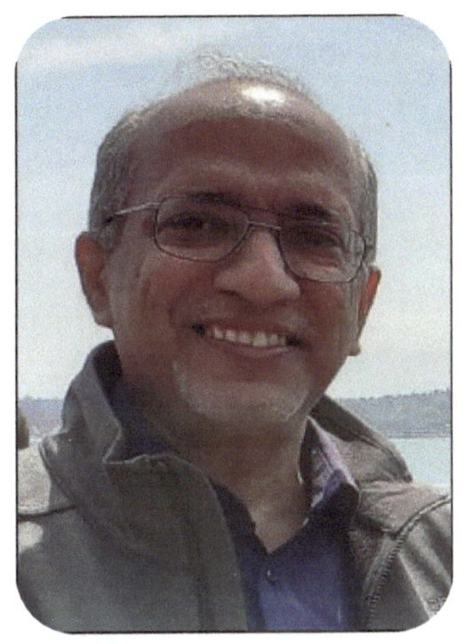

MD Transfusion Medicine is a relatively new postgraduate course in the country, having started only as recently in 2000. Dr. Abhishekh, himself being one of the first postgraduates to earn a degree in the country from a state medical college, is well versed in tribulations and the challenges a trainee in this field has to face. The growth of the Transfusion Medicine practice has been exponential in the past two decades. This is reflected in the growth of the Department at JIPMER as well, ever since it became an independent department in 2009. Dr. Abhishekh has been an integral part of the development of the department, which now boasts of having trained more than 20 postgraduates to date. It is also the training ground for MD Pathology, BSc Blood Banking, fellowship in Apheresis and other clinical postgraduate and super-speciality courses.

With all these years of teaching and clinical experience, the author has put the essential elements of the subject in a student-friendly manner. From its inception, the manual has been intended to fulfil the needs of a trainee in Transfusion Medicine to understand the basic principles governing the subject in a simple language and concise format. It covers all the aspects of Transfusion Medicine. The first section, Introduction to Transfusion Medicine Residency, where the words of a trainee have been included, is an apt way to start a manual. The manual also discusses in detail topics ranging from General Skills of educational science, Specific divisions of Transfusion Medicine, Applied Transfusion Medicine and allied specialities, Exam Preparation, Documentation, Biomedical waste management, Equipment Maintenance, Irradiation lab and safety to Career path after postgraduation. It covers almost all the essentials of blood banking, from donor counselling, and blood grouping, to the complex technical procedures of flow cytometry and apheresis. Another exciting aspect of the manual is the selection of authors who have contributed to the book, ranging from eminent academicians in the field to postgraduate students themselves.

The enormous time and effort to put together the essential elements of the subject are laudable. The manual will be handy for the MD trainees as a resource material for enriching their knowledge and practice of the subject.

Prof. Debdatta Basu

Former Professor and Head,
Department of Transfusion Medicine
JIPMER

PREFACE

Manual for Immunohematology and Transfusion Residents is intentionally abbreviated as "MITR." "Mitr" is a Sanskrit word "मित्र", which means a friend or companion. This book will serve as a companion/friend for all the residents in the field, which will always be with them right from entering the residency till completing it and after that.

Why this book

This book is not intended to be a reference book but a book every resident should carry with him for daily routine work as a quick guide.

Motivation and Inspiration

When I started my journey as a resident in Transfusion Medicine in 2008, it was not an era of information technology or e-resources. It was when we had to go to internet centres to access mail. As I belonged to the first batch, it was a tough challenge to get resources, and we entirely relied on the old copies of Petz, and Rossi, which were available in the library. None of the bookshops was selling any of the Transfusion Medicine books, which are postgraduate level, as there were hardly any buyers. Most of the things which are of practical importance were given in minor detail in those books.

Process: It all started when I was a postgraduate resident student, wherein I had made notes for myself while studying. As things started getting outdated and needed to update, I converted those to soft copies for easy updating.

Challenges and how long

My wife, Dr. Nalini YC, has been the constant support of motivation and support not only for writing this book but for me taking up this field due to her prior exposure as a resident in clinical pathology. Having already authored a book, she constantly kept me pushing and timely advised me many times when I had paused pursuing the completion of this piece.

The book has been divided into six sections with about 40 chapters. The section I introduces you to getting into residency, what you expect out of it and what is expected of you. Section II introduces you to a few general skills required for residents in any field but here with particular reference to this field.

Section III consists of the core topics of the typical rotation of a resident in Transfusion Medicine, like donor section, Immunohematology, Components, TTI, QC etc., with primarily practical tips and not as a replacement to either a theory book or technical manual of Transfusion Medicine.

Section IV consists of the topics from allied departments that are directly relevant to Transfusion Medicine, which the residents usually cover in their residency as part of their peripheral rotation.

Section V covers the topics relevant to managerial aspects of blood transfusion services. Furthermore, finally, section VI consists of topics that will be helpful throughout your career with an insight into what would be ahead of you after completing residency.

The book has been organised and written to cover the aspects covered by guidelines for the competency-based postgraduate training programme for MD in immunohematology and blood transfusion by the Medical Council of India.

Wishing you all the Best

I would urge you to be the best, not good or great, but the Best Dr. Abhishekh B

Contributors

Dr. Esha Toora Senior Resident Department of Transfusion Medicine JIPMER, Puducherry	**Dr. Shahida N** Senior Resident Department of Transfusion Medicine JIPMER, Puducherry	**Dr. John Gnanaraj** Senior Resident Department of Transfusion Medicine CMC, Vellore
Dr. Charumathy A Senior Resident Department of Transfusion Medicine SGPGIMS, Lucknow	**Dr. Anuragaa S** Fellow Department of Clinical Haematology CMC, Vellore	**Dr. Ketan P** Assistant Professor Department of Microbiology AIIMS, Patna
Dr. Ajai R Senior Resident Department of Emergency Medicine JIPMER, Puducherry	**Dr. Sujaya Mazumder** Assistant Professor Department of Pathology AIIMS, Kalyani	**Dr. Dibyajyoti Sahoo** Assistant Professor Department of Transfusion Medicine JIPMER, Puducherry
Dr. Manu Assistant Professor Department of Emergency Medicine JIPMER, Puducherry	**Dr. Prabhu M** Associate Professor Department of Pathology JIPMER, Puducherry	**Dr. Soumya Das** Assistant Professor Department of Transfusion Medicine AIIMS, Nagpur
Dr. Satyam Arora Associate Professor Department of Transfusion Medicine PGICH, Noida	**Dr. Nalini Y C** Associate Professor Department of Physiology Mahatma Gandhi Medical College, Puducherry	**Dr. Veena Shenoy** Associate Professor Department of Transfusion Medicine AIMS, Kochi

Dr. Uday Krishna Associate Professor Department of Radiotherapy Kidwai Memorial Institute of Oncology, Bengaluru	**Dr. Rafi M** Associate Professor Department of Transfusion Medicine Jubilee Mission Medical College, Thrissur	**Dr. Shaiji P S** Associate Professor Department of Transfusion Medicine Government Medical College, Kollam
Dr. Arun R Additional Professor Department of Transfusion Medicine AIIMS, Bibinagar	**Dr. Mohandoss M** Additional Professor Transfusion Medicine(Division) Malabar Cancer Centre, Thalassery	**Dr. Yogesh S** Additional Professor Department of Anatomy JIPMER, Puducherry
Dr. Remi R Consultant in Transfusion Medicine Lisie Hospital, Kochi	**Dr. Puneet Jain** Specialist in Transfusion Medicine Ministry of Health, Saudi Arabia	**Dr. Srikanth U** Lecturer Department of Paraclinical Sciences The University of West Indies, St. Augustine, Trinidad
Dr. Shamee Shastry Professor Department of Transfusion Medicine Kasturba Medical College, Manipal	**Dr. Sajith Menon** Professor Department of Transfusion Medicine Government Medical College, Wayanad	**Dr. Zayapragassarazan** Professor Department of Medical Education JIPMER, Puducherry

Section I

Introduction to Transfusion Medicine Residency

Stepping into the Shoes of a Transfusion Medicine Resident

–Dr. John, Dr. Esha

TRANSITION FROM UG TO PG RESIDENCY

Knowledge, skills, and performance:

"Oh, O Negative blood group is the universal donor; probably, we can transfuse O plasma to any blood group."

"Cryoprecipitate! Is that a new fancy blood product?"

"Mam, can I get 4 SDPs for this bleeding patient? Oh, right. Is it RDPs? What is the difference"?

"Sir, his Hb is 9.6g/dL. We want to transfuse one PRBC because the patient has tachycardia and blood pressure slightly on the lower side...."

These were some of my thoughts as I walked down the corridor, collecting blood for the entire ward as a young, naive intern with ever-burning hope and fiery eyes. The World was not enough; **I felt like House MD most of the time**, walking around the hospital in my tired shoes and pale apron.

We shall live without repercussions for the first and last time in our lives and shall not be held responsible for any action or blunder we make. Most of us agree that undergraduate days and internships were the best time of our lives. Most of the time, we had the comfort of our friends and colleagues, who stood by us no matter what and made us feel that we belonged somewhere in the World. No signs and symptoms of an existential crisis or degree, not even a single day. It felt like you were on the path of adulthood but were still caught up inside your bubble of close company and thoughts.

The slow transformation from an undergraduate to a postgraduate- what changes......?

The transformation from an undergraduate to a postgraduate and the responsibilities that came with it **were unforgiving yet so much fun**.

It was no longer carefree days and blurry nights; instead, it was adventurous and lifesaving.

Residency is more like an educational stepping stone to real life, where you face harsh realities and crucial decision-making skills. Residency prepares you for life. Looking back at my residency in transfusion medicine, I can confidently say I have learned more in the 2-3 years than in my entire life and continue doing so.

The shift from Spinal reflex towards corticospinal reflex

UG days:

We would have spent more time as mindless chilled-out interns waiting for the blood products at the blood bank. It was more than a haven in times of stress and everyday let-downs and a second home to most of us. Our movie dates were planned as the packed red blood cells were cross-matched.

The blood bank is the heart of any hospital, the life-giver. Many memorable friendships were made at the blood bank; we caught up with our batch mates at the blood bank. "Where are you posted? Been a long time?" It was the chilliest place and the hub of all gossip. Undergraduate life was an excellent time to be a tad ignorant (kind of bliss if you ask me) and alive. There was nothing that could hold us down. "Wake up, work hard, learn something new and party hard!" used to be our motto.

The internship was about learning new skills daily; we were young blood, wanting to get the best out of each day. We learned as much as we could as we went along with each passing day. Life and medical skills were essential, and we always had someone above us, a resident or senior, to guide us through difficult medical situations. We were pampered and spoon-fed throughout the internship.

Most of the time, the work we did was what we call spinal work, as someone above us was giving orders on who should get a blood transfusion and who not to transfuse. Indication for blood transfusion was barely understood. Before a transfusion, we never asked the "why, when and what" questions. The only goal was to finish the blood transfusions at the earliest so that work could get over soon. The phrase "Okay fine, just take one PRBC and make sure the patient attendees donate..." became more familiar than any caller tune. It was a never-ending vicious cycle, arguing with the transfusion medicine resident over a blood transfusion that we knew might not be indicated, producing sometimes real, sometimes fake donation numbers to procure blood as soon as possible, and hasty blood transfusions were going on at a regular pace.

PG days:

The day we enter as a postgraduate student in the Department of Transfusion Medicine after completing the internship, we would first experience considerable responsibilities on our shoulders, more than we could fathom and carry. We realise that the decisions we make are going to have crucial implications and consequences. From then on, the decisions we make must be supported by clinical knowledge and adequate evidence.

Residency feels more about owning up to your mistakes and learning from them than trying to run away, which might look easier, but then you lose up on valuable education at the end of the day. The realisations would be endless; you got to be on your feet all the time to learn something new every day. Yes, the residency is a different ball game, a torpedo you see coming, and you should be well prepared. The learning opportunities are endless if you pounce on them as they knock at your door.

Also, in residency, you must learn that "you are on your own." It entirely depends on your ability and skill to make or break your future and career. It is entirely up to us how we want to spend our time at transfusion medicine residency. There is so much to learn and appreciate in this branch, which most of us would not have realised in our undergraduate days. In particular of all medical sciences, transfusion medicine is a beautiful and exotic branch with a small amount of the best of every other field because everyone needs blood. If there is no blood, there is no life.

Residency should be a combination of the right kind of chill and read. A delicate balance must be achieved to maintain your sanity and get the best education possible from whichever institute you are currently in for residency. These days will be some of the most challenging ones and a fantastic learning experience on their own. There will be difficult days that make you wonder, "What are you doing with your life?" "Have you chosen the right branch of medicine?" and is it all worth it?

Adapting and learning:

Nevertheless, as time goes by and you become comfortable at work, you will eventually realise this was you are calling all the while, and you have indeed chosen what is best for you. You will start loving work and will be thirsty to learn more and more every moment of your life thenceforth.

There is no dearth of guidance and help from the consultants and seniors as they have walked along the same path as you are on right now. If you are prepared to work without complaint and yearn to learn, the World will conspire to make you one of the best transfusion medicine specialists someday. Work is worship. The skills you learn here will stick with you throughout your life. Your performance at work will reflect upon your dedication and hard work. If you are ready to go, reach for the stars.

Importance of proper communications.

"What! Do you know that what you are asking for is not an indication of platelet transfusion? Do you understand?"

I do not know how much I need to emphasise good communication skills. You will work in a professional environment, meeting multiple people for different reasons. Learning the art of talking politely and communicating well is imperative to earn a good reputation and rapport in a professional place. There will be countless situations where it seems the only way out is to argue. There will be times when emotions may get the better of us than actual logical common sense. The thought will often blind us that we are right all the time.

The truth is that this is a learning curve, and we can learn something new only when we readily accept that we might be wrong. There will be situations where we might strongly feel that a blood transfusion is not indicated and might have a heated argument with the clinical departments. However, if we listen carefully to the other side of the story, there might be something important that we missed. Always be open to acknowledging that you may be wrong, and there is something to learn new every time. **Effective communication skills begin only when you start listening.**

You can only acquire a higher sense of right and wrong when you start to listen carefully to your seniors and colleagues who are constantly looking out for you. Work etiquette also is essential to earn grace from your consultants, seniors and co-workers. Becoming a PG, you have to start working your way right from the bottom of the food chain. You can work your way up to the top with sheer patience, good etiquette, skills, dedication, persistence, and the right kind of chill attitude.

"Oh, I can do anything and everything on my own; I do not need anyone's help; I am a resident now!"

This was my thought when I first entered residency; it was a difficult transition leaving all my UG friends behind and preparing for the hostility that comes with life and work. However, I was wrong. If you find one good friend who stands by you and helps you grow personally and professionally, you are lucky indeed in your postgraduate life. Everyone needs someone to hold on to, especially during the tough residency days, to keep you alive.

Residency days might make you feel lost and hopeless quickly. Finding someone you can trust and know got your back when you fall may be challenging. The residency will not be work pressure alone; you will be challenged with betrayal, heartbreak, loneliness, marital pressures, family problems, depression, and existential crises. Hence the saying, "when the going gets tough, the tough get going."

If you feel another human being's vibes are at the same level as you, you know that this partnership will last with the correct sustenance effort. The most important thing to remember during residency is that it is a **learning and self-improvement phase.** Even if you are beaten down with so many difficulties and challenges, you always have people to talk to and help you out of any predicament you might be in. You can get better at what you love doing besides work, be it music, art, dance, critique, debates, or the things that make you a human being. Find resources and places that help you grow into a better person alongside a better physician as well. Moreover, finally, when **you got no one, you always got yourself.**

Social and Psychological changes:

Problems always happen when you work with another human being. There will be creative differences, attitude differences, and, most of the time, plain misunderstandings. Nevertheless, you will learn to put aside your differences and look at the big picture during residency. There will be a necessity always to have a good team spirit.

You might not have realised during your internship; how important it is to have good teamwork to get the best out of your work. During residency, each sub-section of transfusion medicine, such as immunohematology, apheresis, blood donation camps, donor complex, etc., will require an effort of a team of consultants, senior residents, seniors, juniors, nursing staff, helping staff and housekeeping, volunteers, drivers, etc. As you earn more responsibilities, you get to learn to give respect and take respect and earn your rightful place in the team if you want your opinions to be valued and respected.

In that case, you must learn to communicate well and in good spirits and diffuse stressful workplace situations with your leadership and ability to earn trust and respect in your professional workplace. Honing your leadership skills and being one is very necessary for the field of transfusion medicine.

Unlike any other branch of medicine, you will be going to places, camps, meetings, rallies, etc., to spread awareness of the importance of blood donation and blood transfusion.

You will be expected to show maturity and leadership skills very early. Identifying and solving problems will become a daily routine for all of us doing a transfusion medicine residency. Knowing the literature about the subject is essential to establish respect and trust, building your leadership qualities quickly and being comfortable giving opinions and counselling residents of other clinical departments about safe and effective blood transfusion.

Maintaining trust and relations with others:

All good friendships, bonds, and relationships in life are built on trust. First, let me talk about trusting yourself and your decisions before anything else. Always think for yourself; trust your intuition before trusting others. Most of the time, it is never about having all the answers but trusting yourself and learning in the direction of what feels right and learning the best way you can. And then comes all other things.

I remember how I counted on my co-interns, who are also my best friends now, with all my life for, in fact, everything. I always knew they got my back wherever I was and in whatever situation I faced. You must earn your street creds in terms of trust and respect at work so that you will be in a comfortable position to advise other departments about blood-related issues.

Always remember to have the burning yearning to learn something new every day, acquire knowledge, develop new skills and techniques and be at the top-notch of your performance each day. Trust and respect for yourself and others are also significant, leading to personal growth, effective communication, sustained partnerships at work, and better team spirit.

Workload and content

"I do not know how I will handle those hectic residency days; Studying for entrance examinations is one, but working every day for 12 hours will need some next-level determination!"

These were a few thoughts during those cumbersome entrance exam preparation days. Yes, the first day I walked into my department, the realities were told as they were. There will be days where I might have to skip meals; there might be sleepless nights, continuous duties, thesis protocol presentation, departmental work, tests, assignments, seminars, journal clubs and just routine work, which can sometimes go on for 12 hours a day in the first year of residency. Nevertheless, what does not kill you makes you stronger.

There will be good times, too, such as when you work up your first Autoimmune Haemolytic Anaemia case and provide a lifesaving compatible unit for the patient or after your first hematopoietic stem cell collection and cryopreservation. However, you have to strive for these simple moments of joy of learning. The subject is so vast that you can learn something new every day. Transfusion medicine is new and exciting; there is always room for discoveries and eureka moments, especially in your apheresis posting and immunohematology section of transfusion medicine.

The first six months will be difficult. There will be many activities going around you. You might have difficulty getting used to the work, place, environment, long hours, and sometimes food.

However, the silver lining is that the whole universe and everyone around you will conspire only to help you and make you comfortable. Your consultants, seniors, colleagues, technicians, and blood bank staff always look out for you and ensure you are doing well. You have people to talk to about any difficulties you might face. Of course, it might be challenging to get used to the new learning environment initially, but we are all in it together. At some point in life, everyone has walked down the same path as you are currently, and yes, we have all gotten through it together. The question is never if you will be able to cope with work but how you will cope, help is always around.

Coping and competence development

Always remember that the amount of time you spend at work, practically doing things, and getting your hands dirty, correlates to how much you will learn. Work is worship. Being proactive at work helps. Since you are no longer an undergraduate, a significant part of education involves you going around seeking skills, competence, and wisdom. Even if there are times when your work is over, and it was a long day, but your seniors are still at work going for a procedure like plasma exchange or cryopreservation, it will not harm you if you join along for the ride. You might get hands-on during the procedure and extra special training on what it is about. All that matters is grabbing all the opportunities knocking at your door and learning something new every day. Furthermore, it feels good to know that you learnt well that day.

The blood centre is **never a one-man army** but a team of capable people of various disciplines coming together to save lives. There are multiple resources and loads of people from whom you can acquire experience and knowledge. There are experienced technicians, nursing staff, cleaning staff, and office staff, some of them working here for decades, from whom you can learn valuable hacks, tricks and, of course, the subject.

Everyone has got a story to tell and lessons to teach. So one of the most important things is to develop an attitude that embraces learning from people you meet; it does not matter if small or big, rich or poor, educated or uneducated, you can always learn something which can blow your perspectives on life and transfusion medicine too as you move around getting to know people.

Preparation for residency

Talking about how to prepare for post-graduation life, let me tell you things as they are. You can never prepare for post-graduation. It is an experience; a roller coaster rides wherein you have to let go of yourself, trusting yourself and the people around you to smoothen the strenuous PG ride. A simple catch-your-breath at the beginning and end of the day will help you prepare for the day and the next. Have some time to reflect on what happened during the day and appreciate the simple things around you that you are being cared for.

Everything you do is a learning experience; stepping stones on the stairway make you a better human and doctor. Do not forget to enjoy the tiny pleasures of life like music, art, literature, and your passion which makes life better no matter how hard the day is. However, side by side, keep reading books pertaining to your field, so learning becomes more intuitive and fun.

Difficulties

Talking about some of the challenges you will face during your residency, especially the first year, let me say that every problem has a solution. Okay, so we are not exposed to immunohematology work during our UG and internship. It is an exceptional and different kind of work.

Our field involves getting around instruments and machines. In the beginning, you may find it hard during case workup, various apheresis procedures and the vibe in general. Even though we are a clinical field, you will not interact with most sick patients. Instead, you will be involved with screening healthy donors for voluntary blood donation, dealing with devices that prepare blood components, testing for transfusion-transmitted diseases and various apheresis procedures involving intricate programming and functioning machines.

You will have to develop skills that help you grow in both man and machines and sick and healthy people. A versatile branch that specialises in many things and gives you a wholesome two-sides-of-a-coin story. There is no better satisfaction than to realise that you have saved many lives.

HISTORY & FACTs

- The second oldest blood bank in the world was developed under Dr. U.C. Brahamachari at the present NRS Medical College Campus, Kolkata, during the second world war.
- The Bombay Blood or hh blood group is a rare blood phenotype first discovered in Mumbai (then called Bombay) in 1952 by Dr. Y.M. Bhende and Dr. H. M. Bhatia
- India has contributed a few rare blood groups, including the Bombay phenotype, Indian blood group antigens like In(a), In5 and I-i- phenotype by SR Joshi
- Dr. Jai Gopal Jolly, famously known as **Dr. J. G. Jolly** (Father of Transfusion Medicine in India)" is credited with establishing a department of excellence where he introduced postgraduate degrees in Transfusion Medicine for the first time in India in SGPGI Lucknow with the first MD Transfusion Candidate as Dr. Debasish Gupte (1989).
- Prof. R.N. Roy, who later on retired as the Prof. & Director Department of Medicine from Medical College, Kolkata, was involved as a Rockefeller fellow in one of the earliest bone marrow transplantation programmes involving cadaver marrow along with Hugh Chaplin Jr. He also developed a technique of plasma haemoglobin measurement with the same boss and the same technique is used till date.

Roles and Responsibility during Residency

– Dr. Soumya Das

Pillars of excellence in residency (the 3 As) -

availability, affability, and ability, in that order.

Introduction - Transfusion medicine is a field of medicine that is a hybrid of laboratory and clinical practices. A clinical field that encompasses all the fields of the medical field under one roof, with its lifesaving decisions and BLOOD. The field of transfusion medicine is ever-evolving. There is a need for an acceptable and dynamic system to keep pace with the rapidly changing knowledge base and technology. Three years of in-house training ensure imparting skills to perform and oversee routine and specialised tests in blood centres, transfusion services, and reference laboratories. They are also exposed to quality systems, regulatory affairs, and transfusion safety matters. They will also be trained to collect and analyse data and write a dissertation, a theory examination on the content and a clinical examination to test the abilities to recognise signs and symptoms.

The purpose of PG education in Transfusion Medicine is to create specialists who would provide high-quality health care and advance the cause of science through research & training.

This chapter describes the roles and responsibilities of a trainee during a transfusion medicine residency.

Skills to learn: Knowledge, Communication, Practical, Clinical, and Organisational

A typical rotation for a Resident in Transfusion Medicine and the corresponding roles and responsibilities would be as shown in the table.

Table 2.1 Typical rotation of a resident in Transfusion Medicine

	Section	Duration (In months)	Objectives/Roles and responsibilities
1	Orientation	1	• Biostatistics, Research Methodology, and Clinical Epidemiology • Ethics • Medico-legal aspects relevant to the discipline • Health Policy issues as may apply to the discipline • Institute-specific protocols. • Biosafety procedures in case of Needlestick Injuries, Spill management
2	Donor section	5	• Motivate donors and recruit them. • Make sure that the donors from whom blood is collected are healthy and free from diseases. Screening and medical examination of Whole blood, apheresis donation, including donors for special donation like granulocytes and Hematopoietic stem cells(allogeneic). • Examine patients for donations like autologous blood, marrow or stem cells or directed donations. Decision-making for the amount to be blood collected from the screened donor • Donor health advice for donors, including management of deferred donors. • Performing phlebotomy as and when required managing adverse reactions and prevention. • Therapeutic phlebotomy, assessment of the patient, and the management of patient and counselling • Coordinating with colleagues and staff posted in the phlebotomy room, teaching them safe and effective phlebotomy steps. • Learning the art of preventing blood donor reactions in predisposed donors. • Collaborate with the pre-transfusion testing resident for allocating fresh blood or blood with special requirements of donor selection • Identify problems in the blood collection area and offer a viable solution
	Camps		• Organising blood donation camps and motivating blood donors/organisers. • Selection and proper donor care in outdoor blood donation camps and ensuring cold chain maintenance. • Develop communication skills to word reports and professional opinions and also interact with blood donors, outdoor camp organisers

3	Component Laboratory	5	• Understand the principles of component preparation by various methods, and be familiar with preparing modified components such as leukofiltered, irradiated or saline washed, pooled, or volume-reduced components following aseptic conditions. • Instructing and supervising the technical staff on the preparation and storing of various blood components • Performing the QC of various components at regular intervals and ensuring the quality of components is meeting the QC criteria • Collaboration with the pretransfusion testing resident on decisions of maintaining platelet, cryo, FFP and CPP stock • Handling the troubleshooting and maintenance of all equipment in the component lab
4	TTI Laboratory	4	• Learn the principles of blood safety, including testing for various transfusion-transmitted infections (TTI), proper disposal of infectious waste, laboratory safety, and personnel safety. • Handling TTI troubleshooting and learning about the rectification • preparation and use of in-house external controls for the TTI lab • Demonstrate proficiency in preparing and interpreting LJ Chart and learn about root cause analysis (RCA) and Corrective and Preventive Action (CAPA) as and when required. • Perform donor notification and counselling, and referral
5	Pretransfusion lab	5	• Supervise/maintain an inventory of various blood components • Take decisions based on patient priority for issuing / restricting blood component • Transfusion consultation- dose and schedule • Planning and executing pretransfusion testing and customising based on recipient requirements • Modification of blood components as per the requirements of the patient • Evaluating the patient who had a transfusion reaction • Reviewing all the discrepant results noted by the technician during the pre-transfusion testing. • Ensuring proper utilisation of the returned unused blood components

6	Immunohematology Lab	5	• Performing ABO/Rh grouping, cross-matching, and other immunohematological tests as per departmental SOP
			• Performing, interpreting, and resolving discrepancies in pre-transfusion testing, ABO/Rh grouping, red cell antibody screen, antibody identification, elution-adsorption, secretor status
			• Management of various clinical conditions requiring immunohematological and transfusion support, including
			  o Multi-transfused patients such as thalassemia, sickle cell disease etc
			  o Alloimmunized antenatal cases(HDN)
			  o Transfusion reactions
			  o Immune hemolytic anaemias
			  o ABO mismatched transplants (BMT / Solid organ)

7	Apheresis section, including stem cells	3	• The resident should understand the mechanisms of apheresis donation, select apheresis donors, manage and prevent adverse donor reactions, and be able to obtain apheresis products meeting quality standards • Apheresis room management, including logistics • Perform QC of all the Apheresis products collected, including viability testing of stem cells • Be able to identify problems in the apheresis collection area and offer viable solutions

	Therapeutic section		• Selection and managing all patients with disorders requiring therapeutic apheresis, including cyto-apheresis and Plasmapheresis
			• Perform and train others in various therapeutic apheresis
			  o Therapeutic plasma exchange
			  o Erythracytapheresis
			  o Thrombocytapheresis
			  o Leukapheresis
			• Recognise nature, assess the significance and manage the complications related to the procedure and their management, Cryo-preservation of harvested products
			• Communicate effectively with clinicians and patients regarding procedures through conversations and writing of consult notes

8	Quality Assurance	1	• Maintenance of the quality of blood components, equipment, and reagents as per recommended standards and regulatory authorities • Develop skills for how SOPs and quality manuals are used, developed, authored, and reviewed and their importance in mandatory laboratory inspection by various accrediting agencies.

9	Peripheral postings	6	As per departmental necessities, refer table
10	Consolidation and Exam preparation	1	
	Total	**36**	

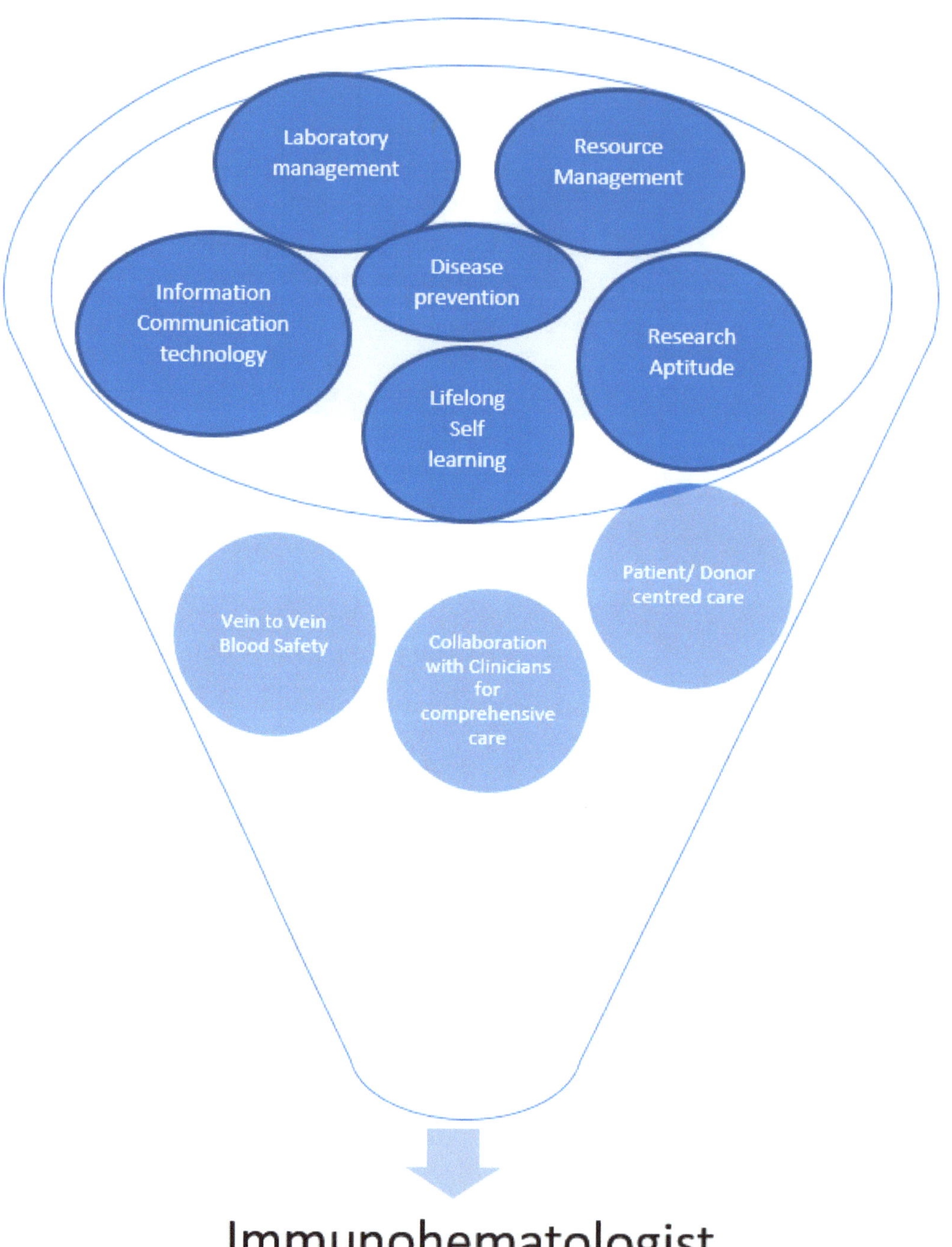

Figure 2.1. Core Principles of training in Immunohematology

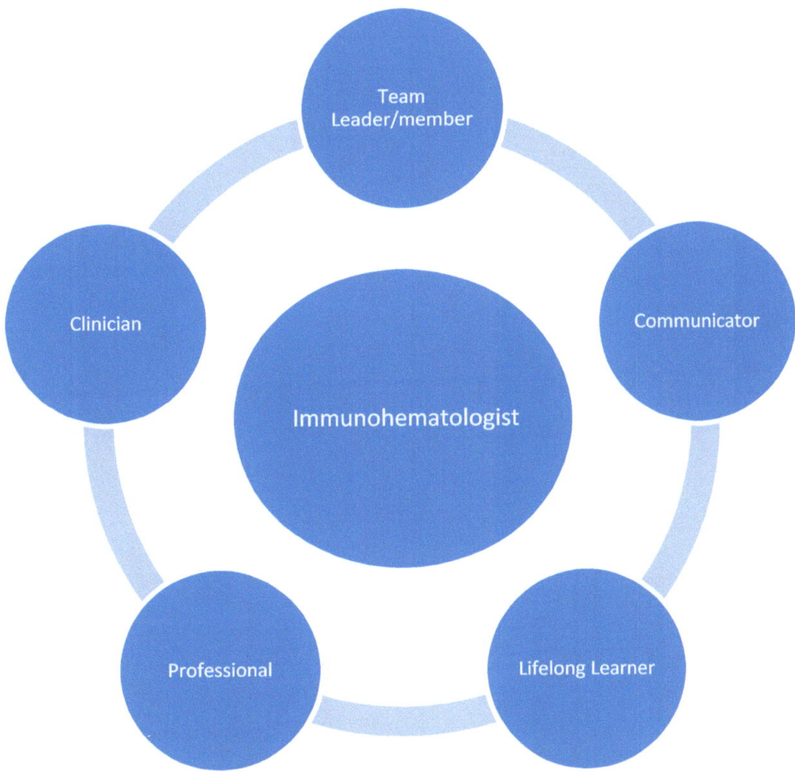

Figure 2.2. Different roles of an Immunohematologist

Periphery Posting:- Residents will get various periphery posting in different departments to understand interdisciplinary approaches and responsibilities. The typical rotation and objectives are mentioned below section-wise.

1. Division Clinical Haematology & Medical ICU

    a. Evaluation and management of various Red Cell Disorders
    b. Approach to a patient with Bleeding, evaluation and management
    c. Hemotherapy for various medical and haematological disorders
    d. Ward rounds, BM aspiration

2. Dept. of Pathology (Lab Haematology & Hematopathology)

    a. Reading and reporting peripheral smears and bonemarrow
    b. Basic Hematological techniques, including advanced haematology (Flowcytometry)
    c. Coagulation lab
    d. Karyotyping (Dept. of Anatomy)

3. Dept. of Microbiology (including ICTC & ART)

    a. Basic culture methods, Sampling for blood culture, staining for bacteria
    b. Serological methods - ELISA, RIA, PCR and other advanced methods for Transfusion Transmitted Infections
    c. Viral culture and serology
    d. Counselling in HIV, Approach to treating HIV

4. Dept. of Nephrology

   a. Approach to Hemodialysis and transfusion management
   b. Pre-transplant workup, donor selection and management

5. Dept. of Medical Gastroenterology

   a. Evaluation and management of Viral Hepatitis

6. Dept. of Clinical Immunology

   a. Diagnostic approach to primary immunological disorders
   b. IV IG therapy, selection of cases and management of adverse reactions
   c. Basic genetics
   d. Investigations for genotyping
   e. PCR, immunoassays
   f. Microarray assays, dot blot assays

7. Dept. of Anaesthesiology & CCU

   a. Transfusion practices in OT & ICU, Cell salvage practices, autologous transfusion, central line access and maintenance
   b. Intraoperative transfusion practices in CTVS, Heartlung machine operation and Hemodynamics
   c. Intubation and airway management

8. Dept. of Emergency Medicine

   a. Fluid management and emergency resuscitation
   b. Massive Transfusion

9. Dept. of Medical Oncology

   a. Transfusion support in Oncology patients
   b. Bone marrow transplantation - Donor/patient evaluation and follow-up
   c. HLA typing

10. Dept. of Obst. & Gynaecology

   a. Antenatal clinic for alloimmunized pregnancy - Evaluation and management, intrauterine transfusion
   b. Transfusion support in the labour ward
   c. Evaluation and management of menorrhagia

11. Dept. of Paediatrics

   a. Exchange transfusion, management of HDN
   b. Neonatal & Pediatric Transfusions

Responsibilities of a Night duty Resident:

- Analyzing blood request forms & samples, followed by decisions regarding the issue, deferring or rejecting the request after communicating with residents of clinical/user departments and physicians for patient transfusions. In case of any problems, obtain clarifications from on-call Senior residents or Consultants.
- Transfusion reaction (includes bedside consultation) and the subsequent immunohematology workup.
- Major transfusion cases (e.g. Exchange transfusion, Massive transfusion etc.) with inputs from Senior residents and Consultant
- Emergency Therapeutic apheresis/plasma exchange, Any other duties as assigned by the Senior resident or Consultant.
- Inventory, equipment supervision

PLANNING YOUR RESIDENCY

– Dr. Charumathy

IHBT, aka Transfusion Medicine, is a field that encompasses treating sick patients and managing healthy donors and running the hospital's transfusion services. We cannot strictly categorise it as a clinical/ non-clinical speciality. On the one hand, we recruit healthy blood donors, manage inventory and run the blood bank; we also deal with critically ill patients requiring therapies such as plasmapheresis, leukocyte apheresis etc. Being in such a grey zone (Pun intended) has its perks.

Junior Residency – the first year

Like in any other department, the first year is challenging. Primarily because we are not introduced to this subject during our undergraduate training, it is like starting afresh, and we need to familiarise ourselves with the basics of theory and practicals. Even those who mastered the bacterial taxonomy in UG's second year will find it hard to remember the major and minor blood group systems, antigens, and their resulting phenotypes. Did you know that there are 40 other blood group systems apart from the ABO and Rh families? Neither did I. Besides, dealing with healthy donors rather than sick patients also takes time. Mind you; you will find yourself calling the donors as patients for the first few months.

As I said, it takes time to get used to. You may not find this stream fulfilling for those who are very much into seeing patients. However, if you are here for the subject, you will love what you are doing and this field's possibilities. So, once I had decided to continue this course, there was no looking back.

The scut work and long hours may stay on for 6-12 months. You learn so much by staying back after work. The immunohematology case workups are good hands-on training. This helps when you start taking on-call duties later. You will be on your own, and one mismatch transfusion reaction or a case of AIHA is enough to keep you occupied for the night. Regular academics help significantly understand the subject and stay up to date.

Doing a thesis is an essential part of postgraduate training. Whatever you had learnt in theory about study designs and biostatistics, you get actually to perform them. It is a learning experience that equips you to implement our ideas and carry out research in future. The research methodology orientation program helps in the introduction of a thesis. Every institute has its protocol for study approval. Departmental review, Institute ethics committee before starting help to give you a good sneak into the protocol. By the end of the first six months, we are good to start your study.

Junior residency – second year

Second-year is unique because one gets to visit other departments as part of the peripheral posting. Learning happens in two ways. We help them understand transfusion science/practices better while we get to learn the clinical aspects and patient perspectives. Transfusion Medicine is ancillary to mainly super speciality departments like Medical Oncology, Hematology, Gastrosurgery, Nephrology and cardiovascular thoracic surgery. OBG and emergency/trauma services too rely significantly on us for timely intervention and blood component transfusions.

The peripheral posting is usually for a total of 6-9 months. In the haematology section of Pathology, the routine consisted of attending the peripheral smear and bone marrow slide reporting. This skill comes in handy during peripheral blood stem cell collection by apheresis. In Anesthesia and critical care, we get to attend the OT and critical care during this period. Using POC investigations to guide transfusions, cell savers, and ECMO are some things we learn here. Utilising the coagulation parameters to decide on the component transfusion comes in handy here.

Medical oncology posting could be overwhelming and equally educative. We get to be with the patient planning for transplants right from deciding the protocol regimen, induction, apheresis collection, conditioning, transplant and the post-transplant phase. Apart from the transplant patients, we also get to attend OPDs and see various haematological malignancies.

Other than the departments mentioned above, we have posting in departments like Nephrology, Medical Gastroenterology, Clinical Immunology, Neonatology, Pediatrics, Emergency medicine and Microbiology.

The second year is when we can attend workshops, CMEs, and conferences conducted at various medical institutes and academic bodies. It helps us get a broader perspective of our speciality. There are a few things like HLA matching and NAT lab for donor TTI testing; you may need to go to other centres as the facilities may not be available everywhere.

One more upside to these peripheral postings is that we may not have departmental call duties during this time. That meant more time to focus on our thesis work, hobbies, or personal life. If you could use this time to study after routine work, you can even present it at national conferences. Voila! That way, you will not be just left with your thesis to publish at the end of your residency.

Junior Residency – final year

The final year means only two things - thesis and exams. Like the first half of my first year, the foremost half would be spent on thesis completion. From winding up the data collection of the past 18 months, analysing the whole data, running around to get hold of a biostatistician to verify the results, writing the manuscript, doing several corrections and proofreading, presenting the data in dept and finally getting them printed once the guide and HOD have given their approval, it was a roller coaster ride. The month of the thesis submission deadline, you can see final year residents from almost every department hovering around the cyber net cafe)

We are officially the EGPGs (exam-going Postgraduates) after thesis submission.

It is time to dive into those books, chapters, and journals we have kept aside until now. By this time, we would have become so good at multitasking (thanks to the thesis work), managing the department work, preparing for and attending the morning academics, doing call duties and preparing for the exams is no big deal. Model exams to prepare us for the finals.

Life on the personal front

Sleep, food, and health – are the three indispensable parts of life. The fourth is some "me time". The first year will have more frequent night duties and 24 hrs shifts which tend to upset the sleep-wake cycle. Hence, I suggest catching up on that sleep as much as possible. We get used to the routine with the passing months, and working up to 36 hrs straight seems like no herculean task. However, we must learn to juggle work, academics and personal time to have a content life. The balance is crucial, neither more nor less of either of those.

Food served in the mess and canteen may be an issue initially, especially when you are across the country or sometimes outside countries. The bright side of this would be the cosmopolitan culture. Yay! However, mess food can still be trouble for those who are too accustomed to home-cooked food. Moreover, there comes the saviour with app-based food delivery and food parcels. And then, there is the option of dining out though it might be heavy on the pocket. Perfect dinner in an ambient restaurant could help end the day on a happy note.

Residency - as gruelling as it can get, one needs time for oneself and the family. No matter how ambitious and focused we are, everybody needs to unwind once in a while. It is what keeps us sane during these tiring times. For some, it is with their kids and family; for others, it could be hanging out with friends or going on a long drive or as simple as spending some time by the places you are comfortable, lost in yourselves. Lucky gets to be day scholars and do their post-graduation, for they get to be with their parents. However, many could be from far-off places and would miss being with family. Even though sometimes the house is near, you may get to visit them only occasionally. This brings us to our next closest thing to family – Friends. They are indispensable, and no matter how busy you are or how many ever power points to do – you need to take time out for them and hang out. Immersing oneself in work totally can take a toll on mental peace. As simple as 30 min chat with them over dinner in the doctor's canteen can cheer you up. Furthermore, they come to the rescue when the days are bad, which are bound to be on some occasions. A Sunday brunch with friends is one of the things that you may look forward to every week.

For most of us who get into the PG program a year or two after UG, it is also that stage of life where marriage is on the cards. I am sure everyone has toiled hard during their internship days and was pretty good at it, but it was different. At that time, we were single (at least technically). We did not have the responsibility that marital life brings with it.

Well, I believe there is no such thing as the right time to get married. If you find the one, you go for it. However, life would be easier for all practical purposes if one gets married in the second year rather than the first or final year. First-year is when we learn the basics and get accustomed to this new field; hence it takes time and effort to understand and excel. Also, the first years get most of the duties, as is always. The final year comes with the added responsibility of thesis and exams. Hence simultaneously starting a new journey on the personal front will divide your attention because even marriage requires work. With the peripheral postings in the second year, it is comparatively easier to focus on the personal life and enjoy marital bliss.

The same goes for planning a family too. Taking a sabbatical of six months will postpone the exams to next semester. However, doing it in the second year would help one get accustomed to managing work while having a baby. One of my seniors had planned so that she had delivered right after her final university exams. That also gives you ample time to spend with your baby as you are done with the exam stress. Ultimately it is one's personal choice, and one must step up to the task.

The three years you spend in residency could be the best years of your life, professionally and personally. The friends you make, the experiences you have, and the training and challenges of embarking on a new career will enrich and give you a new perspective on life.

Residency with Kids:

The residency period sometimes coincides with the time for young doctors when they would like to start families. Undertaking two demanding life events simultaneously can be daunting.

- Plan well and timing: be wholeheartedly ready for it. If possible second or third year would be better compared to the first year
- Please speak to your head/faculty in charge so they can be considerate about it and colleagues so they are aware of it. They can be of great help and support
- Ensure the essential things are taken care of: finances and health insurance.
- Support system: Family support, especially parents, if they possibly can stay with you, would be of great help
- Take good nutrition, take time off when feel stressed whenever possible
- Try enjoying it. Do not try to be perfect
- Be open to options and improvisation
- Prioritise your calls by setting different ring tones, so you do not miss an important call.

TIME MANAGEMENT

– Dr. Nalini Y C

What is time management? What are the benefits?

Time management is "organising and planning the division of your **time** between specific activities. ". Good **time management** enables you to work smarter to get more done in less **time**, even in times of **high** pressure and tight schedules.

Benefits of good time management

- Greater efficiency and productivity
- Better reputation
- Lessens stress
- Better advancements and more significant achievements

How to manage your time effectively?

This is a burning question in everybody's mind. Every individual wants to utilise time to the maximum. It is a prevalent scenario many of us would have encountered where we find it challenging to complete the assigned task in the given timeframe. It is essential to understand that what works for one might not work for the other; nevertheless, I have tried to provide some techniques, tips and suggestions for effective time management.

Note: Try many methods but stick to the method which works out best for you!

Given below is the list of a few grounds' rules for effective time utilisation

- ❖ Start early
- ❖ Make a strategy for long-term projects, including breaks for long-term projects
- ❖ Set goals within the time frame.
  Do not procrastinate
  Keep a diary or a planner
- ❖ Use optimal technology.
  Make a Gannt chart
  Use references management tools
  Learn and adapt to newer techniques from peers and students
- ❖ Identify what works for you and what does not and reinforce the good habits

Learn to say 'no.'
Delegate the work
Work on time trappers
❖ List the activities and classify them based on ABC and VEN principles

ABC & VEN principles of time management

These management principles are ideal for inventory management, but they can be applied to time management and, for that matter, in any aspect of life.

ABC Principle

Categorise the activities based on the time required to complete a job as A, B, or C. ABC analysis helps in identifying activities that require more focus and time.

Table 3.1 The ABC Principle

Activities	% time required to complete the job	Examples
A	70	Writing proposals, and manuscripts, doing research
B	20	Making slides for a presentation
C	10	Checking email

VEN Principle

Based on the quality of the work, it can be classified as

- Vital
- Essential
- Desirable

List out the activities and classify them as mandatory or vital to be performed, essential activities and desirable activities.

Note: combining the VEN and ABC analysis will help us remove our non-essential activities that consume much time.

Tasks can be classified as large, medium, small and very small based on the time required to execute the task.

Table 3.2. Task classification

Size of the task (estimated time)	Description	Examples
Large (>1 h)	Require uninterrupted time and max concentration Schedule this task during alert and productive time	Manuscript writing Clinical research Curricular preparations

Medium (30-60 min)	Concentration necessary Alertness required	Preparing a PowerPoint presentation Clinical work/laboratory work
Small (5- 10 min)	Less concentration and alertness required Can schedule the task as a transition from large to medium	Non-urgent phone calls Patient summaries/reports
Very small (<5 min)	Minimal concentration required It can be used as a fill-in time while waiting for a meeting etc.	Emails Routine paperwork

Recommended techniques for those with short attention spans or low drive.

Swiss cheese technique

It is challenging to complete a task that requires a considerable amount of time in one go. A better way to approach the task is by doing small parts in a limited time.

For example- you cannot write a proposal or a research paper in a day or at one stretch, but you can break it into sub-topics like introduction, methodology etc.. and start working whenever you find time so that when you approach your deadline of submission, all you need to is compile and refine your writings.

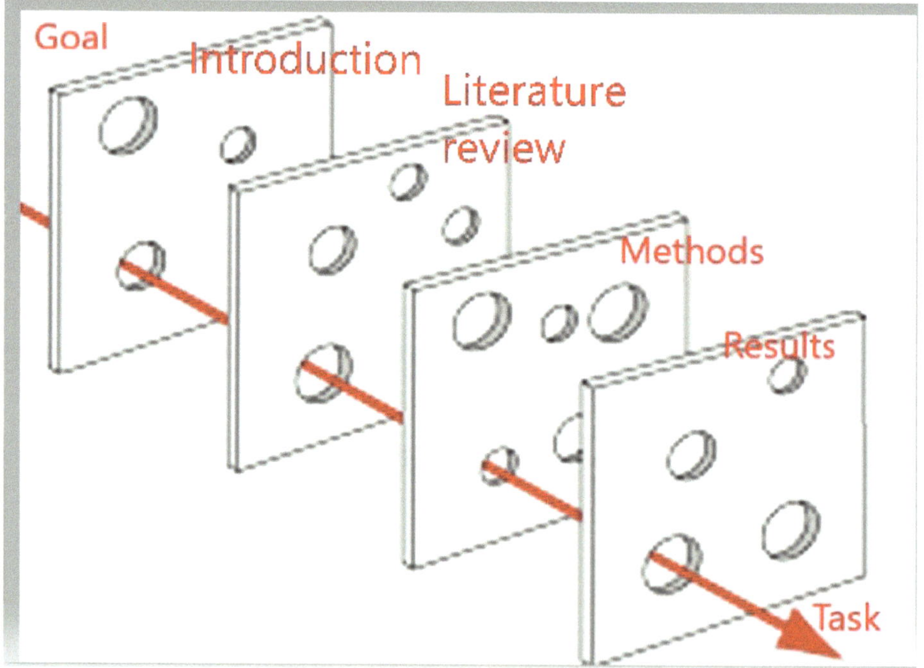

Figure 4.1

Tomato method or the Pomodoro technique

Francesco Cirillo developed this technique, similar to the Swiss cheese technique, which emphasises executing huge tasks as a series of small tasks with adequate breaks to provide motivation.

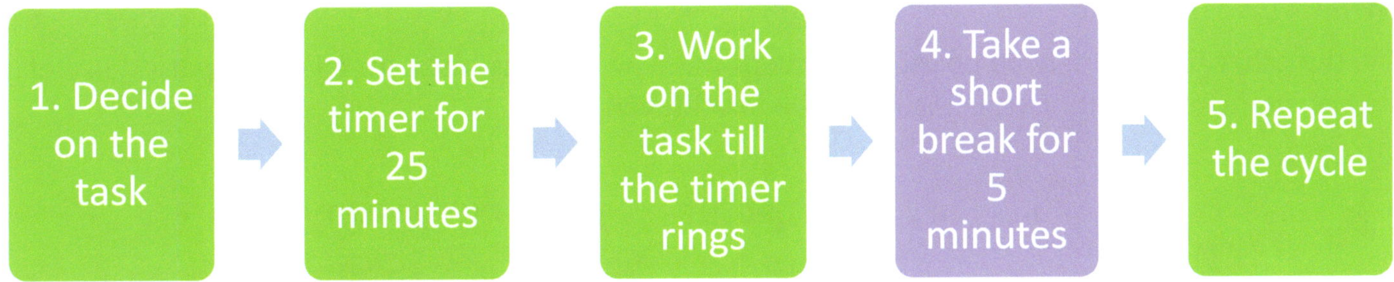

Premack principle & Pareto method

According to this **Premack** principle, always do the unpleasant first. When you have two tasks on hand, but you like task 'A' but dislike task 'B', it is better to complete task B before proceeding to task A. This technique has been used by our parents and grandparents where they coerce the child to eat the fruit(healthy but disliked) in exchange for a cake or television time (unhealthy but liked).

Pareto's method, or the law 80/20, says that 80% of tasks can be solved for 20% of the time spent, and for the remaining 20% of tasks, 80% of the time is spent. This law also describes significant and trivial factors, hidden factors that can affect the outcomes of the tasks either positively or negatively. It says that the ratio of input and outcome is never balanced or equal. For some tasks, the input of 20 per cent can result in an outcome amounting to 80 per cent. So, identifying these tasks helps one maximise the work's efficiency by focusing and prioritising the goal. This rule can be applied to routine activities like buying groceries, clothes etc.

EFFORT	RESULTS
80% TIME SPENT	80% OF THE OUTCOME
20% TIME SPENT	20% OF THE OUTCOME

How to say 'no' or delegate work?

Often, we encounter situations in our personal life or workplace when we want to say "no", but instead of saying it, we end up doing it because we do not know when or how to say "no". When given a responsibility or a job, always ask yourself, will this task help me achieve my long-term or short-term goals? Answering this question will help you decide whether you should devote the time or politely say a "no" to the task allotted.

We all know that saying 'no' is never easy, especially when the task comes as a request from a senior or superior. In such situations, you need to ask yourself

'What must I give up to accept this new responsibility?'

On the other hand, it may be possible to accept the new responsibility for a limited period or delay its acceptance until other vital goals have been achieved.

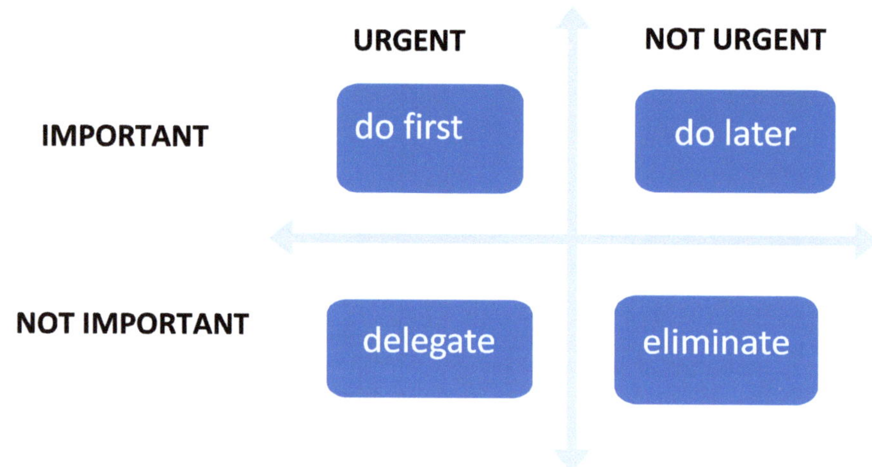

Covey time management matrix technique

Given below are a few examples from our day-to-day life to understand the matrix better

Important	Urgent	Not urgent
	Pressing problems	Exercise
	Deadline driven projects	Relationship building
Not Important	Meetings	Junk mail
	Calls	Time wasters

The advantages of the Application of self-management are

1. Execution of works with a minor time expenditure and efforts
2. Effective organisations of work decrease workload
3. Decrease in haste as well as stresses
4. Increase in satisfaction from the performed works
5. High motivation of the director and workers
6. Achievements of the objectives in a most optimum as well as effective way.

Tips for effective time management

- ✓ List the activities and classify them based on ABC and VEN principles
- ✓ Make a Gannt chart
- ✓ Do not procrastinate
- ✓ Keep a diary or a planner
- ✓ Learn to say 'no 'whenever possible
- ✓ Delegate the work
- ✓ Learn and adapt to newer techniques from peers and students

Table 3.4. 10 common time wasters and potential solutions

Time waster	Proposed solution
Telephone calls	• Check messages and return calls 1–2 times per day*
Email	• Check no more than 3–4 times per day* • Disable auto-alert messages for mail arrivals • Develop a reliable and reproducible filing system for saved messages • Rapidly dispose of unwanted messages at first pass • Accurately identify and discard junk mail
Physical interruptions	• Close the office door and respect when colleagues do the same
Paper	• Handle each piece of paper only once ('When in doubt, throw it out") • Develop a reliable and reproducible filing system • Store publications as electronic PDF files
Repetitive activities	• Automate (e.g., develop patient education handouts) • Create 'quick text' for frequently used phrases in email or electronic medical records • Delegate tasks that others can do
Disorganisation	• Clean and organise the desk and office • Organise paper, mail and electronic files for easier accessibility
Procrastination	• Identify and address reasons for procrastination • Accomplish small increments of progress on a project • Do not allow perfectionism to get in the way of progress
Meetings	• Arrive on time (change the culture of lack of punctuality) • Bring alternative work if others are not punctual
Waiting†	• Perform quick and easy small tasks (clinical or administrative paperwork works well)
Commuting	• Enjoy music, books on tape, quiet self-reflection, and relax • Use audio continuing medical education, or learn a foreign language • Read journal articles if using public transportation

*May not be suitable for specific job descriptions; †Includes waiting for meetings, conferences, telephone hold, etc. This is ideal for completing less important responsibilities (quadrants III and IV in the Covey time management matrix).

ETHICS AND PROFESSIONALISM

Ethics is derived from the Greek word "ethos", which means – "the science of morals."

A - Autonomy

B - Beneficence

C - Confidentiality

D - Do no Harm (Non-maleficence)

E - Equity (Justice)

	Meaning/Explanation	Instances/examples
Autonomy	A clear-sighted individual should be allowed to make an informed, un-coerced decision	Nobody should be forced to donate blood
Beneficence	A known benefit should be accompanied for an action	Transfusion should only be undertaken when the benefits outweigh the risks
Confidentiality	To keep secretive about those things that you came to know as a result of examination/testing to yourself and not share with anybody else unless medically indicated	The TTI results should be revealed to only the respective donor and no one else except the regulatory authority whenever mandatory
Do no harm	Non-Maleficence	When administering drugs for a donor, say G-CSF, it should be made sure that the risk to the donor should be kept to a minimum and should never be driven by the requirements of the recipient
Equity	Justice	Allocation of blood units in constrained inventory should be purely based on the medical urgency of the patient and nothing else

Professionalism is derived from the Latin word "professiō" meaning "public acknowledgement". The term describes the professional attributes required (over and beyond simply having adequate knowledge of medicine and adequate procedural ability) for effective medical practice that the community can trust.

It includes a set of attributes, values, behaviours, commitments, goals and relationships that underpins the public's trust in doctors.

Character:

Develop pride in the profession. If you want to excel in a subject, you should love and develop a passion for it. Initially, it may look unfamiliar and lead to uncertainties in your mind. Speak to your seniors, and do not hesitate to clarify doubts from people already in the field.

Knowledgeable; knowledge is power. It is understandable that compared to residencies in other broad subjects wherein there is enough exposure during the Undergraduate days, you are naïve to Transfusion Medicine, albeit some institutes do allow some exposure during the internship. Nevertheless, start reading small but comprehensive books to get overall exposure to the field. You are free to choose the book, but I would strongly recommend Technical Manual from DGHS because it is concise, easy to grasp, and gives an overall idea of things in a minimal amount of time. Meanwhile, going intensively through the department's SOPs in the sections you are posted is an ideal beginning. NBTC and NACO websites host many resources. Please go through them, especially in line with your posting schedule.

Based on the continuous feedback from the mentors and your seniors, self-awareness and commitment to improvement accept and respond through careful reflection and self-improvement. Make yourself feel by acquiring information and applying it to impact daily proceedings in the department positively.

Developing an affective domain: respect the patients' treatment decisions, or lack thereof, while maintaining a non-judgmental attitude. Doctors are not designed to be machines. We are there to sensitively deliver prognoses and not just mechanically perform tasks and procedures. We need hearts. Patients/donors respond better to a doctor who is empathetic to their needs. Focus on exercising courtesy and compassion with your patients

Service Orientation- place the needs and interests of the patient/donors above your curricular necessities. Once you are through this, believe me, the rest all will fall into place

Develop soft skills: Communication, Empathy, Humility

Attitude- look confident, be a role model

Reliability and Punctuality: consistently meet deadlines without needing reminders

Dressing: Physical impressions are of paramount importance in how people accept you. A clean white coat always looks professional and Respectable. Well-groomed (not overdone) and cleanliness leave a considerable impression. Ladies, do not go too heavy on your makeup or perfume, especially in direct donor/patient care areas. Formals are the one that adds that extra to a doctor.

Being Equipped: A transfusion medicine Resident should always have the following during work hours. Stethoscope, measuring tape, Surface thermometer, a small book, pen torch, a pair of gloves

Be an active listener

Respect Seniors and all your staff. Display humility

There is tremendous scope for innovation and creativity, especially in this field. Stay inquisitive, seek and consider opportunities to improve the care delivered by Transfusion Services

Residents must accept responsibility for their errors and find ways to resolve and/or prevent these from happening.

Leadership skills must be acquired early in this field because they demand them. It has multidisciplinary and multidimensional involvement of people like nursing, technical, social activists and the public in a specialised and unique fashion. Also, given that the medical team's size in most Transfusion services is very small, usually alone most of the time, you tend to assume a headship position early in your career. Transitioning to a leader involves time, experience, and awareness, all of which may be attained by participating in these roles early in your residency. Participating in leadership or observing others in leadership roles as a mentee is a valuable means of gaining exposure to challenges, strategies, and shared visions while establishing meaningful relationships with peers.

Being professional:

Professional competence, effective communication and ethics are the three founding principles of professionalism.

Elements of professionalism
Commitment to competency
Honesty to patients
Improvement in quality of care
Managing conflict of interests
Responsibilities

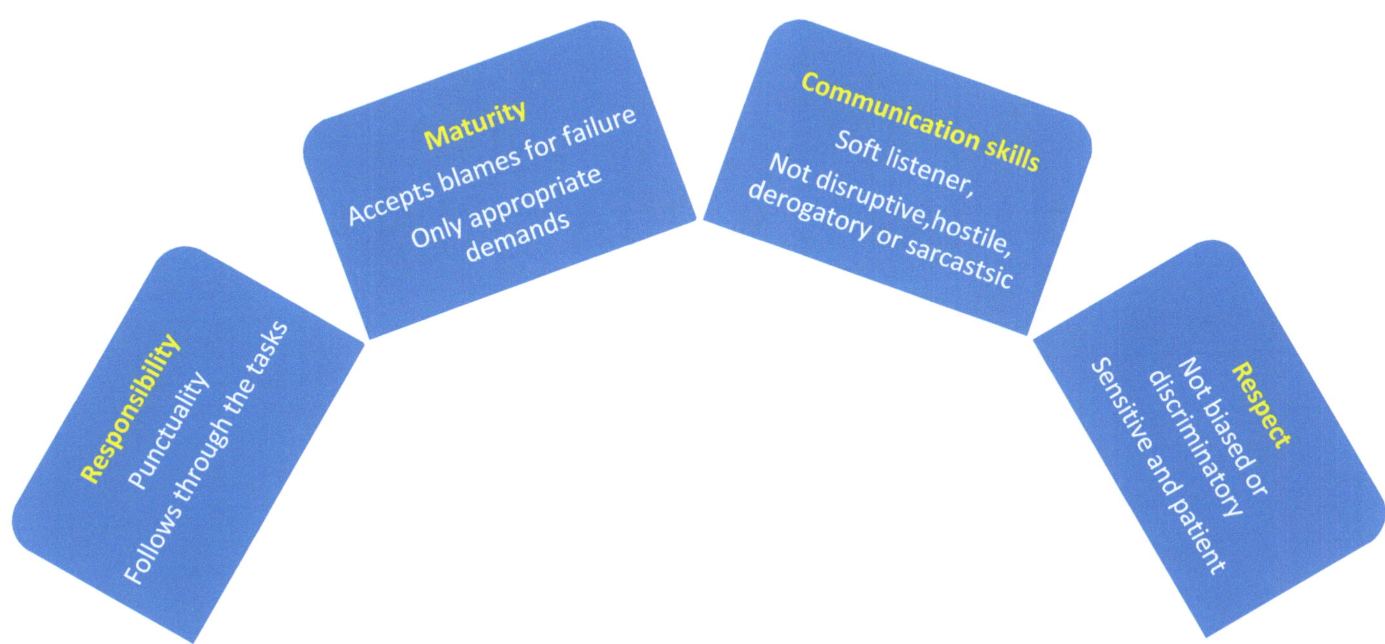

- Show respect, compassion and integrity
- Be responsive to the needs of the patients and society over your self-interest
- Show accountability to the patients, society, and the profession
- Be sensitive and responsive to the patient's age, culture, gender and disability

Expectation from a Resident: Affective Domain
Honesty
Integrity
Responsibility
Trustworthiness
Understand limitations and accept Criticism
Correct deficiencies and improve performance
Commitment to excellence and ongoing professional development
Professionalism
Attitude of cooperation
compassion and sensitivity, respect for their privacy and dignity in the care of patients
Confidentiality
Effective communication- verbal and written
Inquisitiveness
Cleanliness, Punctuality and orderliness
Organisational skills, interpersonal relations, problem-solving ability
Personal safety and working for general work safety

Good Laboratory Practices

– Dr. Sajith Menon

Etiquettes and discipline in the blood centre Laboratory

- Be punctual with regard to timings and duty
- Do not consume food or drinks inside the laboratory
- Stay focused and be aware of your surroundings
- Maintain hygienic practices, including hand hygiene, handling hazardous materials, covering dry/cracked skin, do not apply cosmetics or touching your face, especially around the mouth or eyes
- Keep your personal items separate from lab work
- Wear gloves and wash hands after touching blood, body fluids, secretions, excretions, and contaminated items, whether or not gloves are worn.
- Change gloves between tasks.
- Wear a mask, gown, eye protection, or face shield during activities likely to generate splashes or sprays of blood, body fluids, secretions, and excretions.
- Handle soiled patient-care equipment and linen in a manner that prevents exposure; ensure that reusable equipment is not used for another patient until it has been cleaned and reprocessed appropriately, and ensure that single-use items are discarded properly
- Handle needles, scalpels, and other sharp instruments or devices in a manner that minimises the risk of exposure.
- Use mouthpieces, resuscitation bags, or other ventilation devices as an alternative to the mouth-to-mouth resuscitation methods

Considerations for the Donor Room:

- Gloves may be used by those who want to use them, and their use is not discouraged.
- Gloves are required when you have cuts, scratches, or breaks in skin; when there is a likelihood that contamination will occur; drawing autologous units; performing therapeutic procedures; and during training in phlebotomy

Uniforms and laboratory coats

- Should wear closed laboratory coats or full aprons over long-sleeved uniforms or gowns when they are exposed to blood, corrosive chemicals, or carcinogens. The material of required coverings should be appropriate for the type and amount of hazard exposure.

- Plastic disposable aprons may be worn over cotton coats when there is a high probability of large spills or splashing of blood and body fluids; nitrile rubber aprons may be preferred when caustic chemicals are poured.
- Protective coverings should be removed before leaving the work area and discarded or stored away from heat sources and clean clothing.
- Contaminated clothing should be removed promptly, placed in a suitable container, and laundered or discarded as potentially infectious.
- Home laundering of garments worn in Biosafety Level 2 areas is not permitted because unpredictable methods of transportation and handling can spread contamination, and home laundering techniques may not be effective.

Gloves:

Types of gloves:

i. Sterile gloves: for procedures involving contact with ordinarily sterile body areas.
ii. Examination gloves: for procedures involving contact with mucous membranes and for other patient care or diagnostic procedures that do not require using sterile gloves.
iii. Rubber utility gloves: for housekeeping chores involving potential blood contact, instrument cleaning and decontamination procedures, and handling concentrated acids and organic solvents. Utility gloves may be decontaminated and reused but should be discarded if they show signs of deterioration (e.g., peeling, cracks, or discolouration) or if they develop punctures or tears.
iv. Insulated gloves: for handling hot or frozen material

The following situations require the use of gloves:

- When handling corrosive chemicals and radioactive materials.
- When examining mucous membranes or open skin lesions.
- When collecting or handling blood or specimens from patients or donors known to be infected with a bloodborne pathogen.
- When cleaning up spills or handling waste materials.
- When the likelihood of exposure can not be assessed because of a lack of experience with a procedure or situation.

The safe use of gloves includes the following:

- Securely bandage or cover open skin lesions on hands and arms before putting on gloves
- Change gloves immediately if they are torn, punctured, or contaminated after handling high-risk samples; or performing a physical examination(e.g., on an apheresis donor)
- Remove gloves by keeping their outside surfaces in contact only with the outside and turning the glove inside out while taking it off.
- Use gloves only when needed, and avoid touching clean surfaces such as telephones, doorknobs, or computer terminals with gloves.
- Change gloves between patient contacts. Unsoiledgloves need not be changed between donors

- Wash hands with soap or other suitable disinfectants after removing gloves
- Do not wash or disinfect surgical or examination gloves for reuse. Washing with surfactants may cause "wicking" (i.e., enhanced penetration of liquids through undetected holes in the glove). Disinfecting agents may cause the deterioration of gloves.
- Use only water-based hand lotions with gloves, if needed;oil-based products cause minute cracks in latex

Face shields, masks, and safety goggles

- Full-face shields or masks and safety goggles are recommended when permanent shields cannot be used.
- Masks should be worn whenever there is danger from inhalation. Simple, disposable dust masks are adequate for handling dry chemicals, but respirators with organic vapour filters are preferred for areas where noxious fumes are produced (e.g., for cleaning up spills of noxious materials). Respirators should be fitted to their wearers and checked annually

Hand washing

- Always wash hands before leaving a restricted work area or using a biosafety cabinet, between medical examinations, immediately after becoming soiled with blood or hazardous materials, after removing gloves, or after using the toilet. Washing hands thoroughly before touching contact lenses or applying cosmetics is essential.
- Waterless antiseptic solutions for hand washing as an interim method.' These solutions are helpful for mobile donor collections or areas where water is not readily available for clean-up purposes. However, if such methods are used, hands must be washed with soap and running water as soon as possible.

Eyewashes

- Be aware of how to use them. If a splash occurs, keep eyelids open and use the eyewash according to procedures. You need to go to the nearest sink and direct a steady, tepid stream of water into your eyes. Solutions other than water should be used only in accordance with a physician's direction.
- After eyes are adequately flushed (many facilities recommend 15 minutes), follow-up medical care should be sought, especially if pain or redness develops. Whether washing the eyes effectively prevents infection has been demonstrated, but it is considered desirable when accidents occur.

How to wear sterile gloves

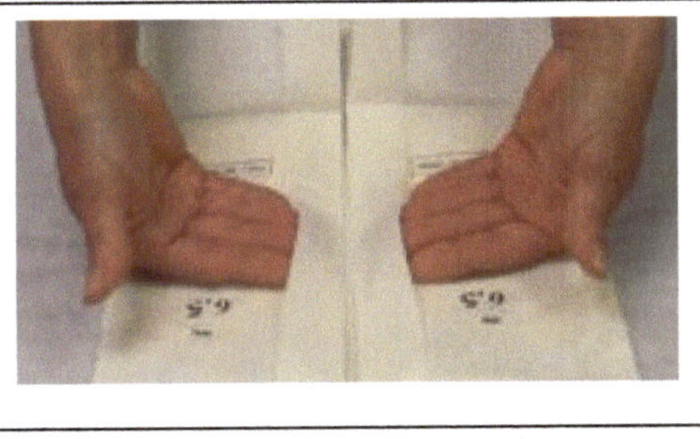	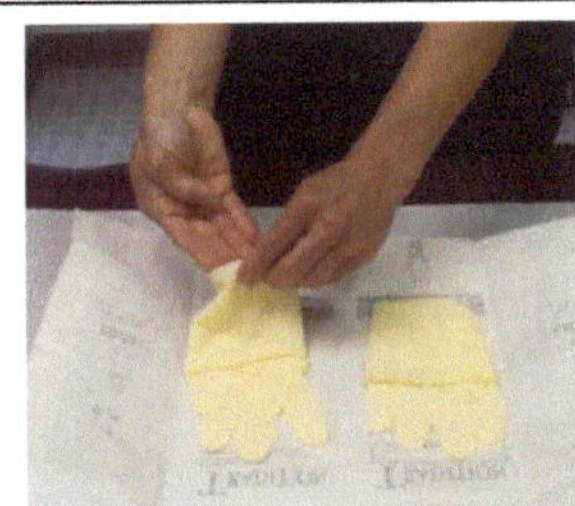	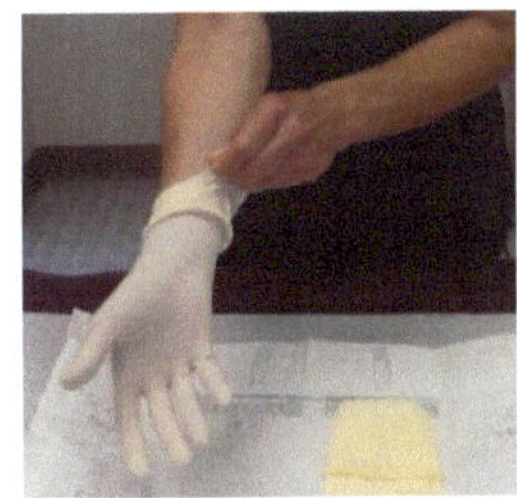
Wash your hands and wipe them dry	Grasp the inside edge of the glove and wear it on your dominant hand	Pull the glove to the end of your fingers and the edge to cover the wrist
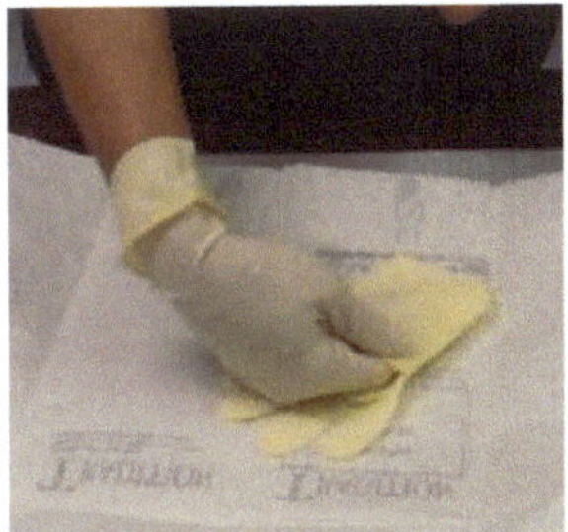	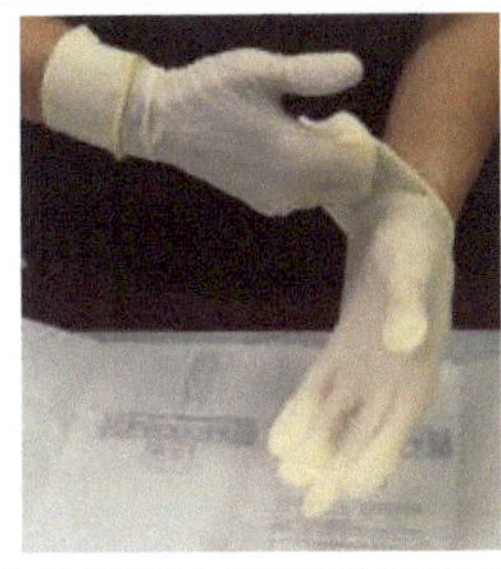	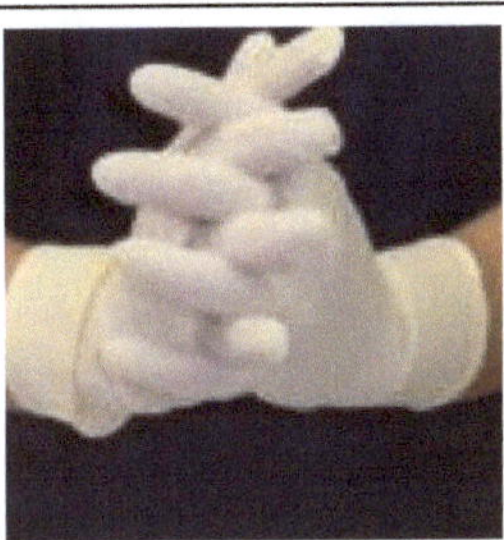
Take the second glove by inserting the fingers in the fold towards the sterile surface	Insert your fingers into the gloves and advance your hand by rolling over the fold by the other hand	

How to remove gloves safely

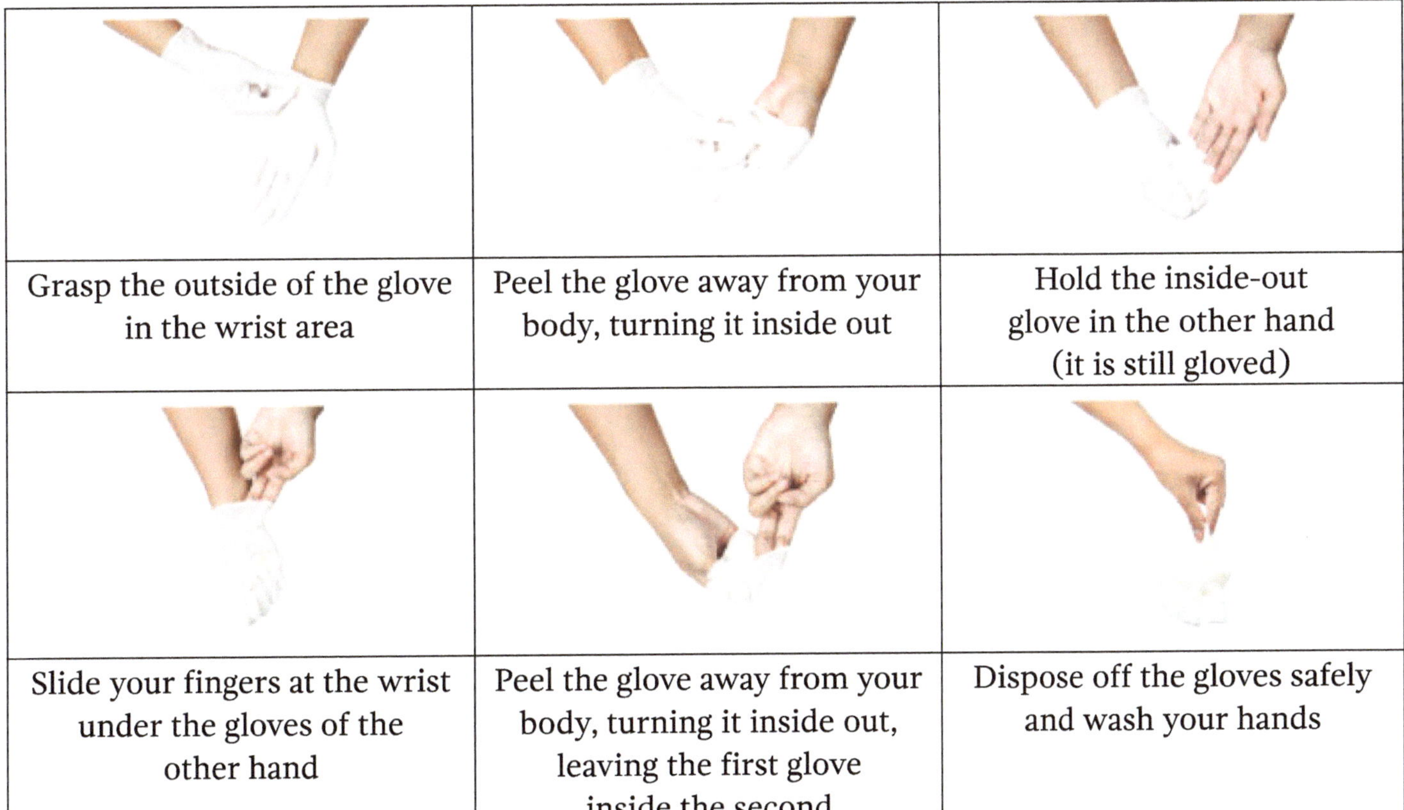

Grasp the outside of the glove in the wrist area	Peel the glove away from your body, turning it inside out	Hold the inside-out glove in the other hand (it is still gloved)
Slide your fingers at the wrist under the gloves of the other hand	Peel the glove away from your body, turning it inside out, leaving the first glove inside the second	Dispose off the gloves safely and wash your hands

Section ll

***

General Skills

COMMUNICATION AND COUNSELLING SKILLS

Counselling is a means by which a person helps another person to clarify his or her life situation and to decide on further lines of action

Blood donor Counseling- "confidential dialogue between a blood donor and a trained counsellor about issues related to the donor's health and the donation process."

It may be provided before, during, and after blood donation.

Confidentiality – "obligation on the part of healthcare professionals and institutions not to disclose personal and sensitive information about their patients or blood donors to third parties."

Privacy refers to a person's right not to be asked about matters of a personal nature.

Informed consent is "A voluntary agreement given by the prospective donor to the donation process, including the donation of blood, the testing of blood for TTI and blood group serology, and, if applicable, the use of blood for additional tests, quality assurance, or research purposes."

Physical setup
- ✓ Switch off/mute the mobile phone
- ✓ Remove all the physical barriers so as to maintain constant eye contact
- ✓ Keep in handy the pen and paper for note-taking
- ✓ Tissue paper to be made available if necessary
- ✓ Some models, e-medias, and pamphlet materials about the anticipated discussion

Don'ts while building rapport: Hostile attitude
Hurrying

A good posture: SHOVLER

Sit Squarely

Head Nods

Open Posture

Verbal following

Lean towards the patient

Eye contact

Relaxed

Counselling skills and techniques	
Type	Means
Careful/positive listening	Body posture
	Minimal encouragers
Attentive behaviours	
Reflective listening	Reflection of content- repeating and paraphrasing
	Reflection of feeling
Information gathering	Open-ended questioning
	Lead/closed questioning
Normalization	
Maintaining focus	
Giving feedback	Identifying strengths and resources

Stages of Counselling for Blood donation:

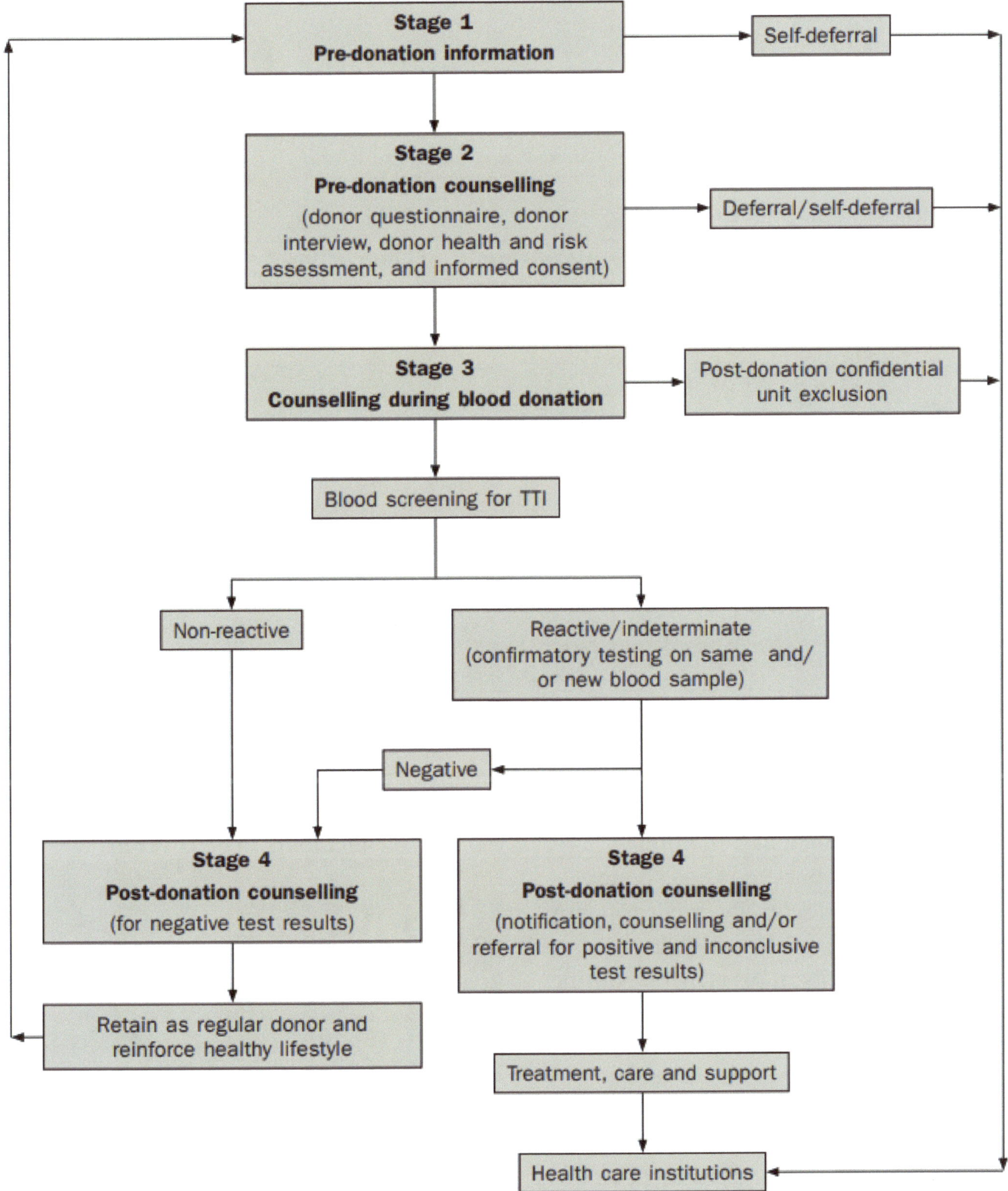

Sociological and Psychological theories of blood donation

- Theory of planned behaviour
- Opponent process theory
- Attribution theory
- Model of Commitment
- Theory of reasoned action

Counselling skills and techniques

No	Essential elements of counselling
1	Explanation of the entire blood donation process
2	Reassurance to allay anxiety and apprehension
3	Promotion of a healthy lifestyle
4	Encouraging to self-defer if the donor might have been exposed to a TTI and referral to voluntary counselling and testing services
5	Information on screening the blood for TTI and the test results
6	Encouraging them to return for future blood donations and become a regular blood donor
7	Explanation of the reason for deferral
8	Clarifying the nature of the deferral (permanent or temporary)
9	Encouraging temporarily deferred donors to return for future blood donations after the defined deferral period
10	Exploration of motivation for blood donation
11	Explaining the reason for deferral and informing on the specific risk for TTI

Situation and Condition	Elements to be covered										
First-time blood donors and young donor	1	2	3	4	5	6					
Donor deferred (temporarily or permanently)		2	3					7	8	9	
A donor with risk for TTI: Self-deferred, Deferred temporarily or permanently during pre-donation counselling			3					7	8	9	10	11
A donor who has: a) Requested confidential unit exclusion (CUE) b) Given post-donation information that warrants temporary or permanent deferral			3						8	9	10	

For donors seeking to ascertain infection status, provide information on voluntary counselling and testing services. Refer them to a healthcare institution for treatment, care and support and provide information on relevant TTI

No	Essential elements of counselling
1	Explaining the reasons for the adverse donor reaction and the treatment given
2	Informing and advising on preventive steps to reduce the risk of adverse reactions, like taking adequate fluids before donation in the case of having a faint during a previous donation
3	Assurance of care for donor well-being
4	Encouragement to return for future donations
5	Reassurance to allay anxiety and apprehension
6	Evaluate suitability for future donations.

Situation and Condition	Elements to be covered
Donors who have experienced an adverse reaction during or after donation or have previously had a reaction to donation	1 2 3 4 5 6
A donor whose donation has resulted in a severe adverse transfusion reaction in the transfused patient	1 3 6

Donors with rare blood groups or unusual red cell serology	1. Inform and explain the nature and importance of the unusual red cell serology, such as rare blood group or an atypical red cell antibody
	2. Advise them to carry this information personally at all times in case the donor ever needs a blood transfusion
	3. Encourage them to return for future blood donations and enrolment in the rare blood donor panel

Situations and conditions		Essential elements of counselling
A donor who shows repeated reactive TTI results on screening and negative results on confirmatory testing	1	Explain the relevance of repeated reactive test results, the need for confirmatory testing, and the results of confirmatory testing
	2	Information about the donor deferral period
	3	Promotion of a healthy lifestyle
	4	Encourage them to return for future blood donations as the confirmatory test results are non-reactive
	5	Reassurance to allay anxiety and apprehension
A donor who has indeterminate TTI test results with unclear confirmatory results, where infection cannot be ruled out	1	Explain the meaning of indeterminate test results, the need for confirmatory testing, and the results of confirmatory testing
	2,3,5,6	Explore all relevant information, including possible TTI risk, repeat testing
	7	Information about the fate of the blood donation

Breaking Bad News

Donors found to have confirmed positive markers for TTI	1. Explanation of the positive TTI test results
	2. Information about the health implications of the positive TTI test results for the donor and the donated blood (discard) and the suitability of the donor for future blood donations
	3. Explore all relevant information, including the possible TTI risk
	4. Reassurance to allay anxiety and apprehension
	5. Information on how to prevent further transmission
	6. Refer for further investigation, management, treatment, and care, if necessary

Protocol for BREAK(S)ing the bad news

Background: Effective counselling depends on in-depth knowledge of the donor's problem. Be prepared with answers to all questions that can be anticipated from the donor. Reasonable doubts of the donors, as well as his relatives/bystanders, should be cleared. An in-depth study on the donor's diseases/conditions, if any, emotional status, coping skills, educational level, and the support system available are all to be reviewed before attempting to break the bad news. The cultural and ethnic background of the donor is essential as well. You have to be sensitive to the cultural orientation of the donor, and it should be respected. His cultural orientation generally governs the individual's thinking and actions.

Rapport: Building rapport is fundamental to a continuous professional relationship. It would be best if you had unconditional positive regard; nevertheless, at the same time, refrain from evolving an attitude of patronization. Establishing rapport is the key to continuing the conversation. Provide ample space for self-disclosure/opening up. The donor should be placed in a comfortable position. The present condition of the donor can be enquired about through open questions. If the donor is unprepared for the bad news, let him finish the well-being talks. Then try to take hints from his conversation to initiate breaking (bad news).

Exploring: While attempting to break the bad news, starting with what the donor knows about his/her illness is easier. Most donors may be aware of the seriousness of the condition, while some may not. You are then in a position to confirm bad news or break it as applicable. The history, investigations, and difficulties you may encounter in the process must be explored. Explore what he/she thinks about the disease or the diagnosis. Identify the potential conflicts between the donor's beliefs and possible conditions. The family dynamics and the donor's coping capacity are of chief interest in delivering the bad news. Other people interested in the donor should be involved in the decision-making process with the donor's consent. Few donors may respond in odd ways to the bad news. Do not jump into premature reassurances before exploring and understanding the concerns. Do not give absolute certainty about longevity to the affected. The prognosis is to be explained in detail; with all available data. A reasonable conclusion based on the facts is to be presented.

Announce: Give a warning shot so the news will not explode like a bomb. Euphemisms are welcome, making sure not to create confusion. The donor has every right to know his condition. Equally, he has the right to refrain from knowing it. So, the announcement of the diagnosis has to be made after getting consent. Your body language is fundamental. It should mirror the affected- the embarrassment, agony, and fear (mirroring the emotions). This will help the donor identify you as one close to himself. Announce the bad news in straightforward terms, avoiding medical jargon. However, sometimes lengthy monologues, elaborate explanations, and stories of people with similar plight may be desirable. Give the information in short, easily comprehensible sentences.

A helpful rule of thumb is- "Do not give more than three pieces of information at a time."

Kindle: People listen and react differently. Some may break down in tears, whereas others remain entirely silent. Few of them may become restless, get up, and pace around the room. Sometimes there may be a complete denial of reality. A scary laugh is also expected behaviour. Give adequate space for the free flow of emotions. Most of the time, people will not actively listen to what you say after revealing the status. At this time, they may ignore further explanations and narratives from you. It is advisable to ensure that he/she listens to what you are saying. Ask them questions like, "are you there?" "do you listen to me?" etc. Ask them to recount what they have understood.

Ensure that the person understands the nature of the disease, the gravity of the situation, or the realistic disease course with or without treatment options. While kindling the emotions, taking care not to utter unrealistic treatment options. The affected and their relatives will cling to it and subsequently feel embarrassed because of its unrealistic nature. Tailor the answers to the question, and you should stay away from lecturing the affected. (Lecturing is when you deliver a large chunk of information without giving the person a chance to respond or ask questions). Beware of "differential listening," i.e., a person will listen to only the information he/she wants to hear. Dealing with denial is another difficult task. In such situations, attempts to break the defence without mutilating the ego should be attempted.

Summarise: Summarize the session and the concerns expressed by the donor during the session. Highlight the main points of the conversation. Put the treatment/care plans for the future in a nutshell. Stress on the necessary adjustments that must be made emotionally and practically. A written summary is appreciable, as the anxious person usually retains significantly less of what is told. Offer availability whenever required, and encourage them to call for any reason if required. Maintain an optimistic outlook. Volunteer if asked by the affected person to disseminate the information to the relatives. Fix the review date before concluding the session. Make sure that the donor's safety is ensured even after they leave the room. Make sure they are not all alone when they go back. Find out if someone at home can provide support. People may even try to commit suicide if he/she feels exceptionally desperate. Assure them that you will be actively participating in all ongoing care plans.

Aspect	Donor	Non-Donor
Affect	donation made them feel generous, assured, relaxed, and useful	feel uncomfortable and ill
Cognition	cite that blood donation is worth any inconvenience and is an essential civic duty	believed that blood donation was dangerous and appeared to know little about the process
Behaviour	behaviours that reflected the donation process were ranked higher and favourably	Ranked unfavourably

Informed Consent

Informed consent is a process of education that occurs over time between physicians and patients or their surrogate decision-makers and others who provide or reinforce different aspects of disclosed information using different education formats (e.g., written, oral, and video).

Thus, people obtaining consent in transfusion medicine should have sufficient knowledge in the field to provide accurate and timely information and answer questions/doubts. You also need to provide education to other healthcare professionals who participate in the consent process

Usually contains the following significant elements

Disclosure: sharing of relevant and available information

Comprehension: make sure what has been told is understood by the patient/donor

Voluntariness: allow them to make the decision instead of coercing them

Competence: ascertain that the patient/donor is capable of making a decision and understanding its consequences and implications

Consent: final decision and authorising it

TAKING AN EFFECTIVE LECTURE

– Dr. Nalini Y C

As a resident of Transfusion Medicine, you will be required to take various lecture classes either for undergraduate courses medical/paramedical, or for interns and residents in orientation classes, or other health care workers on transfusion safety etc. In this chapter we will introduce on few tips to make the lecture more effective and interesting. As it is usually said, the best way to take a lecture is "not to lecture...!!"

What is a lecture?

The word "lecture" is derived from the Latin word *"lectura"*, meaning to read; it originated in the 15th century. A lecture is a careful presentation of facts with organized thoughts and ideas by a qualified person. It is the most commonly used teaching-learning method in medical colleges, even though its role as a primary is questionable. Lecture **per se cannot be good or bad**. The effectiveness of a lecture is dependent on how it is used as a communication tool among students.

Advantages and Disadvantages of Lecture

Advantages	Disadvantages
Preferred mode to introduce a new topic	Learner is passive
Economical in terms of usage of staff and time	Difficult to evaluate how much is understood
It can be used for a large number of students	Not suitable for individual learner needs
Uniformity of content can be maintained	Too much content is delivered
Clarify complex concepts and stress essential points	Difficult to sustain attention span for 50-60 minutes
Provides an updated summary of a topic	Difficult to teach problem-solving exercises

Is it important to know your learners?

Remember, your students are adult learners, thus enjoying a relevant, practical, and exciting learning experience and are interested in learning when learning benefits are highlighted.

Importance of planning for a lecture

Teaching is a skilled professional activity executed by one complex person (teacher) to another more complex person (student) in highly complex situations like classrooms, wards, and outpatient departments. So, **planning is critical.**

A lesson plan is usually made for a conventional class that lasts **40-60 minutes**. A lesson plan **is not the** notes teachers write, emphasizing content from various sources. It would be best if you had a more detailed lesson plan at the beginning of your career, and with experience, a less detailed lesson plan may be enough. **It is desirable that all teachers do lesson planning.**

Broadly these are the **KODES** (steps) you need to work on before you step into the classroom.

Know your students – note to which year or stream of medicine, like M.B.B.S or allied courses, your student belongs! What is their existing knowledge? Try to arouse interest in the topic by providing a good induction or introduction to your class by correlating with clinical-based scenarios or a newspaper clipping relevant to the topic; for example, while taking a class on the hazards of blood transfusion, you can introduce the topic by share your own experience or projecting a newspaper article.

Objectives of the class- spend time working out how many minutes you will spend on each of the specific learning objectives of the class.

Didactic/non-didactic components – will you conduct any activity to complete specific learning objectives? Remember, the average adult's attention span is less than 20 minutes. Try to plan your class so that every 20 minutes, you break the monotony by asking questions, showing a random picture, or solving a riddle. You can even break your monotony with simple activities like asking the students to stand up and raise their hands on your instructions.

E- resources/ other resources – what will be your audio-visual aid- chalkboard, PowerPoint, overhead projectors.

How to communicate effectively?

Delivering a lecture is a skill; practice helps you to sharpen this skill for perfection. Attitude and communication skills are the most critical component of a lecture. Both **verbal and nonverbal modes of communication play an essential role in making your lecture effective.**

- Your voice should be loud and clear.
- Try to maintain a balance between the correct and the prevalent local pronunciation.
- Practice what you want to tell before you tell.
- Maintain your pace throughout the class- do not rush over the topic as you realize you are short of time!

Non-verbal communication: it plays a very role in the teaching-learning process in a classroom. It leaves an **impact on the students,** which ultimately results in better learning and understanding of concepts.

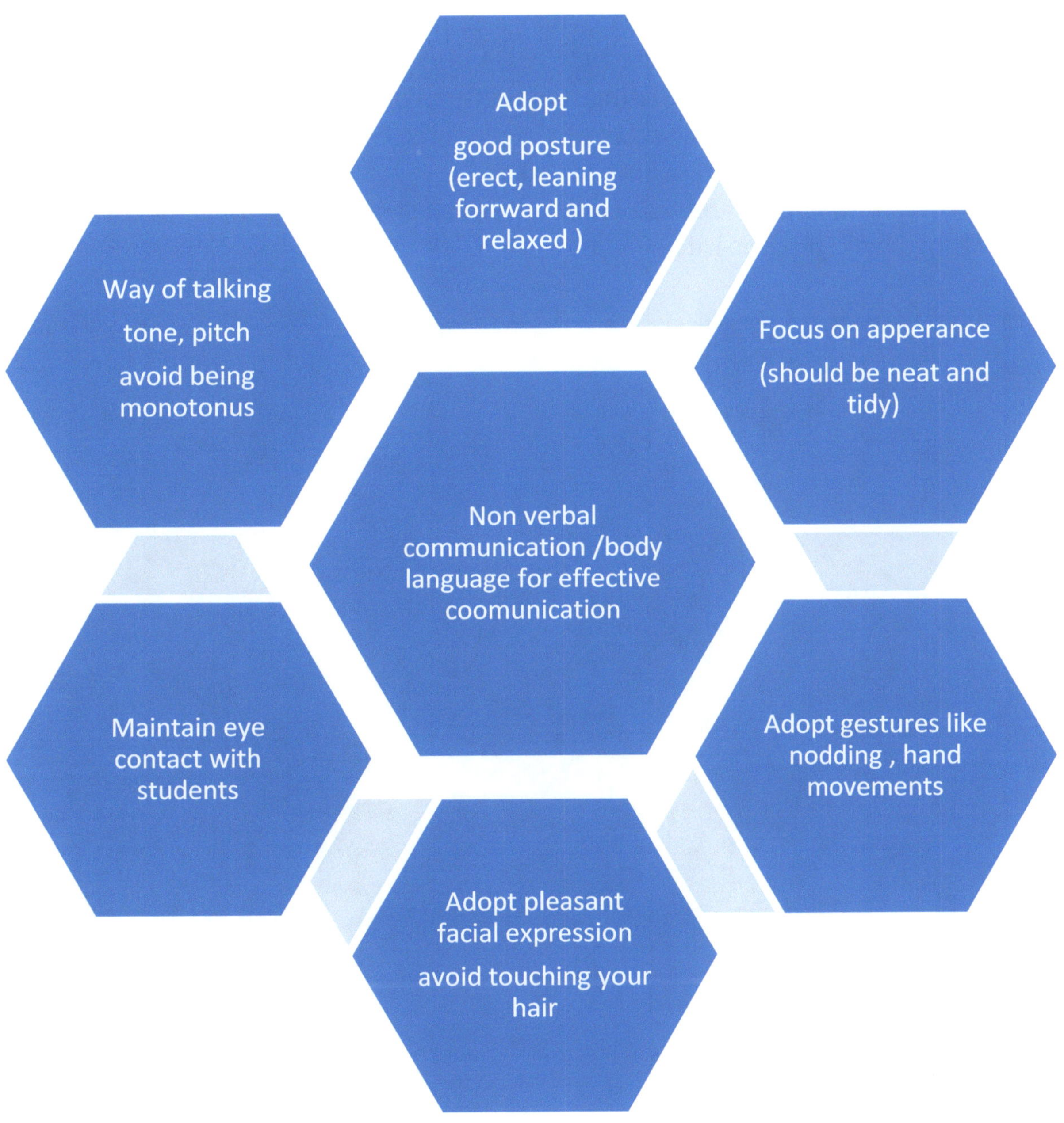

Common modes of non-verbal communication

Common Aids used for lecture

- **Blackboard/whiteboard/green board:**
- It is the oldest, inexpensive tool available, giving a teacher opportunities for creativity. It requires less planning and preparation than PowerPoint, and different colours can emphasize important points.

  Rules to be followed for effective use of the blackboard during a class are listed below
  - ➢ Write in capital letters (when you do this, you do not worry about your handwriting)
  - ➢ Do not write every word on the board – be concise and write keywords.
  - ➢ If you use a whiteboard, use the colour visible to all, like blue or black.
  - ➢ Preferably use the board when you want the students to follow the steps sequentially.

- It is advisable to divide the board into a minor (non-erasable) and a major(erasable) section, as shown in the picture below. Dividing the board into sections helps organize your class better to avoid rewriting frequently used side headings.
- Make sure you do not block what is written on the blackboard.
- Check what you write for spelling mistakes.
- Always erase the board after the class (move the duster in the top to down direction if you are using chalk/blackboard)

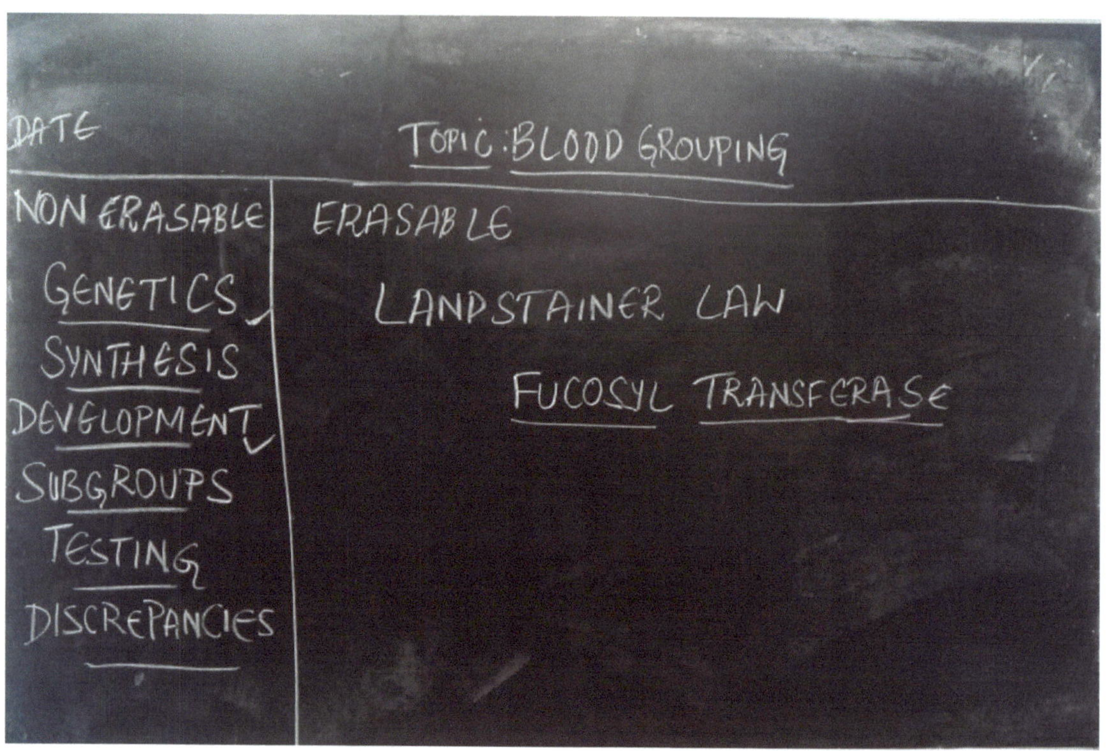

Disadvantages of using a blackboard

- You cannot maintain eye contact with students when writing on the blackboard.
- You cannot retain the written content.

PowerPoint presentation

- Do and don'ts of PowerPoint presentation are shown in the table

Do	Don't
☑ Use sans serif fonts like Arial or Tahoma	☒ Use all caps or italics
☑ Stick to seven by seven or five by five	☒ Underline all words
☑ Make sure the background is white in a dark room	☒ Use decorative fonts.
☑ Spell check	☒ Use irrelevant images
☑ Vary font size, colour or style to draw attention but **avoid doing it all** in one slide.	☒ Use many graphics
☑ Use 2 or 3 colours to emphasise the keywords	☒ Use too many bullets
☑ Keep 1.5-2-line spaces between lines	☒ Vary the starting point for each lie

Common aids for small group teaching

Overhead projector (OHP)

Before the arrival of LCD projectors, OHPs were commonly used during lecture and instruction classes during practicals. It can still be used for small-group teaching.

How to prepare a transparent sheet for projection?

- Put a margin on the transparency sheet
- Use a blue, black permanent marker pen. Red colour can be used for highlighting keywords
- You can write on the transparencies or photocopy the content
- Follow seven by seven rule- seven words per line with seven lines in a transparency sheet
- Use a pencil as a pointer to highlight a particular word or sentence.
- Image

Flip chart:

- Effective tool
- It can be used when you are building a sequence.
- Use colours like blue or black, which are visible to all the students

Flipped classroom:

The flipped classroom is defined as "shifting direct learning out of the large group learning space and moving it into the individual learning space, with the help of several technologies."

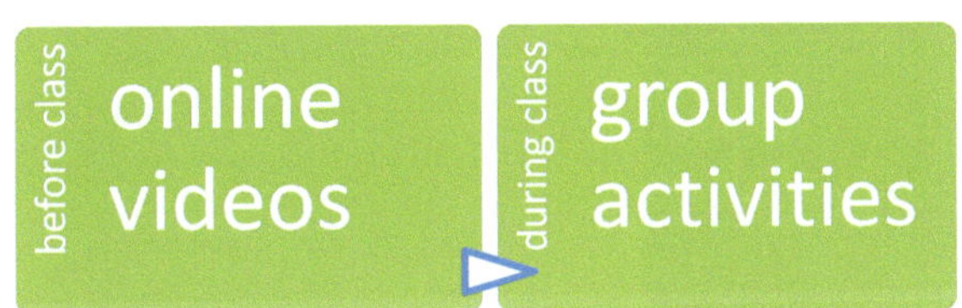

What is a flipped classroom model

Outside class or before class- students read the learning resources provided to them (text, video or audio) chosen by the teacher, followed by small online activities like a

- Short quiz
- Online discussion
- One paragraph summary
- Concept map

Students should be asked to engage in concepts by participating in individual and/or group activities with the instructor's guidance. Given below is the table list of individual and group activities

Individual classroom activities	Group activities
Polling	Think-pair-share
Designing concept maps	Fishbowl discussion
Individual problem solving	Affinity grouping
	Critical debate

Think -pair-share – ask the student to think and share the thought with the adjacent person and discuss with the class

Fishbowl discussion- it consists of two groups, inner and outer groups. The inner group discusses a topic like, for example, "methods that can be adopted to prevent hazards of blood transfusion" Outer group observes and listens to the discussion.

Affinity grouping: like-minded students are grouped and brainstorm ideas

Critical debate: this strategy involved assigning students a problem on a given topic and one group arguing for the topic and the other group against the topic.

How to make it interactive?

The lecture should be planned, so students are **engaged** and involved in the class right from the **beginning**. Below is a list of strategies you can adopt in your lecture according to the students and topics.

Questioning

You can ask students some questions, promote the use of hand gestures when they hear a specific word during your lecture or allow students to respond by using clickers (when you want to take the opinion of the whole class) or use colour cards/polls as audience response, especially in an online class

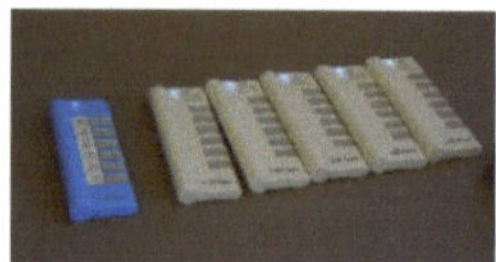

iClickers can be used to take polls

Use rhetorical questions that students are not expected to answer but should stimulate a thought process in their minds.

For Example: What would happen if RBCs were not there and Haemoglobin was freely present and soluble in the plasma

Demonstrations/ videos

Visual stimuli and animations will help in arousing interest in the students and reinforce complex concepts or teach a concept which is to be taught sequentially, like, for example, blood component preparation.

Roleplaying

There is a saying, "I hear, and I forget. I see, and I remember. I do, and I understand."

For example – how to identify the source of error in mismatched blood transfusion.

Problem-solving / Case-based examples

You can give your student's history and clinical investigations in sequential order and ask them the next logical step.

E.g., Investigating a transfusion reaction.

Pre-test and post-test

You can frame questions like true or false or MCQ related to the topic of the day and use them to conduct a pre-test before and after the class.

One-minute paper

You can ask the student to write one aspect of the class which worked for him and one aspect of the class which not work for him on a piece of paper and leave it on the table as he exits the class.

Repetition

Always repeat essential concepts for better retention among learners. "Move from known to unknown and simple to complex."

How to promote retention among students

Summary/take-home message: last five minutes try to give to bird's eye view of what is learned in the last 40 minutes, or you can ask a student to summarize it for you (this trick will enhance student engagement)

Use a variety of stimuli: we usually have the majority of learners in a class who use multiple modes of learning, as some learn by listening, some by writing, some by watching videos and some by doing. Of course, we cannot use all stimuli like visual, auditory, reading, and kinaesthetic in all our classes; try using at least two kinds of stimuli for effective learning among students.

Physical environment: always ensure your students are in a comfortable environment for a better learning process. A too-hot and humid environment is a prevalent environment we encounter in this part of the country.

How to modify your class for online teaching

Considering the current situation of the COVID-19 (Coronavirus) pandemic, e-learning has gained more popularity and is an inevitable method to ensure the continuity of classes. It is important to prepare ourselves for this new mode of teaching. Among the huge list of pros and cons between taking a conventional class and an online class, one factor that plays a key role is that all the students are not in one place, and you do not have control over their behaviour. Here I have tried to give some tips regarding modifying a traditional class into an effective online class.

Use polls: you can conduct a pre-test and post-test using polls or take their opinion on a prevalent topic. The results of the polls will instantly be displayed to the students.

Put questions: modify the content of the presentation in such a way that you are stimulating your student's thought process by asking more questions.

Do not put everything on the slide: put only keywords, diagrams, flow charts and images so the student listens to you primarily to understand the slide's content.

Be prepared for technical issues: there might be network connection issues, so always prepare a class for a shorter duration than the allotted time.

Always give assignments based on the class: if you are taking a module or series of classes, it is good to give a small assignment to your students, which can connect your previous class and the upcoming one.

Use graphs that require student interaction: put a graph on the slide and ask a student to point a point/activity on the graph during your presentation. It will promote active learning among students and increase focused learning.

E.g., an image of a blood product with a label – pick the expiry date, wrongly mentioned contents etc.

Is it necessary to take feedback?

It is crucial to take feedback on your classes. Ideally, feedback should be taken for all the classes we take, but since it is practically impossible to do that, try to take it as frequently as possible and always take feedback from students when introducing new teaching-learning methods or assessments.

From whom and How to take feedback?

Students- the aim of delivering a lecture (a process) is to transfer the information from a teacher to the students (product). Using a quantitative tool, you can ask the students to give feedback on the lecture. You can use a tool that contains simple questions like did you enjoy the session, were the objectives of the class met, etc.? to more complex questions like what you liked about the class, what you did not understand, the teacher allowed the students to ask questions etc.

Peer feedback – ask a colleague of yours to sit through the lecture to give feedback to your class. This will help you to **limit your limitations** during class.

Skills of good lecturing
Preparation:
Take account of the learner's current knowledge
Specify the purpose or outcome
Provide a structure or sequence
Opening
Gain attention, build rapport, and generate interest by giving examples or situations relating to a real-life scenario
Explanations
Clarity in concepts
Providing Information:
Cover the essential facts/theories

Narration: Provide case histories, experiences, patient stories, celebrities with diseases, etc.
Optimal usage of media
Responsiveness to the audience Give them enough time, and do not embarrass them even if doubts may seem silly
Keep them **involved** in some activity
Summarise Provide summaries. They need not always be at the end; points can be summarised after important subtopics

PREPARING AND PRESENTING JOURNAL CLUB

Good journal clubs end with good food or at least a great snack!!

Why read and discuss journal articles?

- Motivates participants to seek and keep up-to-date new medical literature
- Sharpens participants' critical appraisal skills by providing a space to discuss
- Embracing evidence-based practice and translating forefront knowledge to guide clinical practice
- Stimulates academic debates, Make It a Routine
- Helps in interdepartmental social and professional networking
- Stimulates research ideas and generates interest in publications (letter to editor etc.)

How to prepare and present at a Journal Club?

Preparing for a journal club can be a daunting task for a trainee resident, but critically appraising and presenting an academic paper is a competency that is a must for the trainee doctor. Let us know some tricks of the trade.

i. Read the paper thoroughly, making good time and probably repeatedly on parts of the paper you did not understand clearly
ii. Circulate the article to all participants well in advance
iii. Read relevant citations and literature
iv. Either prepare a ppt or project the article directly highlighting the necessary portions you intend to discuss with the participants. If the group is small, handouts also would be a good idea
v. Rehearse the presentation to combat nerves and familiarise the contents

Do not worry, as initially, it may not be easy. The more you do them, the more familiar and comfortable you will become

The presenter will be evaluated based on the following:

Presentation Content: Clear and logical flow of information, Background information and hypotheses, Conclusions and critique of the paper

Presentation style: capturing attention and keeping the audience's interest throughout the presentation

Discussion: generate interesting and lively discussion with the audience

Checklist for Critical Review of Journal Articles
Title:
Is it appropriate for the objectives of the study?
If not, what modifications would you suggest?
Introduction (Background and rationale):
What is interesting about this work?
What circumstances lead to this research?
What are the socio-economic, biomedical and ethical issues?
Is the hypothesis supported?
Is the argument convincing? Is the evidence valid?
Research questions:
Is it likely to add to the understanding of the subject?
Is it a locally specific question?
What are the objectives?
Were the target population and sample size appropriate?
Was the selection unbiased? Was the control group appropriate?
Methodology:
Was the study design, population, randomisation, inclusion & exclusion appropriate?
Was there any bias in information collection?
Are the results convincing, comprehensive and thorough?
Analysis:
Was the test used appropriately?
Is it the aptest test? Were there any alternatives and their discussion?
Results :
Were the experiments done appropriate with respect to the objectives of the study?
Do the results obtained make sense?
Do the legends of the figures clearly describe the data obtained?
Are the data presented in tabular form clear?
Are the legends of the tables clear?
Has an appropriate statistical analysis been performed on the data?

<table>
<tr><td>Discussion</td></tr>
<tr><td>Is it comprehensive with no citation bias?</td></tr>
<tr><td>Are the findings presented clearly with plausible explanations?</td></tr>
<tr><td>Could it be interpreted in any other way?</td></tr>
<tr><td>Conclusions:</td></tr>
<tr><td>What questions remained unanswered?</td></tr>
<tr><td>Are they applicable to the general population?</td></tr>
<tr><td>Are the conclusions justifiable?</td></tr>
<tr><td>Are the limitations discussed?</td></tr>
<tr><td>Does it add to our knowledge or contribute to the field?</td></tr>
</table>

Citation: A later document (with time) referencing a previous document

Citation Index: The number of citations an article has received.

h-*index* is a form of citation index wherein **h** is equal to the number of papers (N) in the list with N or more **citations.** E.g., Say an author has 10 publications, and 5 of his publications have at least 5 citations, then his h-index would be 5. Even if 3 of his articles have more than 10 citations, his i-10 index will be 3, whereas his h-index would still be 5. If his h-index has to increase to 6, then 6 of his articles must receive at least 6 citations.

i10-Index- the number of publications with at least 10 citations

The journal Impact Factor is the average number of times articles from the journal published in the past two years have been cited in the Journal Citation Reports (JCR) year. It is calculated by dividing the number of citations in the JCR year by the total number of articles published in the two previous years. The "JCR Year" refers to the Journal Citation Report year, the individual year for which a metric is provided.

Few essential and well-known Journals in Transfusion Medicine and Immunohematology				
Journal	**Publisher**	**Frequency**	**Society affiliation**	**Impact factor (As on 2022)**
Blood Transfusion	Edizioni SIMTI	Bimonthly (6 issues a year)	Società Italiana di Medicina Trasfusionale e Immunoematologia(SIMTI)	3.662
Transfusion Medicine Reviews	Elsevier	Quarterly	-	3.328
Transfusion	Wiley	Monthly	American Association of Blood Banking	2.8
Vox Sanguinis	Wiley	Monthly	International Society of Blood Transfusion	2.347

Transfusion Medicine	Wiley	Bimonthly (6 issues a year)	British Blood Transfusion Society	2.159
Transfusion Clinique et Biologique	Elsevier	Quarterly	French Society of Blood Transfusion (SFTS)	1.126
Transfusion and Apheresis Science	Elsevier	Bimonthly (6 issues a year)	World Apheresis Association, Turkish Society of Apheresis, European Society for Haemapheresis	1.285
Journal of Clinical Apheresis	Wiley	Bimonthly (6 issues a year)	American Society for Apheresis	0.94
Asian Journal of Transfusion Science	Wolters Kluwer - Medknow	Biannual (twice a year)	Indian Society of Blood Transfusion and Immunohematology	0.662
Global Journal of Transfusion Medicine	Wolters Kluwer - Medknow	Biannual (twice a year)	Asian Association for Transfusion Medicine	
Indian Journal of Hematology and Blood Transfusion	Springer Nature	Quarterly	Indian Society of Hematology and Blood Transfusion	0.925
Immunohematology		Quarterly	American National Red cross	0.69
ISBT Science series	Wiley	Quarterly	International Society of Blood Transfusion	0.48
International Journal of Clinical Transfusion Medicine	Dove Press			

RESEARCH IN POSTGRADUATION

Research is to see what everybody else has seen
And
to think what nobody else has thought

– Albert Szent-Györgyi

Introduction:

Biomedical research in Transfusion Medicine provides a unique opportunity wherein experimental research can encompass a range of opportunities, from basic research on the bed/lab side to patient-oriented clinical research and blood donor research, which is common to none in the field of postgraduate Medicine. Here, there is scope for applying scientific principles to understand the physiological basis and therapy to alleviate or limit pathological illnesses. It is diverse, usually interdisciplinary, and regularly proposes innovation throughout the whole transfusion chain from the vein (of the donor) to the vein (of the patient). Each step provides loads of opportunities, from blood collection through screening, preparation, storage, and transfusion to the patient and outcomes. It includes inquisitiveness and an array of borrowings from animal experiments, cell studies, biochemical, material science, immunology, genetic, hematopoietic stem cells, in vitro production of blood products, as well as logistics, hemovigilance, regulations, physiological investigations, and clinical studies wherein you can look at the benefits of hemotherapy on patients.

Timeline: Though there are subtle variations, usually, the postgraduate student is expected to prepare a protocol and take necessary approvals from the Institute Research Bodies, including clearance from the Ethics committee and be ready to start the study by around six months from the date of joining the Postgraduate course

How do you choose a topic?

Especially in Transfusion Medicine, it happens so that most residents do not have exposure in undergraduate as to what this field has in its womb. Hence it would not be easy to choose the topic on your own. However, nothing should stop you from glancing at what the seniors and others have already taken up the dissertation to get an idea of what you are getting into. However, please do not take up a thesis similar to one before unless it is an epidemiological-based study and you expect a geographic and locoregional aspect for the same. If you are taking something done in the remote past and expecting things to change drastically since that study, make sure you add some novel aspects. Most of the time, the guide chooses the topic for you. However, keep the undermentioned points in mind while committing yourself to the thesis topic.

Points to consider before committing to a thesis topic
• It should be appropriate to your workplace, facilities, and expertise available (*A bird in the hand is worth two in the bush*) • It should be in both the interest of you and your guide • It should be possible to complete the study ideally in a time frame of 18-20 months (*Do not bite more than what you can chew*) • Avoid taking up seasonal issues, as sometimes you may not be able to achieve enough sample size

10.1 PREPARING A RESEARCH PROTOCOL:

Usually, each institute has its format for protocol writing. Throughout this chapter, we will try to take an example of this research topic.

"Comparison of the effect of Irradiation on biochemical parameters of PRBCs stored in SAGM versus those stored in CPDA at the end of **4 weeks**: A prospective experimental study."

However, the main contents would consist of the following.

Title

Make sure your title has the following: **PICOTT**

Population	In whom you are doing the study	E.g., donors, cancer patients, neonates, blood products
Intervention	What is the intervention/test/method you are performing or using in the study	E.g., Irradiation, survey, measurements
Comparison	What is the comparator arm/ population you are using, if any?	E.g., control population, comparative group
Outcome	What is the outcome you are studying for	E.g., improvement, symptoms, levels of various parameters
Time	Mention the duration, retrospective, prospective, etc.	E.g., Follow up period- a few weeks, months
Type of the study	Is it a survey, observational, experimental, etc.?	

Aims and Objectives: Aims are usually the **statement of intent**, what you hope to **achieve** at the end of the project. Objectives are specific statements that define measurable outcomes.

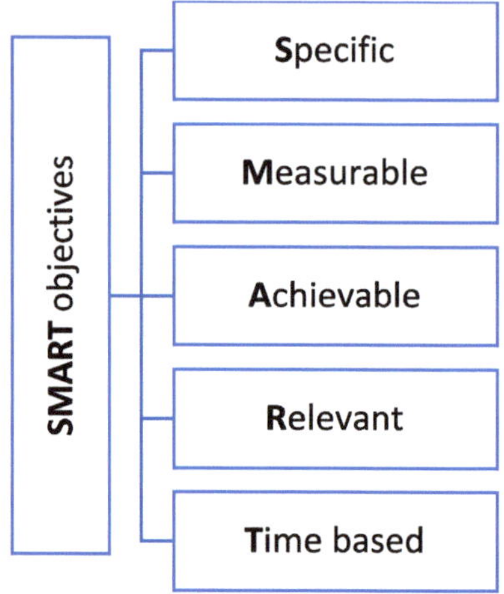

Verbs that are generally used for writing aims and objectives in Biomedical Research			
To analyze	To develop	To estimate	To predict To explore
To compare	To devise	To identify	To summarize To enumerate
To describe	To differentiate	To measure	To observe

Research question and research hypothesis

What is the question that your research is **going to answer?**

Research Hypothesis:

What is the **assumption** on which your study is based?

Introduction:

- ❖ Write briefly about what is already known about the study you are doing.
- ❖ What is the need for such a study?
- ❖ Write about what is **new in the study or what is not known regarding the study topic.**
- ❖ Write what you expect from this study and how the outcome will add to the knowledge or change/modify the ongoing practice.

Review of Literature

The literature review includes a literature search and a comprehensive review of existing literature in the research area of your interest. It is written to have solid background knowledge about the subject/topic you plan your thesis on. Search for the literature using the keywords of your thesis topic. Usually, it is **better to go in reverse chronological order** (from the most recent ones published backwards), download and store the publications, or save them to your account in Pubmed or any other search engine.

Methodology

- ❖ Who are the participants/subjects? If there is a comparison group/controls, mention them as well.
- ❖ What is the study design?

- ❖ Duration of the study.
- ❖ Mention the inclusion and exclusion criteria.

Make sure that the exclusion is a subset of inclusion. For example, if one of the inclusion criteria is "donors who have diabetes and are on treatment for less than five years," then your exclusion criteria should include "subjects without diabetes or diabetics on treatment for more than 5 yrs." It must explicitly state that amongst the people you have included, probably the ones who are asthmatic or hypertensive or, say, people who are on a combination of Insulin and Oral Hypoglycaemics, etc., among the donors who are on treatment for less than 5 yrs, are the subjects to be excluded.

Sampling

- ❖ Mention the type of sampling that will be used.
- ❖ Mention the sample size and the basis for arriving at such a size

Methods:

- ❖ Details of the drugs, devices, and procedures that will be used in detail
- ❖ Variables that will be studied or measured and the methods that will be used.
- ❖ Independent variables that would be collected.
- ❖ Dependent variables are also called outcome variables.
- ❖ List the interacting or confounding variables.
- ❖ Write in detail the data collection methods and periodicity if any follow-up is involved.

Statistical analysis plan

Write how the various analysis performed, the methods used, and how the variables and outcomes will be reported.

The data collection proforma is to be attached

The questionnaire must be attached if it is a questionnaire-based study.

If the questionnaire is in a language other than your local language, search for if the local language has a validated questionnaire. If not available, get it translated into the local language. Check for validity by back-translating it to the original language.

Add a few references. Each institute has different requirements for the number of references to be added. Generally, **10-20 references are ideal.**

Ethical approval

Each Institutional Ethics Committee has its requirements and proforma. However, the general principles are the process or procedure of taking the **study participants' informed consent** after mentioning the risk, if any, of participation in the study. Also, the benefits of participating and the duration the participants must spend in the study are mentioned to the participants.

If exemption from taking informed consent is required, it must be mentioned by giving justification.

Budget

Add a note on how you intend to get the funds to perform the study if necessary. Also, give a short description as to how the funds will be utilized and for what purpose (reagents, consumables, human resources, or any other logistics)

10.2 BASICS IN BIOSTATISTICS

– Dr. Mohandoss M

The chapter briefly discusses the commonly used statistical methods.

The scale of measurements: There are two data types – constant and variable. A constant is a value that does not change in any situation with respect to time, place or person. Variable can take different values concerning time, place or person, e.g. Weight, BP etc. There are two types of variables – Qualitative and Quantitative

Qualitative: also known as Categorical variable. If the study variable is classified as category, class or group, it is a qualitative variable. E.g., the Blood group of the patient (A, B, AB, O) and the severity of donor reactions (mild, moderate and severe). There are two types of Qualitative variables- Nominal and Ordinal.

- **Nominal** – refers to variables where no order is possible in classification (Eg: Sex: Male or Female)
- **Ordinal** –when there is an order in classifying a group of variables (Eg: Disease status – stage I, II, III, IV or strength of agglutination – 0, 1+, 2+, 3+, 4+).
- Dichotomous refers to variables with only two categories (Male or Female), and Polychotomous refers to variables with more than two categories.

Quantitative: also known as Measurable variable. If the study variable is measurable in units and carries numerical value, it is a quantitative variable. In quantitative also, two variables are available – discrete and continuous.

- Discrete has distinct numerical values (Values without decimals).
- Continuous variables are two types – Interval and Ratio.
- *Interval scale:* When the variable has *no valid zero point* and the unit of measurement is arbitrary, it is called an interval. E.g., Temperature in Fahrenheit or Celsius is an interval type of continuous variable as these are two different types of measurement but contain the same information and are linearly related. Celsius start from zero while Fahrenheit starts from 32.
- *Ratio scale:* If the variable has a true zero point independent of the unit of measurement. E.g., weight measured in kg or pounds, both start with zero.

Ratio: describes the relationship between numerator and denominator, where the numerator is not part of the denominator. E.g.: patient/doctor ratio.

Proportion: describes when the numerator is included in the denominator. Usually expressed in percentage. Eg: Transfusion reaction (%) = number of transfusion reactions/number of blood transfusions *100

Distribution:

A normal (Gaussian) distribution is classically a symmetrical bell-shaped curve. If a variable is normally distributed, then the mean and the median values will be approximately equal. While many variables may not follow a normal distribution and show a deviation from normality, it is referred to as a non-normal (non-Gaussian) distribution. Mean, median, and mode will not be equal in non-normal distribution.

Before beginning statistical analyses of a continuous variable, it is essential to examine the distribution of the variable for skewness (tails), kurtosis (peaked or flat distribution), spread (range of the values) and Outliers (the data values separated from the rest of the data)

It will not be normally distributed if a variable has significant skewness, kurtosis, univariate outliers, or any combination.

Information about these characteristics determines what parametric or non-parametric tests need to be used and ensures that the results of the statistical analyses can be accurately explained and interpreted.

Tools for assessing Normality

- Histogram and Box plots
- Q-Q Plot
- Statistical test for normality
  - Kolmogrov- Smirnov test
  - Shapiro-Wilk test

Transforming skewed data

- Various mathematical formulae can be used to transform a skewed distribution into normality. A logarithmic transformation of scores is often effective if a distribution has a marked tail to the right-hand side.
- Other common transformations include square roots and reciprocals.

Commonly used statistical tests

- **Dependent (Outcome) Variable:** This is the main factor that you are trying to understand
- **Independent (Predictor) Variables:** These are the factors you hypothesise to impact your dependent variable.

Chi-square Test (x^2): The chi-square statistic is a non-parametric test used to test the statistical significance of association between two or more categorical variables.

The distribution of a categorical variable in a sample often needs to be compared with the distribution of a categorical variable in another sample.

 Fisher Exact Test is an exact method for testing the hypothesis of independence in the 2*2 table and is applied when one or more of the expected frequencies in a cell is ≤5. The test is usually preferred for smaller sample sizes.

McNemar's Chi-squared Test: The McNemar test is a non-parametric test for paired categorical variables. To use this, the dependent variable must be a nominal variable with two categories (i.e. dichotomous variables) and one independent variable with two connected groups. These two groups in the dependent variable must be mutually exclusive, i.e., participants cannot appear in more than one group.

Comparison between two independent quantitative samples

Student t-test (normally distributed) **and Wilcoxon's Rank Sum Test or Mann-Whitney U test** (not normally distributed) compares two independent quantitative samples. In simple terms, it compares whether the means (student t-test) or medians (Mann Whitney) of two samples tend to be equal or not.

Comparison between two correlated or paired quantitative samples

A paired t-test (normally distributed) **and Wilcoxon's Signed Rank Test** (not normally distributed): It compares whether the differences observed in values of quantitative variables between two correlated samples (before and after) are statistically different or not. It compares the means (paired t-test) or median (Wilcoxon's signed-rank test) of samples tested at two different time points.

Comparison among several (>2) independent quantitative samples

ANOVA (normal distribution) or Kruskal Wallis Test (not normal distribution): Tests whether or not several independent samples of quantitative variables come from the same population.

Comparison among paired (>2) quantitative samples

RM-ANOVA (normal distribution) or Friedman's Analysis (not normal distribution): tests whether differences observed in the values of quantitative variables between different time periods are statistically significant or not.

Correlation (r): Correlation is a statistical technique used to determine the degree to which two variables are related. Correlation analysis shows us how to determine the nature and strength of the relationship between two variables.

- Correlation lies between -1 to +1.
    - A zero correlation: no relationship between the variables.
    - A correlation of -1: a perfect negative correlation.
    - A correlation of +1 indicates a perfect negative correlation.
- Positive correlation:- If two related variables are such that when one increases (decreases), the other also increases (decreases).

    Negative correlation:- If two related variables are such that when one increases (decreases), the other decreases (increases).

    No correlation:- If both the variables are independent.
- **Correlation coefficients (r^2):**-A correlation coefficient describes how closely two variables are related. That is the amount of variability in one measurement explained by another.

- **Pearson Correlation Coefficient:** It is a parametric correlation coefficient. The variables must be approximately normally distributed to measure the linear association between two continuous variables.
- **Spearman's Rank Correlation Coefficient:** It is a non-parametric measure of correlation and could be computed in the following cases:

  1. At least one of the variables is non-normal
  2. Both variables are qualitative ordinal.
  3. One variable is quantitative, and the other is qualitative ordinal.

Regression analysis

- Regression analysis is a set of statistical processes for estimating the relationships among variables. Here the focus is on the **relationship** between **a dependent variable** (outcome or response variable) and **one or more independent variables** (predictor variable).
- It helps one understand how the value of the dependent variable changes when any one of the independent variables is varied while the other independent variables are held fixed. It is also used to understand which independent variables are related to the dependent variable and to explore the forms of these relationships.
- **Simple linear regression** is a model that assesses the relationship between a dependent variable and one independent variable.
- **Multiple linear regression** analysis is similar to the simple linear model, except that multiple independent variables are used.
- **Logistic regression** is one dependent variable (binary or only two categories), one or more independent variable(s) (interval or ratio or dichotomous)
- **Ordinal logistic regression** is one dependent variable (ordinal), one or more independent variable(s) (interval or ratio or dichotomous)
- **Multinominal logistic regression** is one dependent variable (nominal and more than two categories), 1+ independent variable(s) (interval or ratio or dichotomous)

Analytical methods when the outcome variable is quantitative

Desired analysis	Rank, score or Measurement (From normal distribution)	Rank, score or measurement (From non-normal distribution)
Describe one group	Mean, SD	Median, interquartile range (or) Median, range
Compare one group to a hypothetical value	One-sample t-test	Wilcoxon test
Compare two unpaired groups	Unpaired t-test	Wilcoxon's rank-sum test/ Mann-Whitney U test
Compare two paired groups*	Paired t-test	Wilcoxon's signed-rank test
Compare three or more unmatched groups	One-way ANOVA	Kruskal –Wallis test
Compare three or more matched group	Repeated-measures ANOVA	Friedman's Test

Quantify the association between two variables	Pearson's correlation coefficient	Spearman rank correlation coefficient
Predict value from another measured variable	Simple linear regression or non-linear regression	Non parametric regression
Predict value from several measured or binomial variables	Multiple linear regression	

*Paired: if the variables are correlated, i.e., like before and after the design

Analytical methods for binomial outcome variables

Desired analysis	Binomial(Two possible outcomes)
Describe one group	Proportion
Compare one group to a hypothetical value	Chi-square or Binomial test
Compare two unpaired groups	Chi-square for large sample (Fisher's exact test for small samples)
Compare two paired groups	McNemar'schisquared test
Compare three or more unmatched groups	Chi-square test

Analytical methods for binomial outcome variables

Desired analysis	Binomial (Two possible outcomes)
Compare three or more matched groups	Cochrane's test
Quantify the association between two variables	Contingency coefficients
Predict value from other measured variables	Simple logistic regression
Predict value from several measured or binomial/non-binomial variables	Multiple logistic regression

Analytical methods for the time-to-event outcome variable

Desired analysis	Time to event
Describe one group	Kaplan Meier survival curve
Compare two unpaired groups	Log-rank test or Mantel-Haenszel test
Compare two paired groups	Conditional proportional hazards regression
Compare three or more unmatched groups	Cox proportional hazard regression
Predict value from another measured variable	Cox proportional hazard regression (Hazard or survival models)

CMEs/Conferences/ Workshops in Transfusion Medicine - A Resident Perspective

– Dr. Satyam Arora

1. Introduction

Residency is one of the most crucial periods for training and learning in the medical field. This period involves many unique experiences, both academic and non-academic, which shape the future of a candidate. Academics and exams hold an essential part. Another traditional part of the training involves medical conferences and continuing medical education (CME). Residents should try to attend these meetings, present their work and learn from their colleagues and seniors.

2. Type of Academic meets

The academic meetings may be of different types. They may be focused at an Institutional level, State level, National level, or even an international level depending on the scope of the meeting, the delegates and the speakers presenting. For a transfusion medicine resident, the options available for such a meeting may be as follows:

Transfusion Medicine and Blood Banking Related

These scientific meetings are focused on the core subject of Transfusion Medicine and Blood Banking. These are often organized by a local body (such as state organizations) or by, a National body (such as the Indian Society of Transfusion Medicine (ISTM) and Indian Society of Blood Transfusion and Immunohematology (ISBTI)) or even an International body (such as American Association of Blood Bank (AABB), International Society of Blood Transfusion (ISBT) and Asian Association of Transfusion Medicine (AATM)).

These meetings focus on the core subjects of transfusion medicine, such as blood donors or donation, immunohematology, transfusion-transmitted infections (TTI), apheresis medicine, blood components and clinical transfusion with haemovigilance. One should always attend at least one of these meetings during the residency period and present their work (thesis). This helps in exchanging the work and gaining from the experience of other residents in transfusion medicine from other institutions across the country. This also helps in updating the latest developments in the field.

Some of the essential workshops include "HOTS" (focused on HLA-related advancements) by the Department of Transfusion Medicine, Transplant Immunology and Molecular Biology, Indraprastha Apollo Hospitals, New Delhi; "CASCADE" (focused on coagulation-related advancements and blood management) organized Jubilee Mission Medical College and Research Institute, Thrissur in Kerala. Many pre-conference workshops to learn closely about the topics of interest. JG Jolly teaching program by SGPGI/MAHE or JHAKAAS from JIPMER helps, especially exam-going postgraduates, to get the hang of the exams and preparation. Attending these workshops helps a resident get a hand on experience in many topics and an opportunity to interact and network with the experts in the field. Some travel support opportunities are also provided by some organizations based on the quality of the abstract submitted by the resident. These opportunities include "Dr. Harold Gunson" by ISBT, AATM Travel fellowships and ISTM postgraduate (PG) fellowships. These fellowships are a great way to attend the meeting, get recognition for your hard work and manage your travel and stay.

Allied Subjects to Transfusion Medicine

As transfusion medicine is an allied field and works in close association with many other branches for effective patient care hence attending a meeting of allied subjects such as basic sciences, genetics, haematology, paediatrics, neonatology, obstetrics, and oncology may also help the resident learn the newer developments in the allied fields. This is very important for residents as it helps them learn communication skills with other departments and helps in better communication with the clinician.

Presenting work during these allied clinical meetings helps convey your work and provides an opportunity to explain why having transfusion medicine specialist consultation on exceptional cases is essential and your availability to help them in such challenging cases. Networking with clinical counterparts is a significant part of attending these meetings.

Professional Development

Professional training of any physician in medicine deals not only with his field but also some important ones, such as Ethics in Medicine, Research Methodology, Information Technology and Social Media Communications. These are vital sessions that the resident should always try to attend. With evolving times and newer treatment modalities, medical ethics is a vital area to be exposed to during residency. Similarly, information technology, basic use of computers and Internet application with social media communication skills are becoming the need of the hour. Appropriate use of social media/Internet during residency may go a long way in interaction with others in the field and networking with many more. The resident should be aware of the responsibilities as well as duties as a medical professional, and a brief introduction to medicine and its applicable laws are also essential in today's time

3. Why should residents attend the conference

Transfusion medicine residents should try to attend at least one conference during his/her residency time. There are the following advantages to attending these academic meetings such as:

a. Gaining experience in presentation (either poster or oral presentation)
b. Getting feedback on your work
c. Exposure to a variety of research being conducted by others
d. Opportunity to critique and learn
e. Low registration fee
f. Familiarizing yourself with the business in your speciality

4. How should a resident prepare for a meeting or a conference

Academic enrichment, social interaction and travel are some goals for a resident while attending a conference. Preparation for a meeting should focus on all of them, as they are equally important.

a. Academic

Residents should carefully go through the conference's scientific program, which often comprises workshops, lectures, and demonstrations. One should carefully pick the topics of interest and try to attend to them. Oration lectures are often the highlight of the meeting, and a very senior scientist presents them. Oration lectures or academy day sessions should be on top priority to attend. Attending parallel sessions may become very challenging; hence priority should be given to the topic of interest and newer advancements.

b. Socializing

Socializing with colleagues from other institutes and seniors should also be focused while attending these meetings' breakfast, lunch, and dinner. Residents should focus on meeting mentors working primarily in the area of your interest in the field during the conference. These are excellent opportunities to know your colleagues and seniors and interact unofficially with them. ISBT and ISTM provide a unique "breakfast session" exclusively for interacting young professionals with seniors and mentors (one of the must-attend sessions for residents!).

c. Travel and vacation

Travelling around the destination of the conference and exploring a new city or a country is an essential part, as often these are the only opportunities a resident gets during the residency to travel. Stay during this meeting should always be near the conference meeting venue as it saves time and keeps your itinerary flexible. One should do a complete analysis of the places one can visit during the stay. Keeping some time (pre or post-meeting) apart from the academic feast, one should also include all the opportunities to explore the city. Planning the trip with a colleague or a senior is always better as it gives you company and offers an opportunity to know to interact better. *Always keep comfortable footwear for the conference as you might end up wearing the same shoe in the conference hall and on a beach!*

5. How to present during a conference

Conferences and CMEs often allow the resident to present their work in a poster or an oral presentation. Irrespective of the mode of presentation, residents should give their best.

Poster presentation involves summarizing the study in a poster (layout may differ in each conference). Posters (which are often neglected part) provide a great learning experience. One of the most challenging parts of preparing a scientific poster is managing the space to share your findings. One should try to include the following features in a poster

- Plan your poster based on the display settings (portrait or landscape)
- Use uniform colours and fonts (size and style)
- Make sure that your content is not too much (makes it messy) or too little (looks incomplete)
- Try to include all your details in the headings provided
- Try to place more relevant pictures, tables and charts
- Do not repeat information in text and tables or tables and charts
- Try to highlight the uniqueness of your work
- Always prepare well, compare with what is already published
- Keep the interest alive

A poster session involves evaluating your poster by an expert in the field and some questions about your topic. A resident should also find time to read other posters, as it gives an idea of all types of work other people are doing. People look for talent for hiring based on your work, so staying at your poster can sometimes earn you positions.

The oral presentation involves presenting the study in a PowerPoint presentation (ppt) to a group of delegates. The presentations should always be professionally presented. These presentations involve cross-questioning on your topic, which is essential to the whole learning experience. Residents should try to attend other colleagues' oral presentation sessions, irrespective of whether they are presenting or not.

6. Young Professional Forum or Council

This is a relatively new concept introduced by ISBT in 2018 to have some of the young fellows from the field on board with them. This has helped guide society to move with time and keep note of the young generation's interest or the next generation in the field. Similarly, in 2020, ISTM introduced the Young Professional Forum to engage more and more residents and early career researchers with ISBT activities. This is a very significant way to increase awareness of the field. Residents should take part in such activities and increase their participation in the same.

Final Advice

a. Do not let the opportunity pass by (Unless you need to)
b. Pick the sessions you are interested
c. Attend Lectures
d. Pack smart (the lesser, the better)
e. Present a poster or a paper (always try to present something)
f. Network, Network, Network!

Tips for a good poster presentation

- **Plan:** Read the instructions to presenters carefully – size, location/venue, display/view time, layout suggestions and any other additional information requested
- **Content:** limit to 2-3 key ideas and convey them effectively
- **Know your audience:** steps of a standard immunohematology test may not be required for a transfusion medicine audience but may be required in a general conference. Physicians would be interested in clinical applications of the test.
- If planning to include tables, include the part of the table which has significant findings only. The whole table may not be required. (Graphs are preferred over tables)
- Pictures are always more appealing than text
- First, write the methodology and results. Introduction and discussion receive minor importance in a poster.
- The most important finding should be at the eye level of the audience! Not at the bottom.
- Text as bulleted points rather than complete sentences
- **Rule of 10:** 10 or fewer panels/sections, ten or few lines and ten words, and visible from a distance of 10 feet
- Ideal fonts are – Arial, Helvetica, Tahoma, and Verdana (No horizontal extensions or tapering ends)
- Avoid using "italics" or "underlined fonts". Use "bold" judiciously
- Show it to your peers and take comments
- **Preparation:** Use pleasing colour combinations, and add borders and institutional logos. Use consistent colours for all figures/tables
- **Transport:** special package if required (cylindrical tube or poster carrier). If travelling by flight, carry hand baggage. Carry tape, Velcro, pins, scissors
- **Display and presentation:** visit the poster area well before the scheduled display. Be available during the complete duration of the allotted time. Invite experts and peers in the area of your poster to give feedback.

Tips for an excellent Oral presentation

Abstract preparation and Submission: if your study is complex, concentrate on only one aspect of it. Choose whether appropriate for the forum (Clinical work may not be of interest in the society of basic scientists and vice-versa).

Use active voice and past tense.

Presentation:

Length: Generally, one can speak 100 words per minute (do not confuse with words in ppt).

Usually, one slide per minute. (Simple pictures may take less whereas complex ones may need more time)

70% of your talk to be dedicated to methods and results (roughly equal amongst them)

15% each for introduction and discussion/conclusion

If you wish to show a slide twice in your presentation, have it twice rather than going back on the presentation.

Look for typographical errors.

Make sure your presentation is also loaded for remote access if required, along with carrying it on your device

Use appropriate animations

The talk:

Rehearse well before the actual talk. Can ask peers to observe and give feedback

Opening and closing statements are to be the most appealing. Leave a take-home message

Use speech modulation, pausing during the talk

Stick to the time

Please think of the possible questions that may be asked and be prepared for them. A fantastic presentation may become bland if you cannot answer the questions sufficiently.

Let the answers be brief. If you cannot answer something beyond your scope, admit it graciously.

Writing case reports

Writing case reports is one of the initial steps in medical writing, especially for postgraduates, who are expected to do it in their residency either for journals or in conferences/interdepartmental meetings.

What to publish?

1. Recognition and description of a new blood group variant
2. Recognition of a rare entity antigen
3. A novel way of resolving discrepancies or different immunohematological approaches to known discrepancies or problem
4. Detection of adverse or beneficial side effects of component therapy not described or noticed with an unusual presentation, happening with a blood component not usually known to cause that event, or a combination of adverse events
5. Education and audit, Impact of change of policy or SOP/ step
6. A new indication for a known blood component, a novel modification of the component
7. Illustrations/demonstrations of novel techniques or modifications to existing ones

Structure:

Title	PICOT (Patient, Intervention, Case report/series, Outcome, The condition)
Abstract	Introduction: what is unique about the case, and what it adds to the scientific literature Main symptoms and essential clinical findings, diagnosis, intervention and outcome Conclusion: take away message
Introduction	Purpose (why this is unique) Background information: Incidence, the number previously presented Define terms or words that are essential to understand the information in the paper
Case presentation (methods and results)	Patient information, his primary concerns and symptoms, relevant medical, transfusion, family, obstetric, psychosocial, and genetic history. Past interventions with the outcome(Transplant, IVIG, monoclonal antibody therapy etc.). Physical examination and critical clinical findings Timeline, testing, diagnostic challenges, DDs considered and how they were excluded, the complete immunohematological workup with pictures and antigrams whenever applicable Intervention/treatment done Follow-up and outcome, prognosis wherever applicable Adverse and unanticipated events
Discussion	Summarise what the case contributes Opinions Evaluate the case for accuracy, and derive new knowledge and/or applicability to practice Natural history of disease or factors Rationale for management significance or outcome of the case and why the care provided may or may not have been beneficial Limitations and their significance some suggestions for future inquiry into the topic
Conclusion	Take home message/learning from the case

CARE guidelines/checklist is something you follow so that you do not miss anything

Audits in Transfusion Medicine

– Dr. Soumya Das

Introduction: -

Transfusion services must move beyond the after-the-fact quality inspection into blood bank practices that proactively improve each day-to-day operations process. Periodic statistics or audits in the Transfusion Medicine centre are one of the routes through which information is transferred from data producers to end-users or decision-makers. The information is required for multiple purposes, from the development of statistical databases to necessary analytical public health reports and similar information products, with the ultimate goal of ensuring Safe Blood Transfusion for the Patient. Quality indicators are indispensable tools, which various stakeholders in the blood transfusion establishment now demand to adjudge and improve quality performance. Practitioners and policymakers in transfusion medicine must ensure that the quality indicators they institute are appropriately selected and analysed effectively and efficiently monitor quality. Standards are necessary to adequately compare variables of interest across time and units and ensure transparency and accountability in the system.

An audit involves checking a process, the structure, or even the outcome to ensure that it conforms to an expectation of performance. They are valuable, if written, to thoroughly review all the crucial systems within the laboratory. All audits are carried out based on a pre-described method. The audit is a system of investigation, evaluation, measurement, and continuous assessment and improvement. The audit is based on set guidelines but determines the difference between the directions and what has been done. The audit will reveal whether the process is doing what is desired of it and efficiently. Audits of transfusion practice can occur both in the blood bank and in the hospital wards and operation rooms; audits of the latter are generally performed to ensure that clinicians follow the institutional directives or guidelines for transfusion practice. Only by looking at a process can potential areas for improvement be found. This text describes essential monthly audit topics that should be carried out inside the transfusion centre service

Donor Room:

- Total No of Donors screened

Screened Donors	Total	Male	Female
Total Screened	N (%)	N (%)	N (%)
In-House	N (%)	N (%)	N (%)
Camps	N (%)	N (%)	N (%)

- Total No of Donation
- Percentage of Donors deferred =

$$\frac{Total\ No\ of\ Deferred\ Donors}{Total\ No\ of\ Donors\ Screened} \text{ X } 100$$

- Reasons for Donor deferral with no donors deferred for the particular reason
- Donor deferral rate:

  a. Total
  b. Permanent
  c. Temporary

- Quality Control of the Method for Haemoglobin Estimation
- Status of Various Instruments/Equipment in the Screening Area

Phlebotomy Room:

1. Total donors bled - also differentiate the donors bled in-house (Blood Bank) and Outdoor

No of Donations	Total	Male	Female
Total Donation	N (%)	N (%)	N (%)
In-House	N (%)	N (%)	N (%)
Camps	N (%)	N (%)	N (%)

2. Percentage of donations collected from first-time donors
3. Blood bag inventory

Types of Blood Bag available	Opening Stock on the 1st of the month	Used during the Month	Stock available at the end of the month	Critical Stock Based on the centre usage (2 months)
Single, Double				
Triple, etc				

4. Donor Reactions

Donor Reactions	Total			Male			Female		
	Total	Systemic	Local	Total	Systemic	Local	Total	Systemic	Local
Total	N (%)			N (%)			N (%)		
In-House	N (%)			N (%)			N (%)		
Camps	N (%)			N (%)			N (%)		

5. Percentage of Donor Reaction =

$$\frac{Total\ No\ of\ Donor\ Reaction\ including\ Local\ reactions}{Total\ No\ of\ Donors\ Donation} \times 100$$

6. Details of the Donor Reaction should be described as mentioned below

   a. Venepuncture failures (failure to introduce the needle into the donor's vein)
   b. Failed whole blood collections (interrupted blood collection due to slow or inadequate flow, hematoma, donor faintness or collapse, technical factors etc.)
   c. Clots in red blood cell (RBC) components
   d. Poor Yields on blood collection
   e. Inadequate volume collected
   f. Systemic Reaction

7. Therapeutic Phlebotomy

Component Lab

1. No of the Components Prepared

   a. Total WB collections:
   b. PRBCs
   c. FFPs   [kept for cryo]
   d. RDPs
   e. Cryos
   f. CPPs

2. Nonconforming BC due to the inadequate storage conditions
3. Expired platelet concentrate shelf life
4. Expired RBC concentrate shelf life
5. Discard rate

Component/ reason for discard	TTI positive					Less volume	leakage	others
	HIV	HBV	HCV	RPR	Malaria			
Whole blood								
PRBC								
FFP								
RDP								
CRYO/FFP								

6. **Quality Control of Blood Components**

   a. It should be performed on at least 1% of all components prepared. (all parameters to be measured)

b. If fewer than 100 per month, then at least 75% or more of the components monitored must meet specifications

Volume - Volume should be recorded on all units

$$Vol\ (ml) = \frac{Weight\ of\ bag + blood\ components(g) - wt\ of\ empty\ bag}{The\ specific\ gravity\ of\ the\ component}$$

Specific gravity

Packed RBC	=	1.093
Platelets	=	1.035
Plasma	=	1.030
Whole blood	=	1.053

How to sample the blood component for QC

- Non-destructive sampling methods usually involve the use of pack tubing
- Mixing the product and stripping tubes is vital
- The tubing should be stripped thrice before collecting the blood component sample.
- Sampling methods must be validated to ensure that they produce consistent samples, regardless of the operator
- AVOID taking from the last part of the tube
- This section is difficult to strip correctly, and the last 2 cm should be cut off after stripping the rest of the line
- For platelet count, samples should be taken into a dry EDTA tube to induce disaggregation

Points to look for in QC of Platelet concentrate

- **All units should show a 'swirling' effect**
- No pink/red discolouration on visual inspection = insufficient red cells to cause immunisation
- (RDP from 450 ml whole blood) – PRP Method

Transfusion Transmitted Lab

- Total no. of samples tested =
- Total no. of whole blood(WB) donor samples tested =
- No. of reactive WB samples =
- Total no. of SDP samples =
- No. of reactive PR samples =
- Reactive percentage: (Total Positives/Total no of Samples tested)=
- Reactivity of HIV, HBsAg, HCV, Malaria, RPR
- Confirmation for Individual and Donor Notification

1st test results	Our repeat test results	Micro/confirmation results	Donor notification

- Stock Update

Name of the Kit	Opening Stock on the 1st of the month	Received during the Month	Used during the Month	Stock Available at the End of the Month	Critical Stock Based on the centre usage (2 months)

- LJ Chart Plotting

Pre-Transfusion Testing

- No of requests :
- No. of Issues :
  - PRBC: FFP: Platelets: SDP: Cryoprecipitate:
- Department wise Issues
- Returned Blood Components and Reasons for the same
- Discards of Blood Components
- Transfusion Reaction =

$$\frac{Total\ No\ of\ Adverse\ Transfusion Reactions}{Total\ No\ of\ Blood\ Components\ Issued} \times 100$$

- Patient sample nonconformities
- Nonconformities in the requests for pretransfusion testing
- Test turnaround time – urgent requests
- Test turnaround time – routine requests
- C: T ratio
- ABO/Rh(D) discrepancies
- WBIT errors
- RBC units issued under the emergency release procedure
- Traceability of issued units (confirmation of transfusion or discard)
- Wastage rate (Expiry as well as others)

Apheresis Section

- Total Number of procedures:
- Voluntary repeat donors
- First-time replacement
- Donor reactions
  - Hypocalcemia
  - Hematoma
- Kit wastage
- All the Platelet Concentrates collected by Apheresis needs to undergo a Quality Check before the issue

Clinical Transfusion Audits:

1. Appropriateness of Blood component usage (%)
2. Deviation from practices and protocols
3. Blood administration compliance rates
4. Effectiveness of Massive Transfusion Protocol

Type	Timing	Performed by	Advantages	Disadvantages
Prospective	Real-time	The staff of the department Computer analysts	Proactive	Labour intensive Can cause a delay in issue/TAT
Concurrent	12-24 hrs	Transfusion safety officer	Consultative and training opportunity	Labour intensive Needs cooperative clinicians
Retrospective (internal)	Days to weeks	Quality manager Peers from other depts	Easy Provides data for trends and benchmarking	Non-standardised
Retrospective (External)	Days to weeks	Trained outsiders (3rd party)	Objective thorough and standardised	Expensive

CALCULATIONS IN TRANSFUSION MEDICINE

Some useful conversions

1 inch = 2.54 cm

1 Kg = 2.2 lbs

1 g/dL = 0.62 mmol/L (For Hb)

1.1 Blood Volumes:

i.   Preterm neonate = 100ml/kg
ii. Term neonate = 85ml/kg
iii. Infant (1-4 months) = 75 ml/kg
iv. Child (<25 kg) = 70ml/kg

Adults

Table Gilcher's Rule of Fives

Habitus	Obese	Thin	Normal	Muscular
Male(ml/kg)	60	65	70	75
Female (ml/kg)	55	60	65	70

Based on BMI

BMI	< 18.5	- 24.9	25 – 29.9	>30
Blood volume (ml/kg)	80	70	65	55

The most accurate way is to use *Nadler's Formula*

Patient	Formula (To be used only when weight is more than 55 pounds or 25 kg	
Male	$\{(0.006012 \times H^3) \div (14.6 \times W)\} + 604$	$\{(0.3669 \times H^3) + (0.03219 \times W)\} + 0.6041$
Female	$\{(0.005835 \times H^3) \div (15 \times W)\} + 183$	$\{(0.3561 \times H^3) + (0.03308 \times W)\} + 0.1833$
	H=Ht in inches, W= Weight in Pounds	H=Ht in mts, W= Weight in kg

Lindenkamp's Nomogram can also be used for pediatric patients to calculate blood volume when weight and height are known.

$$RBC\ Volume = Total\ Blood\ Volume \times \frac{Hct}{100}$$

$$Plasma\ Volume = Total\ Blood\ Volume \times \frac{(1-Hct)}{100}$$

1.2 Anticoagulant ratio:

An AC: WB of 1:9 means 1 ml of anticoagulant is added to 8 ml of whole blood.

2.2.1

Component	Dose	Expected Increment (Assuming 100% recovery)
RBC	5 ml/Kg to raise Hb by one gm%	3.5 ml per Kg of Pure red cells (100% Hct) raise the Hb by one gm%
Platelets	1 unit of RDP per every 10 Kg Body weight (or) 5 ml/Kg	50,000/µl
FFP	10-15 ml/kg	15-20% rise in factor level
Cryoppt AHF	1-2 units/10 kg	60-100 mg/dL rise in Fibrinogen

2.2.1CCI:

$$\frac{Platelet\ count\ increment/\mu L \times Blood\ Volume(L)}{Number\ of\ platelets\ transfused\ (10^{11})}$$

Problem: A man weighing 80 Kg and a height of 180 cm had a platelet count of 12,000/µL. He was transfused with a standard unit($3x10^{11}$) of apheresis platelets. His platelet count increased to 46,000/µL. What is the Corrected Count Increment?

Solution:

Platelet count increment = final platelet count (after transfusion)- initial platelet count(pretransfusion)

$$46,000/\mu L - 12000\mu L = 34,000/\mu L$$

Body Surface Area = = 2 m^2

No of platelets transfused= 3×10^{11}

Applying,

$$\frac{34,000 \times 2}{3(10^{11})} = 22,667$$

Platelet Recovery:

$$\frac{\text{Platelet count increment/}\mu L \times \text{Blood Volume(L)}}{\text{Number of platelets transfused}}$$

Problem: Consider the same patient in the problem above

Solution: Blood volume (Estimated) would be 80kgx70ml/Kg = 5600ml or 5.6L

Platelet recovery would be $= \dfrac{34{,}000 \times 5.6 \times 10^6}{3 \times 10^{11}} = 0.635$ (or) 63.5%

CCI of less than 7500 is usually considered to be refractoriness

If within one hr. of transfusion, then it is considered of Non immunological cause

If within 24 hr. of transfusion, then it is considered of immunological cause

2.2.2 Plasma Therapy:

Factor-based: The same formula may be used for any factor. Remember that the frequency of transfusion will differ depending on their half-lives.

Fibrinogen:

Fibrinogen Increment $=$ Fibrinogendesired $-$ Fibrinogeninitial

Total fibrinogen to be transfused $=$ Fibrinogen increment $\times$ Plasma Volume

Problem: A patient with haemorrhage post-partum was known to have a fibrinogen level of 70mg/dL and Hematocrit of 33%. How many bags of Cryo is to be transfused to this patient if she weighs 70 Kg?

Solution:

The intention is to raise the Fibrinogen to 100mg/Dl

Required increment $= \dfrac{(100\text{-}70)}{100} = 0.3$

Plasma Volume $= 70 \times 65 \,(1\text{-}\,0.33) = 3049$

Fibrinogen required $= 3049 \times 0.3 = 915$ mg

Each Cryo bag has about 80mg of fibrinogen, So $\dfrac{915}{80} = 11.44$ (around 12 bags)

3.1

$$\text{Number of units to screen} = \frac{\text{Number of desired units}}{\dfrac{(1-\text{Antigen frequency})}{100}}$$

Problem 1: If a patient has Anti-c and Anti-S, how many RBC units will the transfusion service need to test to find two units compatible with the patient?

(Frequency data: c = 80%, C = 68%, s = 90%, S = 55%)

Solution:

Number of units to be tested= No of units required÷ percentage of RBC units compatible

As per the given data, the number of units negative for "c" would be 20%

the number of units negative for "S" would be 45%

The number of units to be tested is $\dfrac{2(\text{No of units required})}{0.2\times0.45}$ = 22 units

Problem 2: The prevalence of various antigen/phenotype frequencies in a population is given below:

Phenotype	Frequency (%)	Phenotype	Frequency (%)
A	20	Fy(a+b-)	15
B	25	Fy(a+b+)	41
O	45	Fy(a-b+)	32
AB	10	Fy(a-b-)	12
DCE	1	DcE	14
DCe	41	Dce	4
CE	1	Ce	2
Ce	36	cE	1
S+s-	10	S+s+	42
S-s-	0	S-s+	48

An O+ve thalassemic patient has developed alloantibodies. His serum contains anti-c, anti-Fy^a, and anti-S. What will be the prevalence of a compatible unit for this patient?

Solution:

Number of units to be tested = No of units required÷ percentage of RBC units compatible

As per the given data, the number of units negative for "c" would be 81%

the number of units negative for "S" would be 42%

the number of units negative for "Fy^a" would be 44%

The number of units to be tested is $\dfrac{1(\text{No of units required})}{0.8 \times 0.44 \times 0.42}$ = 6.8 units

4.1

FMH

$$\text{Fetomaternal Hemorrhage} = \text{Maternal Blood Volume} \times \frac{\text{Number of fetal cells}}{\text{Number of Maternal cells}}$$

A 300µg vial can neutralize 30 ml of whole blood or 15 ml of PRBCs.

$$\text{So number of vials required} = \frac{\{\text{FMH(ml)} + 1\}}{30} \text{ (approximated to nearest whole number)}$$

4.2 Intrauterine Transfusion

The volume of blood to be transfused =

$$\frac{\text{Estimated Fetal Wt.(gm)} \times 0.14 \text{ mL/gm (HctTarget-HctCurrent)}}{\text{Hct of the product}}$$

Problem: An Antenatal mother needs an intrauterine transfusion. The current Hct of the fetus is 15gm%. The estimated fetal weight is 1000gm. The Hct of the given blood product is 85%. The Perinatologist expects to raise the Hematocrit of the fetus to 40%.

Solution:

$$\frac{1000(\text{gm}) \times 0.14 \text{ mL/gm } (0.40-0.15)}{0.85} = 41.17 \text{ ml}$$

4.3 Exchange transfusion:

A double-volume exchange transfusion (170ml/kg for a full term or 200ml/kg for VLBW infants) removes approximately 70-90% of circulating red cells and approximately 50% of total bilirubin.

For Polycythemia: Target Hct is 55%- 60%

$$\text{Volume of replacement fluid} = \text{Blood Volume} \times \frac{(\text{Observed}_{\text{Hct}} - \text{Desired}_{\text{Hct}})}{\text{Observed}_{\text{Hct}}}$$

Problem: A neonate weighing 2.6 kgs was found to have an Hb% of 22.5gm%. It was decided to reduce the Hb% to about 20 gm%. What amount of Blood is to be removed and replaced in this infant?

Solution:

$$\text{Volume to be removed/replaced} = 195 \frac{(0.675-0.6)}{0.675} = 21.7 \text{ ml}$$

Blood volume = 2.6× 75ml/kg = 195 ml

Current Hct = 3 × Hb% = 67.5

RhIG dosage calculation

1. Determine the percentage of fetal red cells in maternal circulation
2. Determine the maternal blood volume
3. Determine FMH (% of fetal red cells × maternal Blood Volume)
4. Dose of RhIG = FMH × 10 µg of RhIG
5. The number of vials = total RhIG dose in µg ÷ dose per vial.

   [Always overcorrect. (if the number of vials is a decimal less than .5, round down to a lower number and add 1 vial, e.g., If we get 2.3 vials, then round down to 2 and add 1 vial, i.e., 3)

   if the number of vials is a decimal more than .5, round up to a higher number and add 1 vial, e.g., If we get 2.8 vials, then round up to 3 and add 1 vial, i.e., 4]

---

5 Apheresis

5.1.1 Conversion of Hb to Hct

$$\text{Hct (\%)} = 3 \times \text{Hb(g/dL)} \text{ or } [\text{Hb(mmol/L)} \times 5] - 2$$

5.1.2 Weight to Volume

$$\text{Volume} = \frac{\text{Weight}}{\text{Density}}$$

5.1.3 Ideal body weight

Males: 48 kgs for first 152.4 cm + 1.1 kg for each additional cm

Females: 45 kgs for first 152.4 cm + 0.9 kg for each additional cm

Example: What would be the ideal body weight of a male and a female patient measuring 160 cm each?

$$160-152.4 = 7.6$$

For males: 48+ (7.6 × 1.1) = 48+8.36 = 56.36 kgs

For females: 45+ (7.6 × 0.9) = 45+6.84 = 51.84 kgs

Adjusted body weight = Ideal body weight + 0.25 (Actual weight- Ideal body weight)

Example: What would be the adjusted body weight of the female patient mentioned above if her actual weight was 60 kg?

Adjusted body weight = Ideal body weight + 0.25 (Actual weight- Ideal body weight)

$$= 51.84 + 0.25 (60 - 51.84)$$

$$= 51.84 + 0.25 (8.16)$$

$$= 51.84 + 2.04 = 53.88 \text{kgs}$$

$$\text{Body mass index (BMI):} \ \frac{\text{Weight(kg)}}{\text{Height}^2\text{(mts)}}$$

Example: A patient is 172 cm tall and weighs 80. Calculate his BMI.

$$BMI = \frac{80}{(1.72)^2} = \frac{80}{2.9584} = 27.04$$

Removal efficiency in Therapeutic plasma exchange:

$$Substance_{remaining} = Substance_{initial} \times e^{-PV\ processed} \qquad (PV = plasma\ volume)$$

Example: A patient with GBS has antibody levels of 5 g/dL. A double volume exchange was performed. What is the expected post-procedural value of the antibodies in the patient?

$$Substance_{remaining} = Substance_{initial} \times e^{-PV\ processed}$$

$$= 5 \times 2.72^{-2} \qquad (e\ is\ a\ constant\ 2.72),\ PV=2$$

$$= 5 \times \frac{1}{(2.72)^2} = 5 \times \frac{1}{7.39} = 0.68\ g/dL$$

Fraction of cells remaining:

$$= \frac{\%\ of\ cells\ present\ Post\text{-}Exchange}{\%\ of\ cells\ present\ Pre\text{-}Exchange}$$

Example: If a patient with HgbS levels at 90% received a Red cell exchange and post-procedure, his HgbS levels were 40%, what is the fraction of cells remaining with the patient?

$$Fraction\ of\ cells\ remaining = \frac{\%\ of\ cells\ present\ Post\text{-}Exchange}{\%\ of\ cells\ present\ Pre\text{-}Exchange} = \frac{40}{90} = 44\%$$

Collection efficiency:

$$\frac{Cells\ in\ product\ bag}{[(Preprocedural\ count + Postprocedural\ count) \div 2] \times (Blood\ volume\ processed - Volume\ of\ anticoagulant)]} \times 100$$

Or

$$\frac{Cells\ in\ product\ bag}{(Preprocedural\ count) \times (Blood\ volume\ processed - Volume\ of\ anticoagulant)]} \times 100$$

Example: If the donor has a precollection platelet count of $2.6 \times 10^9/L$ and his count is reduced to $1.9 \times 10^9/L$ post pheresis. What is the collection efficiency of the equipment if the product had 3×10^9 platelets after processing 2.3 litres of blood utilizing 300 ml of ACD?

$$\frac{Cells\ in\ product\ bag}{[(Preprocedural\ count + Postprocedural\ count) \div 2] \times (Blood\ volume\ processed - Volume\ of\ anticoagulant)]} \times 100$$

$$\frac{3 \times 10^9}{[(2.6 \times 10^9/L) + (1.9 \times 10^9/L) \div 2] \times (2.300 - 0.300)]} \times 100$$

$$\frac{3 \times 10^9}{[(4.5 \times 10^9/L) \div 2] \times (2.000)]} \times 100$$

$$\frac{3 \times 10^9}{4.5 \times 10^9/L} \times 100 = 66.7\%$$

Example: An autologous stem cell donor is undergoing Hematopoietic progenitor cell collection. His preprocedural CD34 count was 35×10^6 cells/L. After processing 12 litres of whole blood using 500 ml of anticoagulant, 280×10^6 cells/L were collected in the product. What is the collection efficiency?

$$\frac{\text{Cells in product bag}}{\text{(Preprocedural count)} \times \text{(Blood volume processed - Volume of anticoagulant)}]} \times 100$$

$$\frac{280 \times 10^6 \text{ cells/L}}{(35 \times 10^6 \text{ cells/L}) \times (12.0 - 0.5)L]} \times 100$$

$$\frac{280 \times 10^6 \text{ cells/L}}{(35 \times 10^6 \text{ cells/L}) \times (11.5 \text{ L})]} \times 100 = 69.6\%$$

$$\text{Blood volume to process} = \frac{\text{Cells of interest needed}}{\text{Cells of interest in Peripheral blood} \times \text{Collection efficiency}}$$

Example: An allogeneic stem cell donor is undergoing Hematopoietic progenitor cell collection. His peripheral blood CD34 count is 40×10^6 cells/L. The recipient's weight is 60 kg. If the Collection efficiency of the apheresis equipment is 45%, what should be the volume of blood processed to achieve a dose of 4×10^6 cells/Kg?

$$\text{Blood volume to process} = \frac{\text{Cells of interest needed}}{\text{Cells of interest in Peripheral blood} \times \text{Collection efficiency}}$$

The recipient weighs 60 kg. At a required dose of 4×10^6 cells/Kg, he would require a total cell dose of $60 \times 4 \times 10^6$ cells = 240×10^6 cells

$$\text{Blood volume to be processed} = \frac{240 \times 10^6 \text{ Cells}}{40 \times 10^6 \text{ cells/L} \times 0.45} = 13.33 \text{ Litres}$$

If the anticoagulant is used in the ratio 1:12, then $13.33 \times 1 = 1.21$ Litres of anticoagulants will be used. So 11

the total amount of anticoagulated blood processed will be 13.33+1.21 = 14.54 litres.

$$(ECV)\text{Extracorporeal volume (\%)} = \frac{ECV}{TBV} \times 100$$

Problem: A male patient underwent apheresis, and a 300ml product was collected by a machine whose volume in the disposable set was 285 ml. 3 blood samples of 5 ml each were also collected for various testing purposes. What is the ECV% if he weighed 60 kg?

Blood volume = 70ml/kg × 60 kg = 4200 ml

Total blood removed = ECV of the machine/disposable kit+ product volume + samples collected

$$= 285 + 300 + (3 \times 5) = 600 \text{ ml}$$

$$(ECV)\text{Extracorporeal volume (\%)} = \frac{ECV}{TBV} \times 100 = \frac{600}{4200} \times 100 = 14.28\%$$

6. Blood Group genetics

In a given population, 17% of women are D-negative. 83% of their partners are D positive, of whom 35 are *DD* and 48 *Dd*. 20% of the pregnancies are ABO incompatible as well.

   i. What number of pregnancies will be Rh incompatible (mothers will conceive in whom the fetus is D positive and the mother is D negative)?

  ii. What number of fetuses will likely be affected?

Solution: All the 35% of partners who are DD and 50% of partners with Dd(48), i.e., 24%, will impregnate their partners with a D-positive fetus

     i.e., 17(0.35+0.24) = 10

so 10 of the 17 mothers will harbour a D-positive fetus in the first pregnancy. But the first pregnancy just leads to sensitization

The number in which a D-negative woman is carrying her second D-positive infant is given by: All the 35% of partners who are DD and 50% of partners with Dd(48) in the first pregnancy multiplied by 50% in the second pregnancy, i.e. (0.5×0.5×48) = 0.12

     17(0.35 + 0.12) = 8

In calculating the frequency of opportunities for immunization to Rh D, account must be taken of the fact that primary immunization to Rh D is rare when the fetal red cells are ABO incompatible with the mother's serum. In the question, it is mentioned that about 20% of pregnancies are ABO incompatible as well.

Thus, figure '8' must be multiplied by 0.8 (80%) to give an estimate of the number, i.e. about 6,

7. TTI

The number of units of blood supplied in 2015 at the Hospital blood bank was 20,000. 60% of these donations were from repeat donors, with seropositivity for HBV being 1%. The seropositivity among first-time donors was 2%. The sensitivity of the assay used is 99%. The repeat donation rate was, on average, twice a year. The assay can detect the infection earliest by 8 weeks after infection. What is the total number of seropositive units which have made their way into the inventory?

Solution:

a. For first-time donors:

No of donations by first-time donors × seropositivity (%) ×(1-sensitivity)

8000 × .02 × .01= 1.6

b. For repeat donors:

[No of repeat donors × seroconversion%] + [duration of window+ {(1-sensitivity) × duration post window}]

Duration of the window is 8/26 weeks (denominator 6 months = 26 weeks)

(12000 × .01x8/26) + (12000 × .01 × .01 × 18/26) = 37.7

Total = a + b = 39.3

8. Inventory management

A 2000 bedded multispecialty hospital collected and utilized 20000 units of blood during 2020. The hospital plans to add another 50 trauma beds and 100 general beds in 2021. The hospital authorities estimate an increase of 2000 patients in the year. Estimate the approximate total blood unit requirement for the year 2021.

Solution:

Estimate the number of hospital beds & multiply by 7 for general beds and by 20 for acute care beds

Add 10% to discard

Add 4% for disasters

0.40 donations for each patient admitted to a hospital

1–2% of the world's population needs blood

The number of additional general Beds is 100. So, the number of units required is 100×7= 700

The number of additional Acute care Beds is 100. So, the number of units required is 50×20=1000

Adding previous years utilization 20000+700+1000= 21700

10% for discard. i.e., 2170

4% for Disasters, i.e., 87

In total 23,957

EMERGENCY RESUSCITATION IN THE TRANSFUSION MEDICINE UNIT

– Dr. Manu, Dr. Ajai R

Emergencies are not uncommon in any unit. Emergencies like transfusion reactions may be seen as anaphylaxis, allergic reactions, or donor reactions like syncopal attacks and panic attacks are common. This chapter introduces you to the zone of resuscitation, which includes basic life support (BLS) measures, resuscitation procedures and a few critical concepts.

Introduction

Improving how we respond with life-saving techniques to emergencies is based on the most current research techniques and is organized into a systematic response called the Chain of Survival, which begins with Basic Life Support (BLS). The Chain of Survival provides the person with the best chance to receive the care needed and return to a healthy life.

- *Taking the right step in an emergency is critical in deciding between the life and death of a patient in cardiac arrest*

Keys for BLS:

- Quickly start the Chain of Survival.
- Deliver high-quality chest compressions to circulate oxygen to the brain and vital organs.
- Know when and how to use an Automatic External Defibrillator (AED).
- Provide rescue breathing.
- Understand how to work with other rescuers as part of a team.

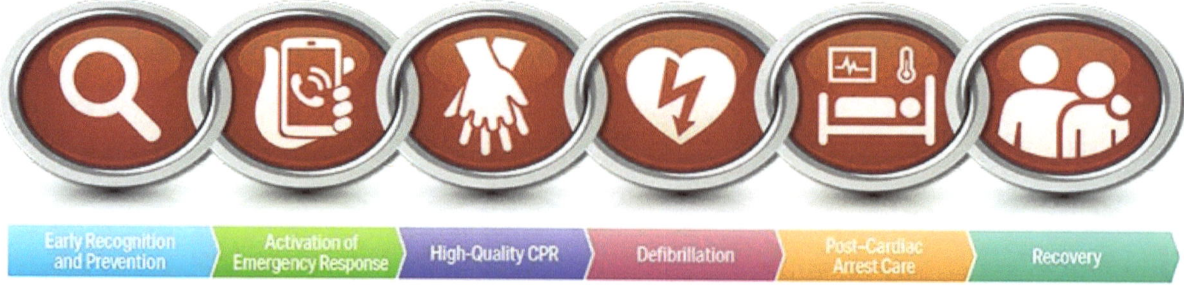

Adult IHCA Chain of Survival

Initiating a Chain of Survival

Early initiation of BLS has been shown to increase the probability of survival for a person with cardiac arrest. To increase the odds of surviving a cardiac event, the rescuer should follow the steps in the Adult Chain of Survival

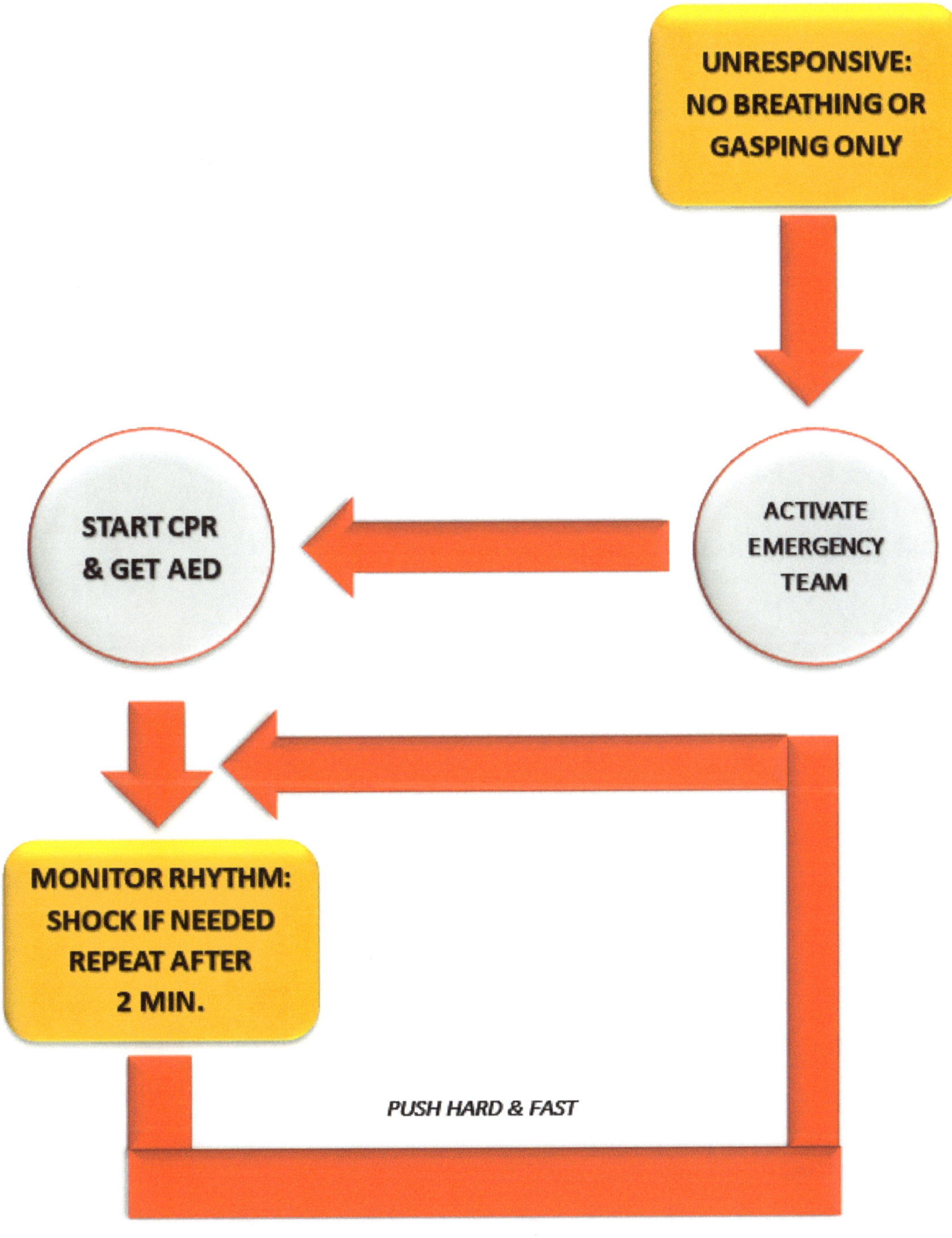

ONE-RESCUER BLS – CPR FOR ADULTS

Be Safe

- Move the person out of harm.

- Be sure you do not get injured yourself.

Assess the Person

Tap the shoulders and talk to them loudly.

Call for help

- Send someone for help.

- If alone, call for help while assessing for breathing and pulse,

  without leaving the person.)

Cardiac arrest or Not?

- Check pulse and breathing simultaneously.

- If no palpable carotid pulse and breathing are noted, the emergency medicine team must get

  an AED and begin compressions.

Defibrillate

- Attach the AED when available.

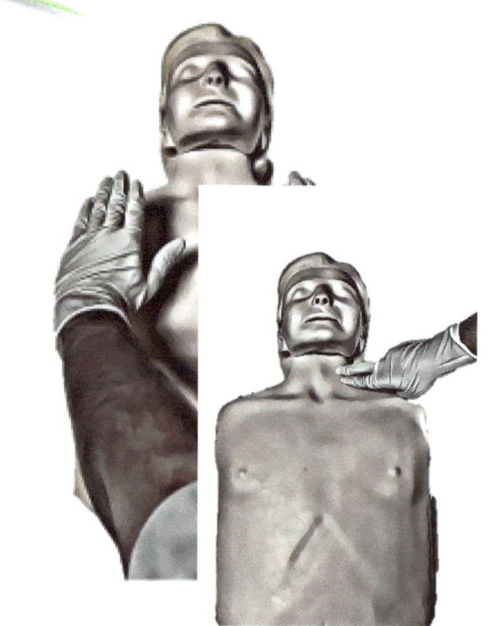

CPR – A Step-by-Step Approach

STEP 1: Check for the carotid pulse on the side of the neck. Remember not to waste time trying to feel for a pulse; feel for no more than 10 seconds. If unsure that you feel a pulse, begin CPR with a cycle of 30 chest compressions and two breaths.

- *Checking the carotid pulse. A, Locate the trachea. B, Gently feel for the carotid pulse.*

STEP 2: Place the victim on his or her back. Make sure he/she is lying as flat as possible and on a hard surface to prevent injury while doing chest compressions to be effective.

STEP 3: Use the heel of one hand on the lower half of the sternum in the middle of the chest. Put your other hand on top of the first hand.

STEP 4: Straighten your arms and press straight down. Compressions should be at least two inches into the person's chest and at a rate of 100 to 120 compressions per minute.

STEP 5: Be sure that you completely stop pressing on the chest and allow the chest wall to return to its natural position between each compression. Leaning or resting on the chest between compressions can keep the heart from refilling between each compression and make CPR less effective.

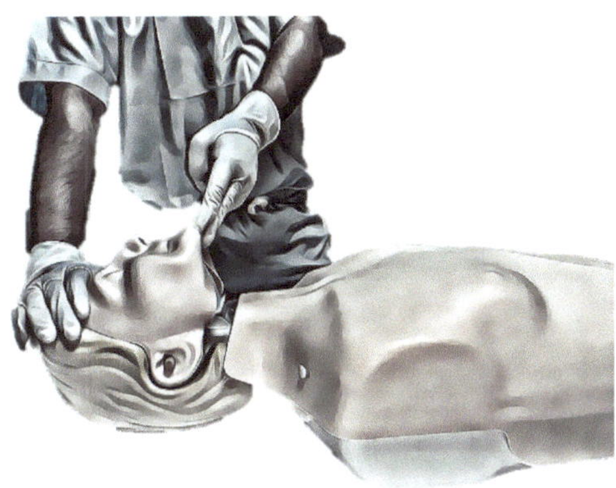

STEP 6: After 30 compressions, stop compressions and open the airway by tilting the head and lifting the chin.

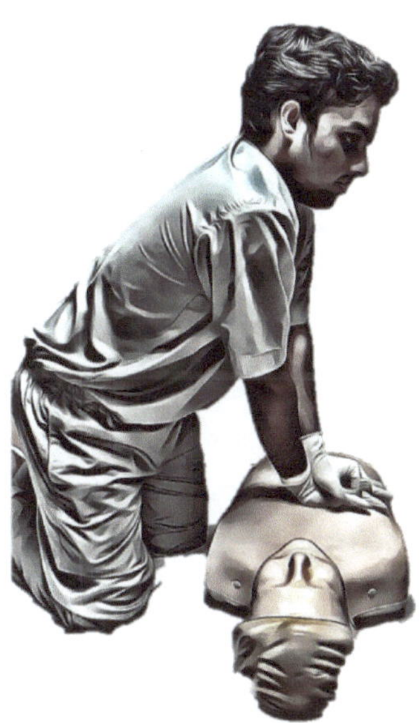

a. Put your hand on the person's forehead and tilt the head back
b. Lift the person's jaw by placing your index and middle fingers on the lower jaw; lift.
c. Do not perform head-tilt/ chin lift if you suspect the person may have a neck injury. In that case, the jaw thrust is used.

B. Jaw thrust manoeuvre

a. For the jaw-thrust manoeuvre, grasp the angles of the lower jaw and lift it with both hands, one on each side, moving the jaw forward. If their lips are closed, open the lower lip using your thumb.

STEP 7: Give a breath while watching the chest rise. Repeat while giving a second breath. Breaths should be delivered over one second.

STEP 8: Resume chest compressions. Switch quickly between compressions and rescue breaths to minimize interruptions in chest compressions.

Two-Rescuer BLS - CPR for Adults

A second person will often be available to act as a rescuer. The AHA emphasizes that cell phones are available everywhere, and most have built-in speakerphones. Direct the second rescuer to call emergency without leaving the person while you begin CPR. This second rescuer can also find an AED while you stay with the person. When the second rescuer returns, the CPR tasks can be shared.

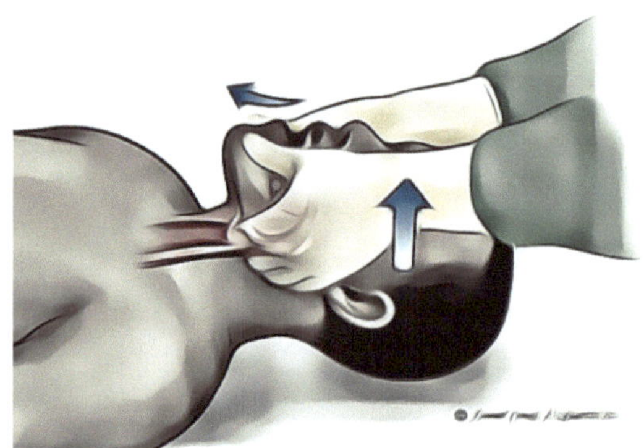

1. The second rescuer prepares the AED for use.
2. You begin chest compressions and count the compressions out loud.
3. The second rescuer applies the AED pads.
4. The second rescuer opens the person's airway and gives rescue breaths.
5. Switch roles after every five cycles of compressions and breaths. One cycle consists of 30 compressions and two breaths.
6. Stop pressing the chest between each compression and allow the chest wall to return to its natural position. Leaning or resting on the chest between compressions can keep the heart from refilling between each compression and make CPR less effective. Rescuers who become tired tend to lean on the chest more during compressions; switching roles helps rescuers perform high-quality compressions.
7. Quickly switch between roles to minimize interruptions in delivering chest compressions.
8. When the AED is connected, minimize interruptions of CPR by switching rescuers while the AED analyzes the heart rhythm. If a shock is indicated, minimize interruptions in CPR. Resume CPR as soon as possible.

Breathing - Adult Mouth-to-Mask Ventilation

In one-rescuer CPR, breaths should be supplied using a pocket mask, if available.

1. Give 30 high-quality chest compressions.
2. Seal the mask against the person's face by placing four fingers of one hand across the top and the thumb of the other hand along the bottom edge of the mask.

3. Using the fingers of your hand on the bottom of the mask, open the airway using a head tilt or chin-lift. (Do not do this if you suspect the person may have a neck injury) .
4. Press firmly around the edges of the mask and ventilate by delivering a breath over one second as you watch the person's chest rise.
5. Practice using the bag valve mask; it is essential to forming a tight seal and delivering effective breaths.

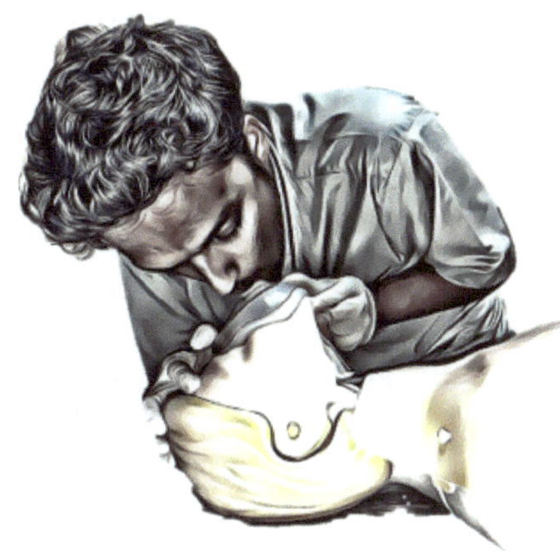

Mouth-to-mask, lateral technique. The lateral technique allows the rescuer to perform 1-rescuer CPR from a fixed position at the side of the victim.

Breathing - Adult Bag-Mask Ventilation in One & Two-Rescuer

If two people are present and a bag-mask device is available, the second rescuer is positioned at the victim's head while the other rescuer performs high-quality chest compressions. Give 30 high-quality chest compressions.

1. Deliver 30 high-quality chest compressions while counting out loud.
2. The second rescuer holds the bag mask with one hand using the thumb and index finger in the shape of a "C" on one side of the mask to form a seal between the mask and the face, while the other fingers open the airway by lifting the person's lower jaw.
3. The second rescuer gives two breaths over one second each.

One rescuer uses the bag mask. The rescuer circles the top edges of the mask with her index and first finger and lifts the jaw with the remaining fingers. The bag is squeezed while the rescuer observes the chest rise. A Mask seal is key to the successful use of the bag mask.

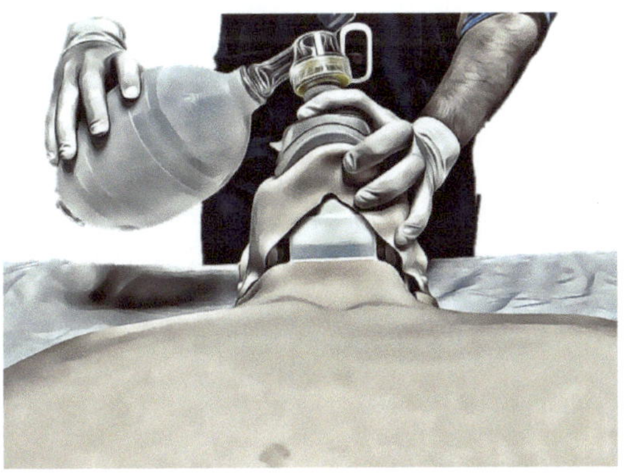
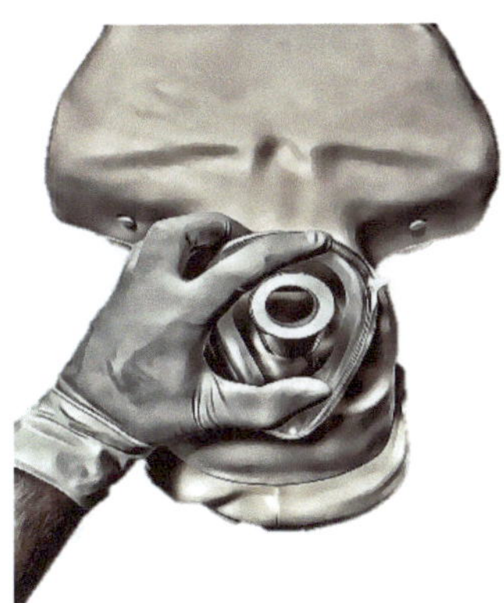

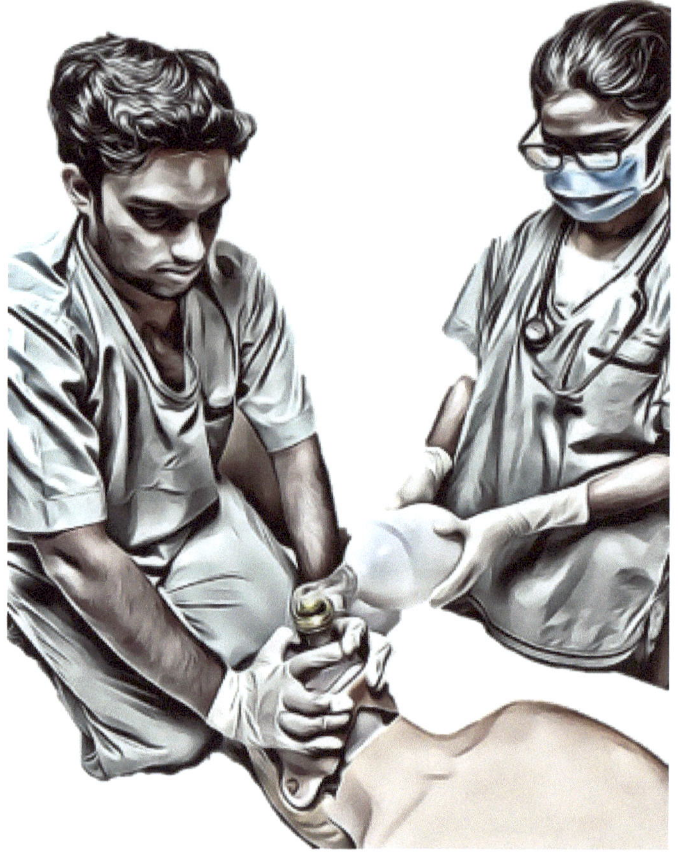

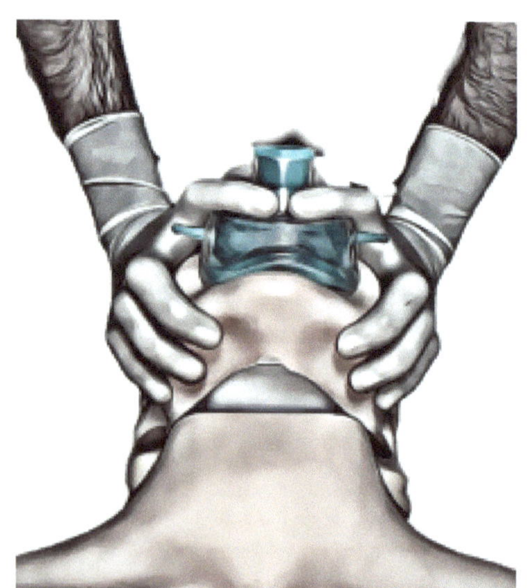

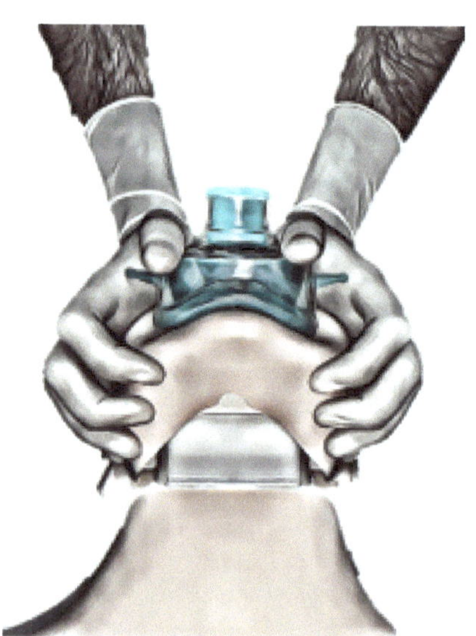

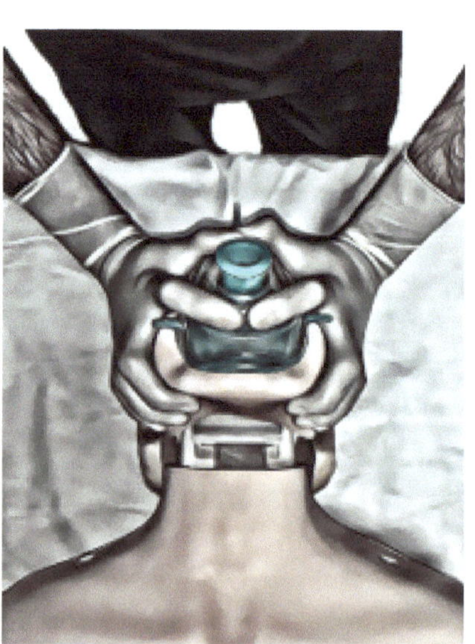

Two-rescuer use of the bag mask. The rescuer at the head uses the thumb and first finger of each hand to provide a complete seal around the edges of the mask. Use the remaining fingers to lift the mandible and extend the neck while observing the chest rise. The other rescuer slowly squeezes the bag (over 2 seconds) until he observes chest rise

PUTTING IT TOGETHER - ADULT BLS ALGORITHM

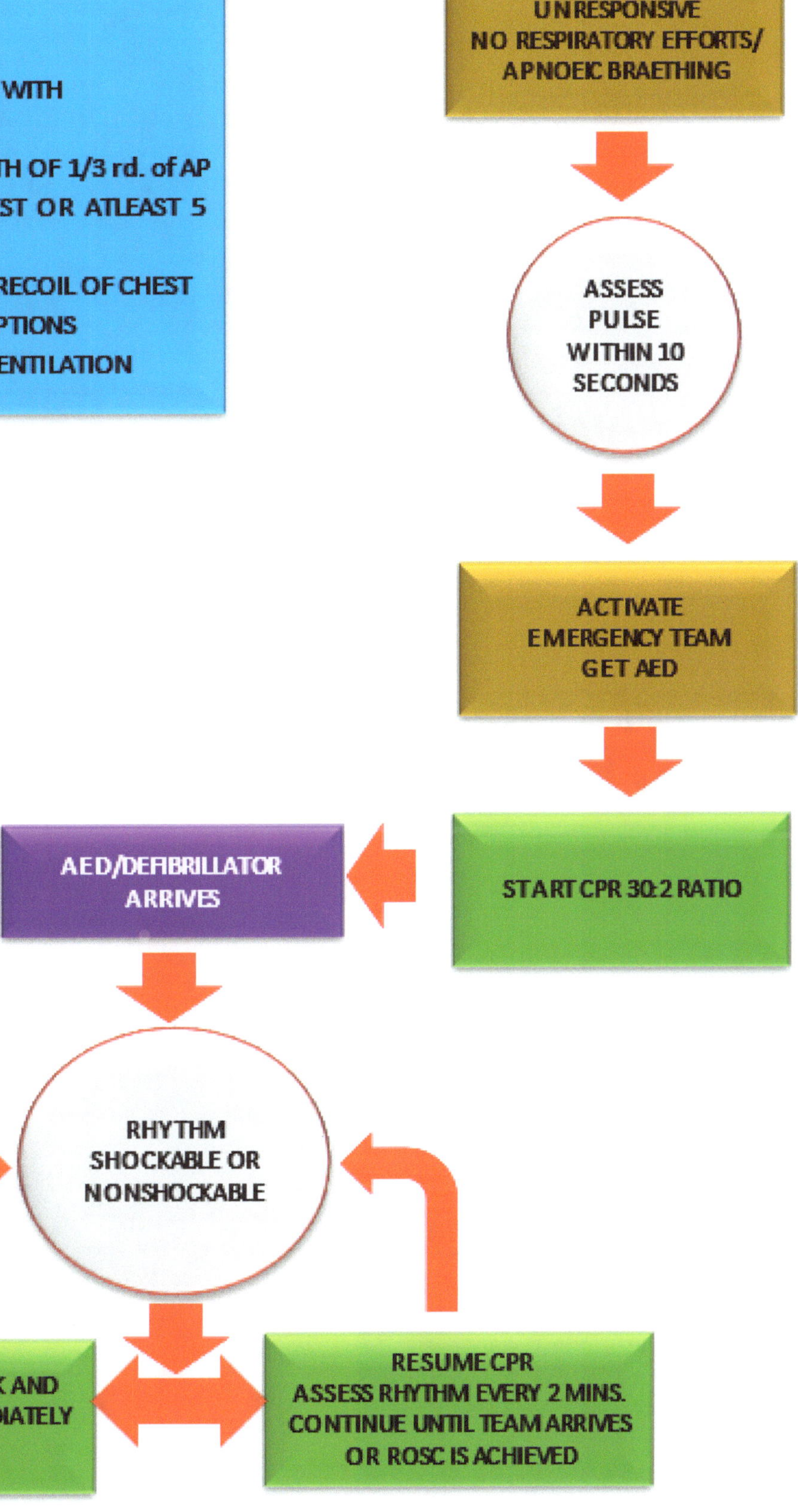

ROSC- Return of normal circulation

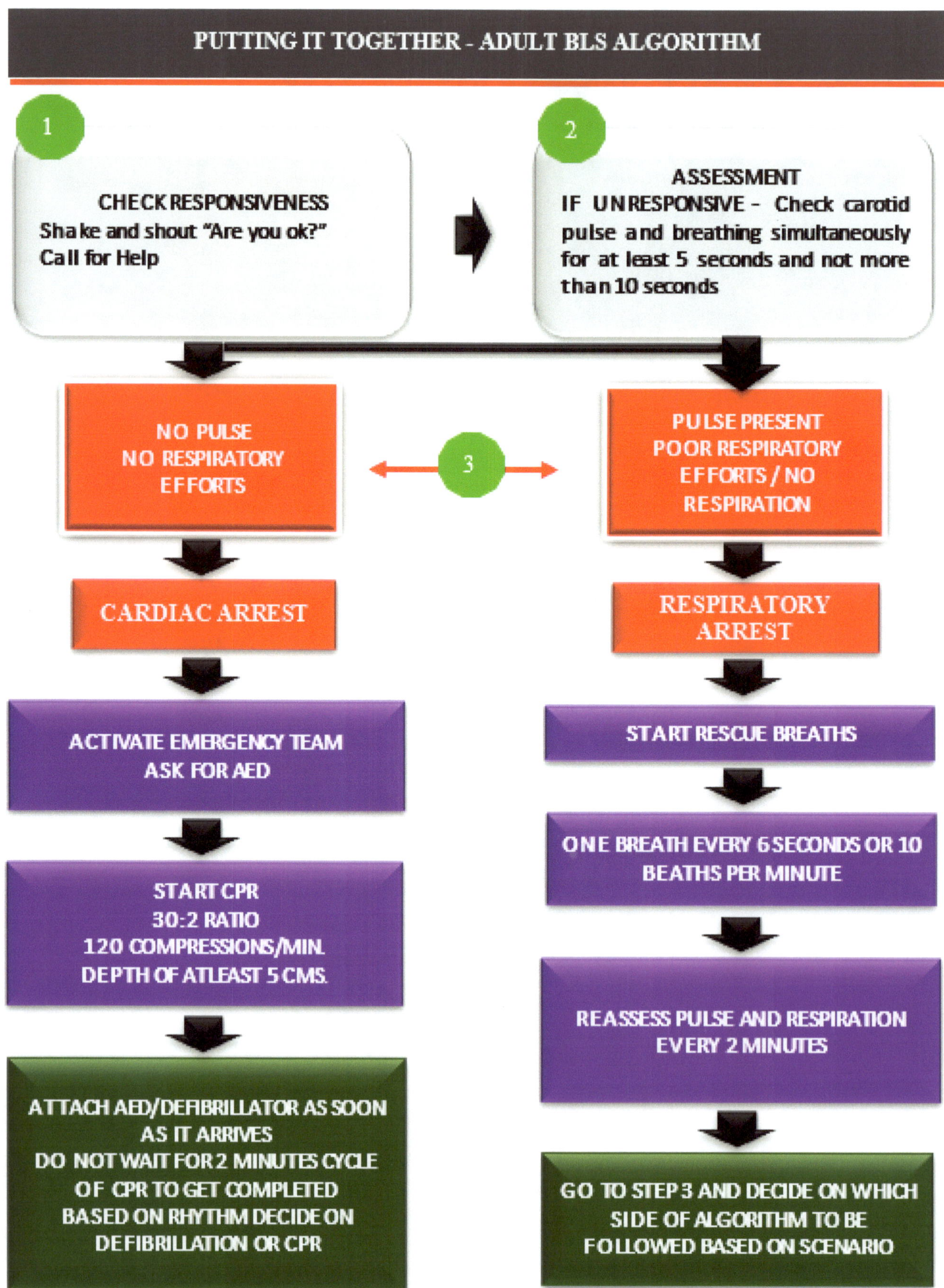

Airway Management

- *The priority is the establishment or maintenance of airway patency*

Until an advanced airway is inserted, the rescue team should use mouth-to-mouth, mouth-to-mask, or bag-mask ventilation. An advanced airway (supraglottic airway, laryngeal mask airway, or endotracheal tube) provides a more stable way of providing breaths and should, therefore, be inserted as early as possible in a resuscitation effort.

Normal Vs Obstructed Airway

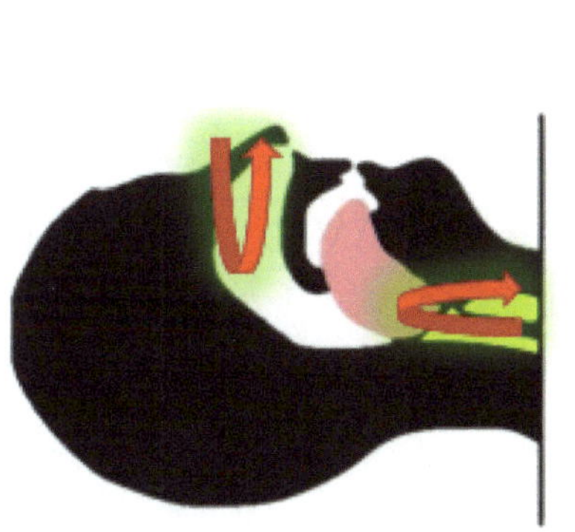
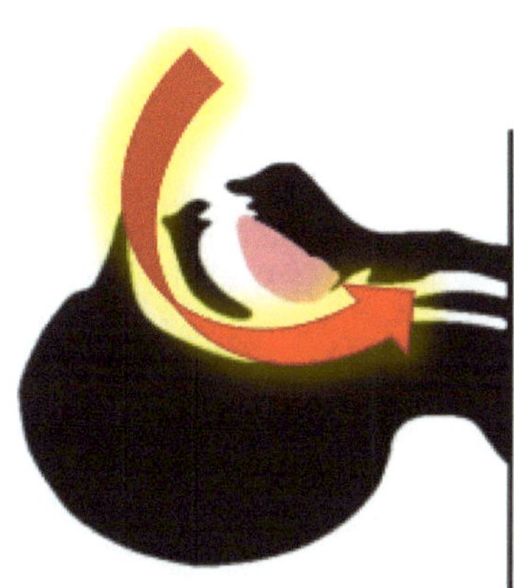

Question	Discussion
How would you commence your patient's airway assessment? *What does snoring indicate, and what are the options?*	- Speak to the patient and ask him his name and what occurred. - If he can speak, his airway will not likely be obstructed. - Listen for noisy airway sounds. - Snoring indicates partial airway obstruction, most likely opposition of the tongue with the posterior pharyngeal wall. - Simple airway manoeuvres should be implemented to open the airway.

Mouth-To-Mouth Rescue Breathing

When a pocket mask or bag mask is unavailable, it may be necessary to give mouth-to-mouth breaths during CPR. Mouth-to-mouth breathing effectively delivers oxygen into the person's lungs without putting the rescuer at high risk. The rescuer's exhaled air contains approximately 17% oxygen and 4% carbon dioxide. This is in contrast to the 100% oxygen available with ventilation with 100% high-flow oxygen.

Adults And Older Children Mouth-To-Mouth

Do not give breaths too rapidly or too forcefully. Doing this may cause air to be forced into the stomach, resulting in distention and less room for lung expansion. It may also cause vomiting.

To deliver mouth-to-mouth breaths, do the following:

1. Open the airway using the head-tilt/ chin-lift manoeuvre.
2. Pinch the person's nose closed with your hand on the person's head.
3. Create a seal when using your lips to surround the person's mouth.
4. Blow into the person's mouth for one full second and watch for the chest to rise. Tilt the victim's head further back if the chest does not rise.
5. Give an additional breath for over one second.
6. If you cannot see the chest rise in two breaths, continue giving chest compressions.

Chest Compressions & Airway – Adult Vs Child

PARAMETERS	ADULT	CHILD	INFANT
Rate	100–120/min.	100 – 120/min.	100 – 120/min.
Depth	At least 5 CMS.	At least 5 CMS. (or) 1/3 rd. Of AP diameter of the chest	At least 4 CMS. (or) 1/3 rd. Of AP diameter of the chest
Compression: Ventilation	30:2	30:2 – One rescuer 15:2 – Two rescuers.	30:2 – One rescuer 15:2 – Two rescuers.
Airway opening	Head tilt & Chin lift	Head tilt & Chin lift	Neutral position
Breathing technique	Mouth - mouth	Mouth - mouth	Mouth – mouth -nose
Rescue breaths	1 breath every 5-6 sec.	1 breath every 3-5 sec.	1 breath every 3-5 sec.

Allergy & Anaphylaxis

Anaphylaxis is a severe allergic reaction with a rapid onset; it may cause death and requires emergent diagnosis and treatment.

Clinical Criteria For Anaphylaxis

Urticaria, generalized itching or flushing, or oedema of lips, tongue, uvula, or skin developing over minutes to hours and associated with **at least 1 of the following:**

- Respiratory distress or hypoxia (or)
- Hypotension or cardiovascular collapse (or)
- Associated symptoms of organ dysfunction (e.g., hypotonia, syncope, incontinence)
- Two or more signs or symptoms that occur minutes to hours after allergen exposure:
- Skin and/or mucosal involvement
- Respiratory compromise
- Hypotension or associated symptoms
- Persistent GI cramps or vomiting

Consider anaphylaxis when patients are exposed to a known allergen and develop hypotension

FIRST-LINE THERAPY

- Emergency management starts with assessing the airway, breathing, and circulation. Assess vital signs and pulse oximetry. Initiate IV access, oxygen administration, and cardiac rhythm monitoring in patients with severe symptoms.
- The first-line therapies for anaphylaxis (airway protection, oxygen, decontamination, epinephrine, IV crystalloids) have an immediate effect during the acute stage.
- Airway and Oxygenation In severe anaphylaxis, securing the airway is the priority.
- Examine the mouth, pharynx, and neck for signs and symptoms of angioedema: uvula oedema or hydrops, audible stridor, respiratory distress, or hypoxia. If angioedema produces respiratory distress, intubate early since any delay may result in complete airway obstruction secondary to the progression of angioedema.
- Provide supplemental oxygen to maintain arterial oxygen saturation >90%.
- Decontamination If the causative agent can be identified, termination of exposure should be attempted.
- Gastric lavage is not recommended for foodborne allergens and may be associated with complications (i.e., aspiration) and delays in administering more effective treatments (e.g., epinephrine).

| RECOGNITION | ➡ | RESUSCITATION | ➡ | TRANSFER |

The outcome of a successful recognition depends upon how early a life-threatening event is and how soon the resuscitation is in place. Early recognition and commencement of resuscitation are vital to a patient's successful cardiac arrest outcome. Even the slightest delay in any of these components can drastically alter the outcome and prognosis.

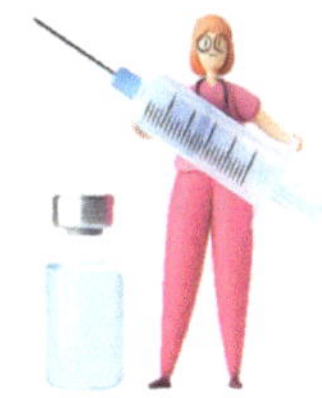

STAFF

Having a trained resident and staff in the bay makes all the difference. Having prior knowledge and experience in basic and advanced resuscitation will make all the difference than, with no one on the team with no prior experience. A team leader who guides the entire resuscitation process, two rescuers (one for CPR and one for airway management) and a staff who is well aware of what is going on and what is the next drug to be kept ready in place is vital for successful resuscitation.

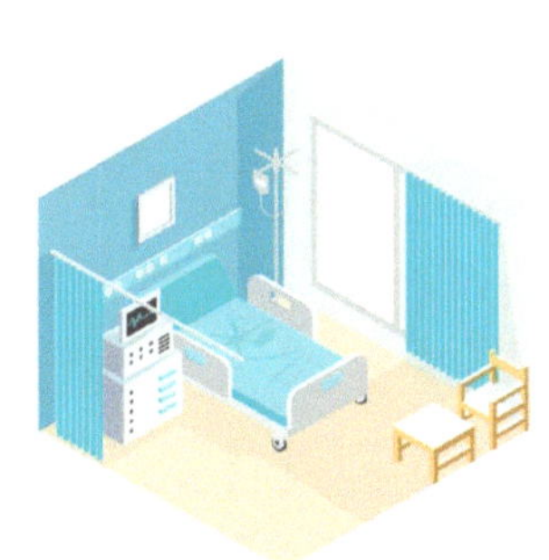

SPACE

A dedicated area for resuscitation is of grave importance in every unit. Resuscitating a patient in the middle of nowhere and the same happening when there is a controlled environment alters and improves the outcome. A dedicated area with the gurney and all necessary equipments, including cardiac monitors, defibrillator, and resuscitation drugs, make resuscitation much easier and practically more feasible.

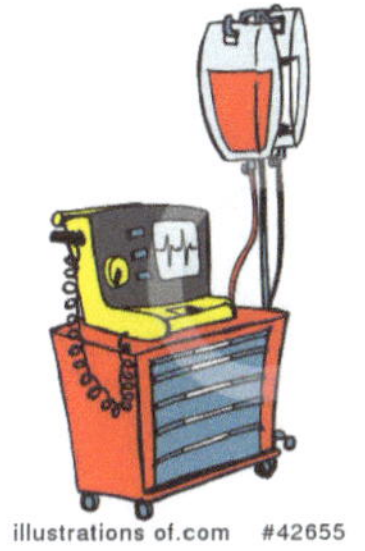

EQUIPMENTS

As much as early recognition of cardiac arrest and initiation of CPR is vital, as resuscitation progresses, airway equipments, intravenous access lines and drugs are equally important. A crash cart with baseline drugs required for resuscitation improves the success and outcome of ongoing resuscitation step by step.

DRUG	ADULT DOSE	PEDIATRIC DOSE
FIRST LINE THERAPY		
Epinephrine	IM: 0.3–0.5 milligram (0.3–0.5 mL of 1:1000 dilution); or EpiPen®0.3mg epinephrine	IM: 0.01 milligram/kg (0.01 mL/kg of 1:1000 dilution) or EpiPen Junior® 0.15 milligram of epinephrine
	IV bolus: 100 micrograms over 5–10 min; mix 0.1 milligram (0.1 mL of 1:1000 dilution) in 10 mL NS and infuse over 5–10 min	-
	IV infusion: start at 1 microgram/min; mix 1 milligram (1 mL of 1:1000 dilution) in 500 mL NS and infuse at 0.5 mL/min;	IV infusion: 0.1–0.3 microgram/kg per min; titrate dose as needed; maximum, 1.5 micrograms/kg per min
Oxygen	Titrate to Sao2 ≥90%	Titrate to Sao2 ≥90%
IV fluid: NS or LR	1–2 L bolus	10–20 mL/kg bolus Second-Line Therapy
SECOND LINE THERAPY		
H 1 blockers		
Diphenhydramine	25–50 milligrams IV, IM, or PO every 6 h	1 milligram/kg IV, IM, or PO every 6 h
H 2 blockers		
Ranitidine	50 milligrams IV over 5 min	0.5 milligram/kg IV over 5 min
Cimetidine	300 milligrams IV	4–8 milligrams/kg IV
Corticosteroids		
Hydrocortisone	250–500 milligrams IV	5–10 milligrams/kg IV (maximum, 500 milligrams)
Methylprednisolone	80–125 milligrams IV	1–2 milligrams/kg IV (maximum, 125 milligrams)
TREATMENT OF BRONCHOSPASM		
ALBUTEROL	**Single treatment: 2.5–5.0 milligrams nebulized**	**Single treatment: 1.25–2.5 milligrams nebulized**
IPRATROPIUM BROMIDE	**Single treatment: 250–500 micrograms nebulized**	**Single treatment: 125–250 micrograms nebulized**
MAGNESIUM SULFATE	**2 grams IV over 20 min**	**25–50 milligrams/kg IV over 20 min**

Essential Equipment Checklist

Oxygen mask with reservoir bag	Pocket Mask and one-way valve
Automated External Defibrillator (AED) with electrodes	Epinephrine/Adrenaline (1:1000)
Oxygen cylinder (of the suitable size to deliver high flow O_2	Atropine
Syringe and needles	Airway devices
Gloves	0.9% Saline
Intravenous cannulas (20G/18G)	Lactated ringer's solution
25% Dextrose	Glucometer with strips
Sharps box	Suction apparatus

Section III

Specific Divisions of Transfusion Medicine

DONOR SCIENCE AND BLOOD DONATION

15.1 APPLIED BASIC ANATOMY

– Dr. Yogesh S

VEINS OF UPPER LIMB.

The veins draining the upper limb are grouped as follows (Fig.1):

Superficial veins

- These are located in the superficial fascia.
- They include

    1. Dorsal venous arch
    2. Cephalic vein
    3. Basilic vein
    4. Median cubital vein

Deep veins

- These are located deep in the deep fascia.
- These include

    1. Venae comitantes that accompany the large arteries such as radial, ulnar, and brachial arteries
    2. Axillary vein

General features of superficial veins

- *Location*: Superficial veins lie in the superficial fascia.
- *Course*: Superficial veins run away from the pressure points. These pressure points include the palm, ulnar border of the forearm, back of the elbow, and back of the trunk.
- *Length*: Preaxial (cephalic) vein is longer than the postaxial (basilic).
- *Communicating channels*: The median cubital vein transmits most blood from the cephalic to the basilic vein.

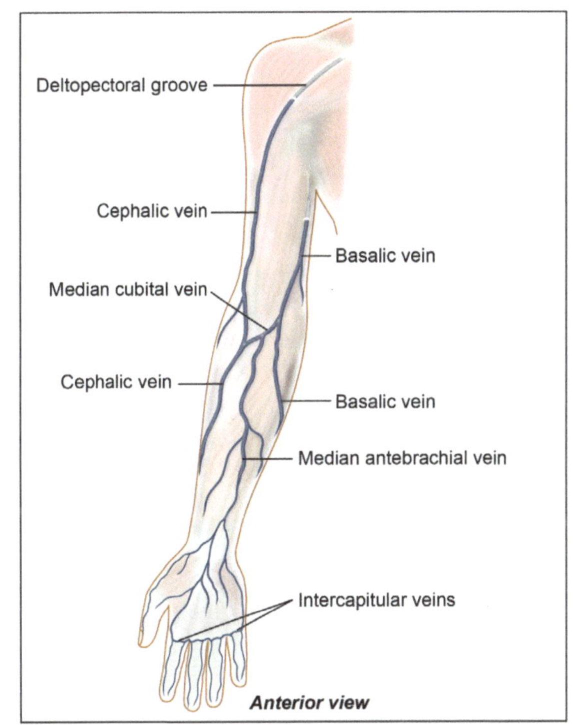

Fig. 1: Superficial veins of the forearm (right, anterior view). Skin is dissected out to visualize the superficial veins of the forearm. (Source: Textbook of Human Anatomy, Yogesh Sontakke, CBSPD)

- *Perforating veins*: They transfer the blood from superficial veins to deep veins. Perforators have valves that allow unidirectional transmission.
- Accompanied by cutaneous nerves and lymphatic vessels.

Dorsal Venous Arch

- The dorsal venous arch is a network of superficial veins that lies on the dorsum of the hand (Fig. 2).
- Tributaries of the dorsal venous arch

  1. Three dorsal metacarpal veins
  2. Dorsal digital veins
  3. Veins of palm that cross the margins of hand
  4. Perforating veins that pass through interosseous spaces

- Continuation of the dorsal venous arch

  Medial end – basilic vein

  Lateral end – cephalic vein

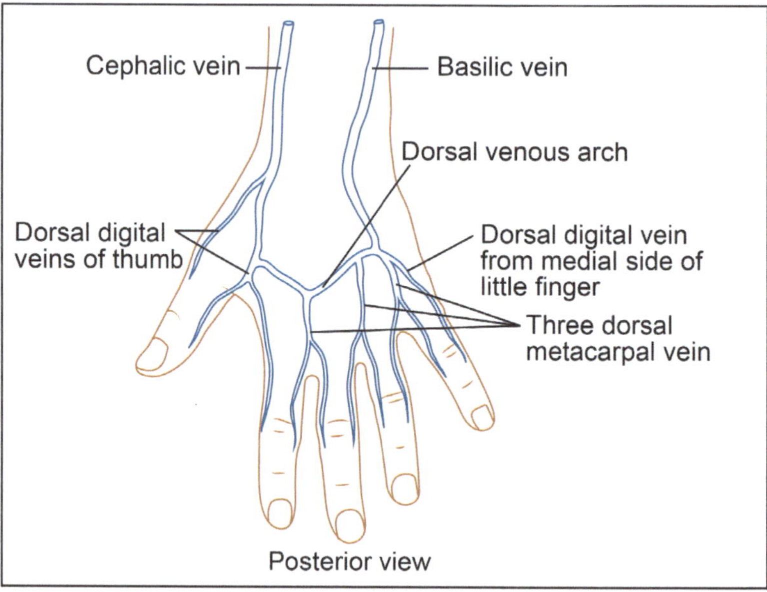

Fig. 2: Dorsal venous arch (left, posterior view). (Source: Textbook of Human Anatomy, Yogesh Sontakke, CBSPD)

Cephalic vein

- It is one of the important superficial veins of the forearm (Fig. 3).

Beginning

- It begins as the continuation of the lateral end of the dorsal venous arch.

Course

- It runs in the roof of the anatomical snuff box. It turns anteriorly along the lateral border of the forearm. It runs upward in the roof of the cubital fossa. It runs upward in the arm and pierces deep fascia at the lower border of the pectoralis major muscle. It then follows the course of the deltopectoral groove. In the infraclavicular fossa, it pierces clavipectoral fascia and joins axillary vein.

Termination

- The cephalic vein opens into the axillary vein.

Some interesting facts

- *Accessory cephalic vein:* It is occasionally present. It passes along the lateral border of the forearm and joins the cephalic vein near the elbow.
- The lateral cutaneous nerve of the forearm accompanies the cephalic vein.
- The basilic vein is accompanied by the posterior branch of the medial cutaneous nerve of the forearm

---

Basilic Vein (Fig. 3).

Beginning

- It begins as the continuation of the medial end of the dorsal venous arch.

Course

- The basilic vein runs upward along the medial border of the forearm to reach anterior to the cubital fossa.
- It runs in the roof of the cubital fossa and then in the front of the forearm.
- It pierces deep fascia in the middle of the forearm and runs upward on the medial side of the brachial artery.
- At the lower border of the teres major muscle, it continues upward as the axillary vein.

Termination

- Basilic vein continues as axillary vein.

Median Cubital Vein

- The median cubital vein is a small communicating channel between cephalic and basilic veins.
- It crosses obliquely in front of the elbow and lies on the roof of the cubital fossa.

Beginning

- It begins from the cephalic vein, 2.5 cm below the bend of the elbow.

Course

- It passes upward and medially in the roof of the cubital fossa.

Termination

- It opens in the basilic vein, 2.5 cm above the bend of the elbow.

Communication

- The median cubital vein communicates with deep veins through a perforator vein. This perforator vein pierces bicipital aponeurosis and thus fixes the median cubital vein (Fig. 3). It has a valve that allows blood to flow from the median cubital vein to deep veins.

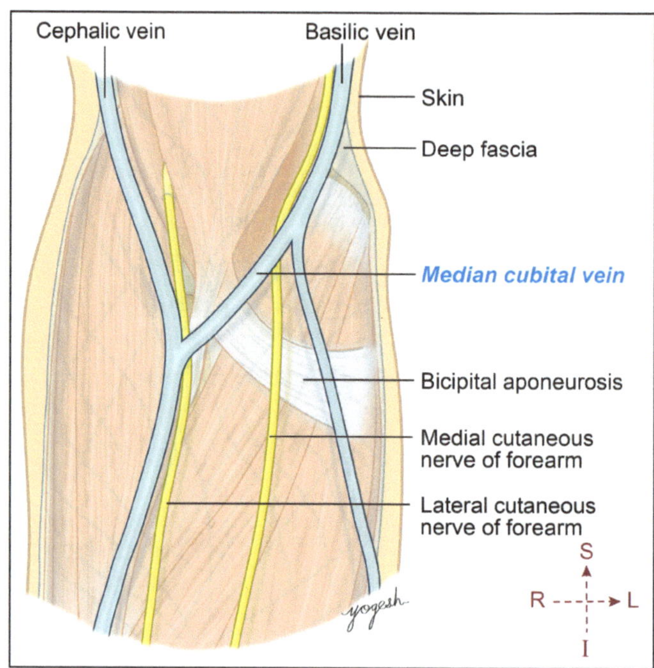

Fig. 3: Median cubital vein in the roof of the cubital fossa (right, anterior view)
(Source: Textbook of Human Anatomy, Yogesh Sontakke, CBSPD)

Median Vein of Forearm

- The median vein of the forearm is present in some individuals. It is also called the *median antebrachial vein*.

Location

- It lies on the front of the forearm.

Beginning

- It arises from the palmar venous plexus.

Course

- It ascends upward on the front of the forearm between basilic and cephalic veins.

Termination

- It opens in the median cubital vein. Sometimes, it may terminate in basilic or cephalic veins.

> *Some interesting facts*
>
> - There are many variations in the pattern of superficial veins of the forearm. Sometimes median vein of the forearm bifurcates to form the lateral median cephalic and medial median basilic veins. In this situation, the median cubital vein is absent.

The pattern of superficial veins and their variations

A different pattern of superficial veins of the upper extremity is reported. Some of them are as follows:

1. M-shaped arrangement or classical type: In the front cubital fossa, the median antebrachial vein divides into two terminal branches, the median cephalic and median basilic vein, which join the cephalic and basilic vein, respectively.
2. Modified M-shaped arrangement: In this pattern, one or two more veins in front of the forearm are present, ending in the basilic vein. Sometimes one or two more veins in front of the forearm are present, ending in the median cephalic or basilic vein. Sometimes in a modified M-shaped pattern, the double brachial part of the cephalic vein is present.
3. An n-shaped arrangement or embryonal type: This pattern resembles elbow veins in infancy. In front cubital fossa, the median antebrachial vein ends into median cubital vein.
4. Modified N-shaped arrangement: In this pattern, the median antebrachial vein ends in the basilic vein. The median cubital vein is present. Rarely, in the modified N-shaped pattern, the cephalic vein continues superomedially as the median cubital vein, and the proximal cephalic vein does not exist.
5. Rarely there is no communication of the cephalic and basilic veins. In this pattern, the median antebrachial and accessory veins drain into the basilic or cephalic vein.
6. Sometimes, two median cubital veins are present over and under the crease of the elbow. The median antebrachial vein ends in the median cubital or basilic vein.

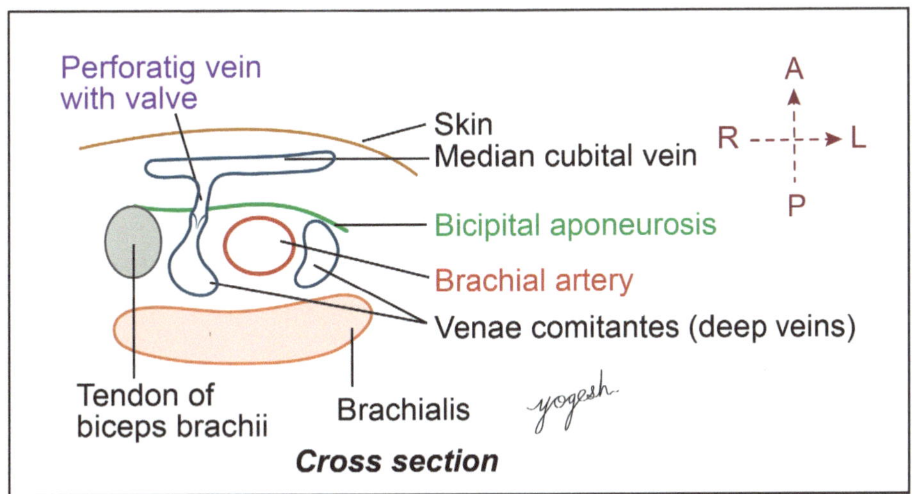

Fig. 4: Relations of the median cubital vein (right, cross-section inferior view)
(Source: Textbook of Human Anatomy, Yogesh Sontakke, CBSPD)

Histology of veins

Histologically, veins are grouped into four groups based on their size as follows (Fig.13–15):

1. Venules (diameter 10–100 µm): They receive blood from capillaries
2. Small veins (diameter 0.1–1 mm)
3. Medium-sized veins (diameter 1–10 mm): They accompany arteries
4. Large veins (diameter >10 mm)

- The smallest veins are called venules. They collect blood from capillaries. The diameter of the venule is 0.1 mm or less.
- Venules are of two types:

    1. Post-capillary venules (10–50 µm diameter) receive blood from capillaries. They are lined by endothelium and pericytes.
    2. Muscular venules (50–100 µm diameter): They are lined by endothelium, 1–2 layers of smooth muscles and surrounded by a thick layer of connective tissue.

Medium-Sized Veins

- Medium-sized veins (1–10 mm diameter) show poorly identifiable three layers of vessels: Tunica intima, tunica media, and tunica adventitia (Fig.14). Tunica intima consists of endothelium, basal lamina, thin subendothelial connective tissue, and discontinuous internal elastic lamina. Tunica media is thin and consists of a few layers of smooth muscle cells. Tunica adventitia is a thick layer of connective tissue containing collagen and elastic fibres. Medium-sized veins accompany medium-sized arteries. For example, radial vein, tibial vein, popliteal vein, and so on. Medium-sized veins show the presence of valves in their lumen to prevent the retrograde (backward) flow of blood. Venous valves are more in veins of the lower limb to counteract the effect of gravity.

Large Veins

- Large vein (>10 mm diameter) shows the presence of three layers of vessels: Tunica intima, tunica media, and tunica adventitia (Fig.15).

    Tunica intima: consists of vascular endothelium, basal lamina, and thin subendothelial connective tissue. Subendothelial connective tissue contains few smooth muscle cells.

    Tunica media: It consists of concentrically arranged smooth muscle cells, collagen fibres, and fibroblasts. The boundary between tunica media and tunica intima is difficult to decide.

    Tunica adventitia: It is the thickest layer of the large vein. It consists of longitudinally arranged smooth muscle cells. It also contains collagen fibres, elastic fibres, and fibroblasts. Examples: Superior vena cava, inferior vena cava.

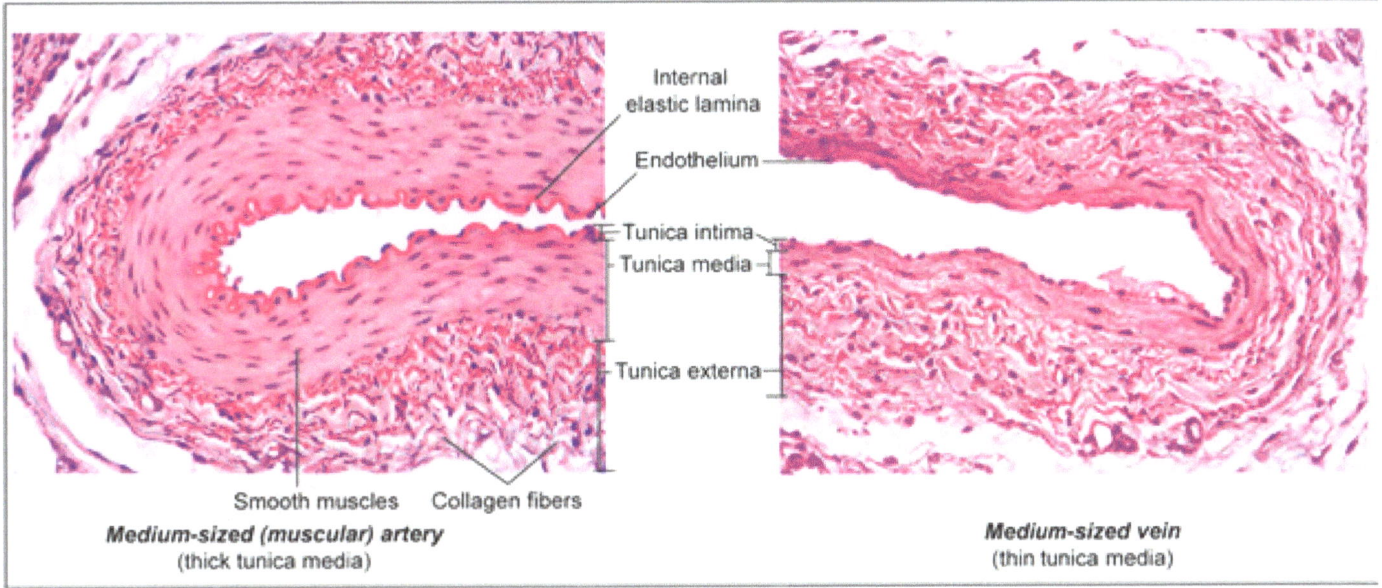

Fig. 14: Photomicrograph. Layers of a medium-sized artery (muscular artery) and medium-sized vein (H&E stain, high magnification). (Source: Textbook of Human Histology, Yogesh Sontakke, CBSPD)

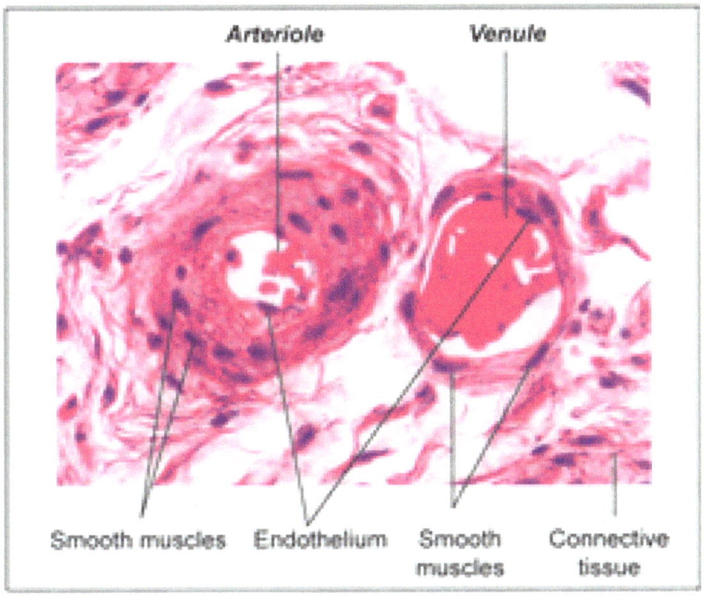

Photomicrograph. Arteriole and venule (H&E stain, high magnification). (Source: Textbook of Human Histology, Yogesh Sontakke, CBSPD)

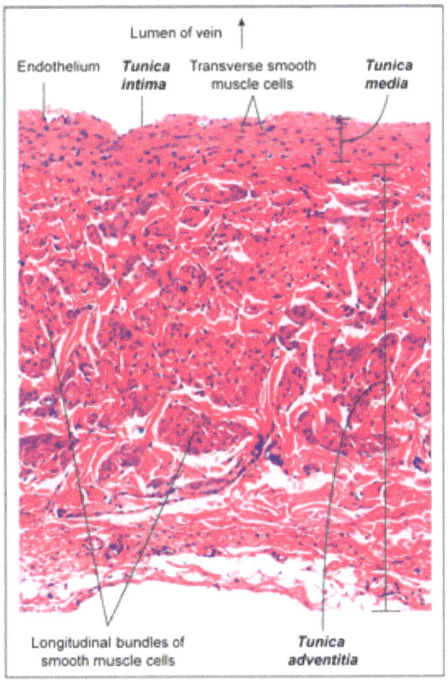

Photomicrograph. Large vein (low magnification, H&E stain). (Source: Textbook of Human Histology, Yogesh Sontakke, CBSPD)

15.2 OVERVIEW OF BLOOD COLLECTION

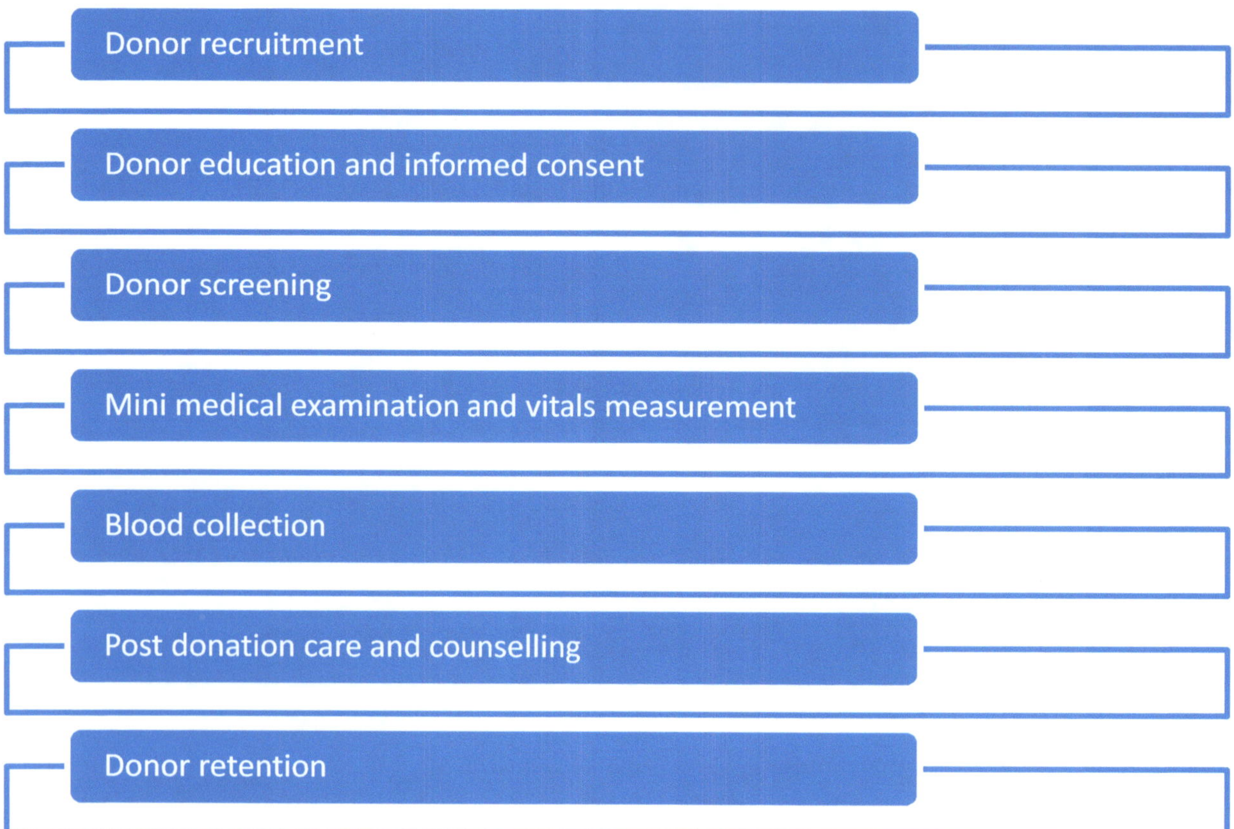

Figure 4. The flow of blood donation

IH Testing	TTI Testing	Others
• ABO and Rh Typing • Antibody detection and screening • ABO antibody titres • DAT	• HIV, HBV, HCV • HTLV, CMV • Syphilis • Malaria • Hepatitis A, Parvovirus B19	• HLA antibody testing • Extended blood group antigen testing • Platelet antigen typing • Haemoglobin S testing • Screening for IgA deficiency

Figure 5. Blood donor testing

15.3 DONOR SCREENING AND SELECTION

– Dr. Anuragaa S

The purpose of blood donor selection is to:

1. Protect donor health and safety by collecting blood only from healthy individuals
2. Ensure patient safety by collecting blood only from donors whose donations, when transfused, will be safe for the recipients
3. To identify factors that might make an individual unsuitable as a donor, either temporarily or permanently
4. Reduce the unnecessary deferral of safe and healthy donors
5. Ensure the quality of blood products derived from whole blood and apheresis donations
6. Minimize the wastage of resources resulting from the collection of unsuitable donations.

Condition	NBTC/DnC Criteria	WHO Criteria	AABB Criteria
Weight	45 Kg for 350 ml 55 Kg for 450 ml 50 Kg for Apheresis	45 kg for 350 ml 50 kg for 450 ml	Maximum of 10.5 mL/kg of donor weight, including samples.
Age	18-60 years for first-time donors. Repeat donors up to 65 years.	18-60 years for first-time donors. Repeat donors 65 years.	Conform to an applicable state law or 16 years
Blood Pressure(BP)	Systolic 100-140 mm Hg* Diastolic 60-90mm Hg	Systolic 100-140 mm Hg Diastolic 60-90mm Hg	Systolic and diastolic BP "within normal limits."
	There should be no findings of end-organ damage or secondary complication (cardiac, renal, eye or vascular) or history of feeling giddiness or fainting made out during history and examination. *The drug or its dosage should not have been altered in the last 28 days.*		
Pulse: beats per minute(bpm)	60 to 100 bpm and regular.	60 to 100 bpm and regular.	No requirement in AABB standards
Temperature	Afebrile,37.5^0 C /98.4^{0}F	Afebrile,37.50 C	37.5 C (99.5 F) *
	if measured orally or equivalent if measured by another method.		
(Whole blood)	12 weeks for males (90 days) 16 weeks for females (120 days)	12 weeks for males 16 weeks for female	8 weeks after whole blood donation.
Time since the last Meal	4 hrs. No fasting		
Travel and residence	History of residence in or travel to a geographical area which is endemic for diseases that can be transmitted by blood transfusion and for which screening is not mandated or there is no guidance in India		

Occupation*	24 hrs. before their next shift Defer if on a night shift with inadequate sleep		
	** The donor who works as an Air Crew, driver of long-distance heavy-duty vehicles and a construction worker on high buildings, either above sea level or below sea level, emergency services or where strenuous work is required*		
Residents of other countries	Accept only after staying in India for 3 continuous years		
Previously donors	Permanently defer donors who have had an unexplained delayed faint with or without injury (or) two consecutive faints following a blood donation.		

	Condition	NBTC/DnC Guidelines	WHO Criteria	AABB Criteria
Respiratory Infections	Cold, cough, sore throat, flu or acute sinusitis	Defer until all symptoms subside and the donor is afebrile	Defer for 14 days	
	Chronic sinusitis	No deferral unless using antibiotics		
	Asthmatic attack	permanently defer	Accept provided asymptomatic and on maintenance dose of non-steroid or inhaled steroids Defer for 14 days after full recovery from acute exacerbation	
	Asthmatics on steroids	Permanently defer	Defer for 14 days after completion of the course of oral or injected steroid	
	Allergy		Accept if symptom-free Defer permanently if a history of anaphylaxis	
	Severe allergic disorder	Permanently defer		

	Bronchitis		Defer for 14 days after full recovery from acute attack and completion of treatment	
Heart Diseases	Any active symptoms (Chest pain, shortness of breath, feet oedema)	Permanently defer	Permanently defer	**Variable** deferral criteria, as defined by the medical director
	Restricted activity			
	Cardiac medication (Digitalis. Nitroglycerine)			
	High blood pressure controlled with medicine	Acceptable if BP normal	Accept BP if the medication was not changed in the last 28 days	Controlled with bp
Cardio-Vascular Diseases	Myocardial infarction	Permanently defer	Permanently defer	Variable deferral criteria, as defined by the medical director
	Coronary artery disease	Permanently defer	Permanently defer	
	Angina pectoris	Permanently defer	Permanently defer	
	Rheumatic heart disease with residual damage	Permanently defer	Permanently defer	
	Structural heart diseases		Accept surgically corrected simple congenital cardiac malformation with no residual symptoms Accept asymptomatic disorder: e.g. functional murmurs, mitral valve prolapse	
Haematological Disorders	Abnormal bleeding tendency or blood coagulation disorder like haemophilia	Permanently defer	Coagulation disorders: carriers can be accepted for haemophilia A or B as long as coagulation factor levels are normal with no history of bleeding or treatment with blood products Defer permanently if coagulation factor deficiencies	Variable deferral criteria, as defined by the medical director

	Thalassemia Trait	No deferral if fitting other donor eligibility		
	Polycythemia Vera	Permanently defer	Permanently defer	
	G-6-PD deficiency	Permanently defer	Accept if there is no history of haemolysis Defer permanently if a history of hemolysis	
	Anaemia	After anaemia, correction can be taken	Accept if a history of iron deficiency anaemia with a known cause, not a contraindication to donation, when treatment completed and fully recovered Accept vitamin B12 or folate deficiency when fully recovered and on maintenance treatment Defer if under investigation or on treatment for anaemia Defer permanently if chronic anaemia Defer permanently if chronic anaemia of unknown cause or associated with systemic disease	
	Haemoglobinopathies and red cell enzyme deficiencies with a known history of haemolysis	Permanently defer		
Neurological Disorders	Fainting, Convulsions & Epilepsy	Permanently defer	Accept if a history of epilepsy or seizures provided off medication and seizure-free for 3 years	
	Migraine	Accept if not severe or occurs at a frequency of less than once a week		

Psychiatric disorders	Schizophrenia	Permanently defer		
Musculoskeletal disorders	**Ankylosing spondylitis**	Permanently defer	Defer permanently	
	Systemic lupus erythematosus	Permanently defer	Defer permanently	
	Psoriatic arthropathy	Permanently defer	Defer permanently	
Endocrinal Disorders		Other than diabetes and hypothyroid disorder on treatment, all other endocrine disorders defer	Defer all conditions Other than diabetes, hypothyroid disorder on treatment	
	Diabetes	Those who are well controlled by diet or oral hypoglycaemic medication, with no history of orthostatic hypotension and no evidence of infection, neuropathy or vascular disease (in particular peripheral ulceration) can be accepted		
	Thyroid disorders	Individuals with Benign Thyroid Disorders can be accepted if euthyroid (Asymptomatic Goitre, History of Viral Thyroiditis, Autoimmune Hypothyroidism) Defer if under investigation for Thyroid Disease or thyroid status is not known Defer permanently if: 1. Thyrotoxicosis due to Graves 'Disease 2. Hyper/Hypo Thyroid 3. History of malignant thyroid tumours		
Kidney diseases	Acute infection of the kidney (pyelonephritis)	Defer for 6 months after cessation of treatment and symptoms free	Accept if fully recovered from acute self-limiting condition (e.g., acute nephritis) provided renal function normal	
	Acute infection of the bladder (cystitis)	Defer for 2 weeks after complete recovery and the last dose of medication		
	Chronic kidney diseases/failure	Permanently defer	Defer permanently	

Gastro-Intestinal system	Stomach ulcer with symptoms or with recurrent bleeding	Permanently defer	Permanently defer	
	Chronic liver diseases with impaired organ	Permanently defer	Permanently defer	
	Diarrhoea	Defer for 2 weeks after complete recovery and the last dose of medication		
	Peptic Ulcer Disease	Those with stomach ulcers with symptoms or with recurrent bleeding should be deferred		
Viral Hepatitis	Unknown hepatitis	Permanently defer	Permanently defer	Permanently defer
	Positive test for Hepatitis B (HBsAg), Hepatitis C (HCV)	Permanently defer	Permanently defer	Permanently defer
	Exposure to hepatitis by tattoos, acupuncture or body piercing	Defer for 12 months	Defer for 12 months	Defer for 12 months
	Worked in renal dialysis	Defer for 12 months	Defer for 12 months	
	Received transfusion of blood and its components	Defer for 12 months	Defer for 12 months	Defer for 12 months
	Close contact with individuals suffering from hepatitis	Defer for 12 months	Defer for 12 months	Defer 12 months
	Hepatitis A or E	Defer for 12 months		
Jaundice	Has ever had jaundice associated with: • Newborn • Rh disease • Gall stone • Mononucleosis	No deferral	No deferral	No deferral

Rheumatological disorders	Systemic lupus erythematosus, scleroderma, dermatomyositis, ankylosing spondylitis or severe rheumatoid arthritis	Permanently defer		
Infectious diseases				
Risk behaviours	Transgender, Female sex workers, Men who have sex with men, Injecting drug users, People with multiple sexual partners	Permanently defer		
HIV Infection / AIDS	High-risk group donors for HIV infection Anti-HIV positive donor Donors having symptoms of AIDS	Permanently defer	Permanently defer	Permanently defer
Malaria:	**Non-Endemic areas:** Travellers who have been in an area considered endemic for malaria	may be accepted one year after returning from the endemic area (if there is no suspicion of malaria)	no symptoms: Defer for 12 months. Those who have had febrile symptoms but were not diagnosed with malaria: defer for 12 months following full recovery or last return from a malarious area, whichever is the longer	Individuals who have lived for longer than 5 consecutive years in a country with areas considered endemic Defer for 12 months after departure
	Immigrants/refugees/citizens coming from a country endemic to malaria	maybe accepted as blood donors, three years after departure from an endemic area, if they have been asymptomatic in the interim	Lived in a malaria-endemic area in the first 5 years of life or for a continuous period of 6 months or more: defer for 5 years after last return	

	Endemic area: Duly treated and free from any symptoms	Accepted 3 months after	Individuals with a recent infection with malaria: deferral for 6 months after completion of treatment or full recovery, whichever is longer	
Syphilis Genital sore or generalized skin rashes	Defer permanently	Defer for 12 months after rashes disappear & completion of therapy	Defer for 12 months or the longest applicable period for the following situations: Following the completion of treatment for syphilis or gonorrhoea	
Tuberculosis	Defer for 2 years following cure (Confirmed)	Defer for 2 years from confirmation of the cure		
Leprosy	Defer permanently			
Babesiosis, Brucellosis		Defer permanently	Defer permanently	
Chickenpox	Defer for 2 weeks following full recovery.	Defer for 14 days following full recovery		
Epstein-Barr virus		Defer until 28 days after full recovery		
Measles, Mumps, Rubella	Defer 2 weeks following full recovery	Defer for 14 days following full recovery		
Gonorrhoea	Defer permanently	Defer for 12 months following completion of treatment and assess for high-risk behaviour		
Campylobacter		Defer for 28 days following full recovery		
Lyme disease		Defer for 28 days following full recovery and completion of treatment, whichever is longer		

Infections (acute bacterial)		Accept 14 days after full recovery and completion of antibiotics Defer for 28 days following full recovery and completion of treatment if symptoms suggestive of infection with salmonella, campylobacter, streptococcus or staphylococcus	
Influenza		Accept asymptomatic individuals with no close contact with those who have an active infection Defer for 14 days after full recovery and cessation of any therapy	
Rickettsial infection		Defer for 6 months following completion of treatment or cessation of symptoms Defer acute Q fever for 2 years following completion of treatment and full recovery, whichever is longer Defer permanently chronic Q fever	
Rubella infection		Defer for 14 days following full recovery	
Salmonella infection		Defer for 28 days following full recovery	
Streptococcus infection	-	Defer for 28 days following full recovery Defer for 14 days following full healing if recent superficial but significant wounds	
Yersinia enterocolitica infection	-	Defer for 28 days following full recovery if recent abdominal symptoms, particularly diarrhoea, suggestive of *Y. enterocolitica* infection	
Zika	Zika infection: Defer for 4 months following recovery. In case of a history of travel to a West Nile Virus endemic area or Zika virus outbreak zone: Defer for 4 months		

Dengue/ Chikungunya	History of Dengue/Chikungunya: Defer for 6 Months following full recovery. Following a visit to Dengue/Chikungunya endemic area: 4 weeks following return from a visit to the dengue-endemic area if there is no febrile illness
Leishmaniasis	Permanently defer
Conjunctivitis	Defer for the period of illness and until on local medication
Osteomyelitis	Defer for 2 years after completion of treatment and cure

Fever	Had prolonged fever or Rheumatic fever	Defer till fully recovered and off medication	Defer until 14 days after full recovery	
Obstetrical causes	Pregnant or recently delivered, Abortion	Defer for 12 months after delivery. 6 months after the Abortion	Defer during pregnancy and lactation Abortion: Defer for up to 6 months	Defer if the donor has been pregnant within the last 6 weeks.
	Breastfeeding	Defer till the baby is on breastfeed	Defer during lactation	
	Menstruation	For the period of bleeding		
Surgical Procedures:	Major surgery	12 months after recovery	12 months following recovery	
	Minor surgery	6months after recovery	Till full recovery	
	GI Endoscopy	Defer for 12 months		
	Open heart surgery, including By-pass surgery	Permanently defer	Permanently defer	
	Cancer surgery	Permanently defer	5yrs for nonhematological solid malignancy	Nonhematologic cancer: Defer for 5 years after completion of treatment. Hematologic cancer (e.g., leukaemia): Defer indefinitely.

	Localized skin cancer that was removed	6 months after the removal	No deferral for in situ skin cancer.	Local skin cancer, in situ cancer: No deferral if treated completely with excision and healed.
	Tooth extraction or dental manipulation	Defer for 6months	Accept 24 hours after simple procedures and 7 days after extraction or endodontic procedures	12 months
	Dental surgery under anaesthesia	Defer for 6 months		12 months
Acupuncture			Defer for 12 months following last procedure	
Transplantation		Permanently defer	Defer for 12 months following transplantation of allogeneic tissues Defer permanently if transplanted with allogeneic cells or tissue sourced since 1980 from a country in which the risk of vCJD has been identified Defer permanently following stem cell or organ transplantation, dura mater graft, corneal transplant or xenograft	12 months. Permanent deferral for dura mater from cadavers

Dermatological conditions				
Acne			Accept provided venepuncture site is unaffected	
Vitiligo			Accept	
Any skin diseases at the phlebotomy site		Defer till it heals Defer if skin punctures or scars indicate professional blood donors or addiction to self-injected narcotics.	Accept mild common skin diseases (e.g. acne, eczema, psoriasis) if lesions not infected, the venipuncture site is unaffected Defer if generalized skin disease and on systemic medication Defer if contagious skin disease Defer permanently if systemic disease affecting the skin (e.g., scleroderma, SLE, dermatomyositis, systemic cutaneous amyloidosis)	
	Herpes		Accept cold sores and genital herpes provided no active lesions Defer symptomatic individuals for at least 28 days following full recovery Defer individuals with HHV8 infection and current or former sexual contacts permanently	

Vaccination and Medications:

No deferral unless the donor has any symptoms
Paratyphoid Rabies as prophylactic Prophylactic Hepatitis B

Two-weeks deferral from the time of vaccination	
Smallpox (two weeks after the scab falls off)	Mumps
Polio Injectable (Salk vaccine)	Yellow fever, Influenza, Swine flu
Measles (rubeola)	Meningococcal
Typhoid, Cholera, Papilloma	Diphtheria, Pertussis, Tetanus
Pneumococcal	Plague

Four-week deferral from the time of vaccination	
Anti-tetanus serum Anti-venom serum Anti-diphtheria serum Anti-gas gangrene serum	Live attenuated vaccines: Polio oral, Measles(rubella), Mumps, Yellow fever, Japanese encephalitis, Influenza, Typhoid, Cholera, Hepatitis A

<table>
<tr><td>Twelve-months deferral from the time of vaccination</td></tr>
<tr><td>Anti-rabies vaccination (post-exposure)
HBIG (hepatitis B immune globulin), Gamma globulin</td></tr>
</table>

<table>
<tr><td>Defer Permanently</td></tr>
<tr><td>Anticonvulsants, Pituitary growth hormones of human origin
Anticoagulants, Sedatives or tranquillizers in high doses
Antithyroid drugs, Vasodilators
Cytotoxic drugs Etretinate (e.g.Tegison), Digitalis Vasodilators, Dilantin</td></tr>
</table>

Drug	NBTC/D&C Criteria	WHO Criteria	AABB Criteria
Oral contraceptives	No deferral	accept	accept
Analgesics	No deferral	48 hrs	accept
Allopurinol	No deferral		
Vitamins, Mild sedatives and tranquillizers	No deferral	No deferral	No deferral
Ketoconazole, Anthelminthics	If the donor is well, Defer for 7 days after the last dose		
Salicylates(aspirin)	3 days.	5 days	36 hours
Isotretinoin (Accutane)	1 month from the last dose	28 days	3 years
Finasteride (e.g. Proscar)	1 month	28 days	1 month
Oral anti-diabetic drugs Acceptable with no vascular complication	No deferral medication has been not altered/ dosage adjusted in the last 4 weeks	No deferral	N0 deferral
People with diabetes on insulin	As long as receiving	defer	defer
Antibiotics (oral)	3 days	Accept 14 days after completion of treatment Accept if on long-term antibiotics for acne	
Antibiotics (injection)	4 days after the last dose		
Cortisone	7 days		
Ticlopidine, clopidogrel		Defer for 2 Weeks after the last dose	
Piroxicam, dipyridamole		Defer for 2 Weeks after the last dose	

Radioactive contrast material	Defer for 8 weeks		
Dutasteride	Defer for 6 months after the last dose		
Cardiac medication (digitalis, nitro-glycerine)	Permanently defer		
Medicine to treat hypercholesterolemia	No deferral		
Alcohol intake	Should not be a regular heavy drinker	Accept if there are no signs of intoxication	
Any medication of unknown nature	Defer till the information is available		

15.4 PHLEBOTOMY AND ADVERSE DONOR REACTIONS

3 vital **C**'s to put the donor at ease

Confidence

Care

Concern

<u>6 Ss of a good vein</u>

Superficial- palpable   Straight

Smooth/Scarless   Shine- tells about the turgor

Supported   Sufficient Diameter

<u>Treatment of Hematoma/bleeding from phlebotomy site 4Ps</u>

Position the donor's arm: Help the donor hold his arm in a non-dependent position.

Packing: Place gauze or cotton on the phlebotomy site or apply a tight bandage. Cold packs are also helpful by causing vasoconstriction

Pressure on the phlebotomy site: Stops the progression of the hematoma.

Procedure: Rarely in case of arterial puncture or so, ligation or surgical stopping is required

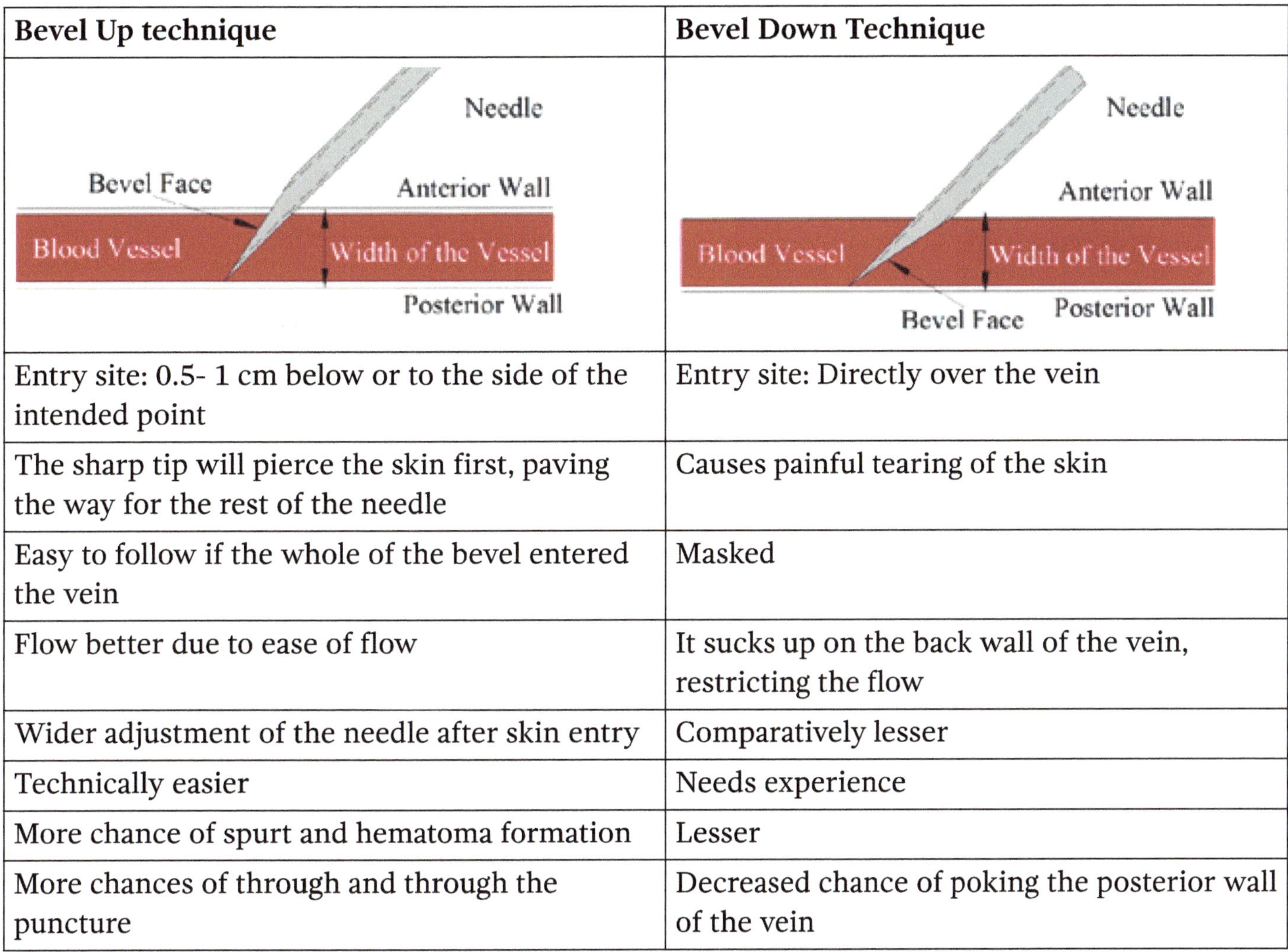

Bevel Up technique	Bevel Down Technique
Entry site: 0.5- 1 cm below or to the side of the intended point	Entry site: Directly over the vein
The sharp tip will pierce the skin first, paving the way for the rest of the needle	Causes painful tearing of the skin
Easy to follow if the whole of the bevel entered the vein	Masked
Flow better due to ease of flow	It sucks up on the back wall of the vein, restricting the flow
Wider adjustment of the needle after skin entry	Comparatively lesser
Technically easier	Needs experience
More chance of spurt and hematoma formation	Lesser
More chances of through and through the puncture	Decreased chance of poking the posterior wall of the vein

Table- 1: Factors influencing successful venipuncture

Donor factors	Anatomy of the vein
Environmental Factors	Blood drive, Number of donors
Phlebotomist factors	Knowledge, Attitude, Experience
Others	Quality of the needle

Vasovagal Syncope

1907: The term "vaso-vagal" was used by Sir William Gowers, who described a constellation of "vagal" symptoms, including epigastric, respiratory, and cardiac discomfort associated with vasomotor spasm.

1932: Sir Thomas Lewis, a British cardiologist, redefined vasovagal syncope along pathophysiological lines of a fall in blood pressure as an added phenomenon to a slowing in ventricular rate

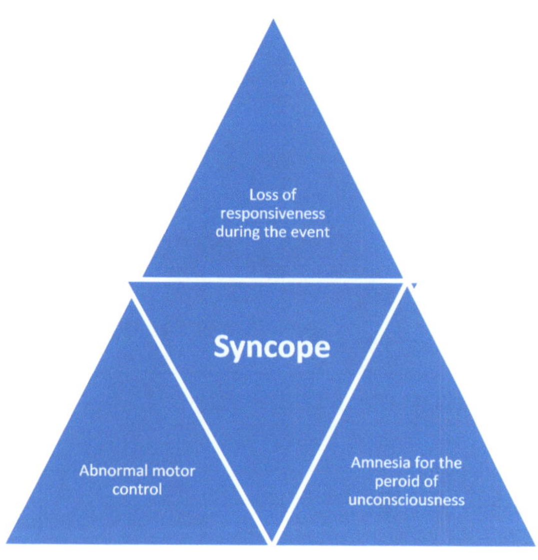

Triad of syncope/T-LOC

Syncope is defined as a Transient Loss of Consciousness(T-LOC) due to transient global cerebral hypoperfusion characterized by rapid onset, short duration, and complete spontaneous recovery

Pathophysiology:

Reflex syncope: (vasovagal)

Reflex syncope is an episodic disturbance of BP regulation involving reflex and environmental and physical effects.

Reflex effects include

a. Cardio inhibition (by increased vagal outflow)

b. Vasodepression: loss of vasoconstriction (decreased sympathetic outflow)

Presyncope (30-60 seconds)	**Syncope**	**Postsyncope**
Abdominal discomfort/nausea Palpitations Lightheadedness Unclear thinking Visual disturbances Buzzing in the ears	Gasping, snoring , apnea	Amazement Fatigue
Sweating Yawning	Fainting Eye movements Incontinence of urine/feces	Early -Flush , Late - pallor Incomprehension Hypotension

Blackout

Staring

Freeze

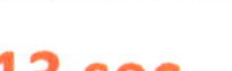

Eyes: Midline fixation, upwards turning

Loss of muscle tone, Loss of consciousness

Period 1

Fainting Rate: 0.04%

- Prior to introduction of the needle

Period 2

Fainting Rate: 1.1%

- Needle introduction
- Blood removal
- Needle removal
- Standing up(upto 4 minutes of needle removal)

Period 3

Fainting Rate: 1.4%(On site)

0.3% (off site)

- On site: refreshment area

- Off site: after leaving donation site

Donor Reactions and their pathophysiology	
Symptoms	
Weakness and Tremulousness, Dizziness, light-headedness, confusion, Nausea, Abdominal pain	
Signs	**Pathophysiological basis**
Pale skin and lips (Facial pallor- first sign)	Vasoconstriction (sympathetic) and reduced BP or blood flow. Increased vasopressin due to hypotension leads to vasoconstriction. The epidermis contains melanin and carotene
Head dropping	Loss of muscle tone
Apnoea/Gasping	Cerebral hypoperfusion
Urinary or faecal incontinence	Loss of sphincter tone due to hypoperfusion of the brain
Flush	Overshoot of BP post syncope due to the flow of well-oxygenated blood into the vasoconstricted bed

Sweating	Sympathetic activation of sweat glands, adrenaline
A feeling of sudden warmth/cold	Sweat release + cutaneous vasoconstriction
Palpitations	Sinus tachycardia
Sighing or yawning	When carbon dioxide increases, yawn provides an influx of oxygen (or expulsion of carbon dioxide). It helps increase a person's alertness and is a way of controlling brain temperature
Pupillary dilation	sympathetic activation and adrenaline, parasympathetic (pupillary constriction) is inhibited
Restlessness, Social withdrawal (becomes quiet), Loss of Consciousness	
Hyperventilation or rapid shallow breathing	the reflex response to increase venous return and to reduce abdominal pump
Vomiting	digestive "vagal" activation
Jerky movements	Cerebral hypoperfusion

DDs for Syncope
Reflex: Situational, Carotid sinus hypersensitivity, vasovagal
Cardiac: Arrhythmias, structural cardiac abnormalities, MI
Orthostatic Hypotension: Initial, classic
Others: Epileptic seizure, Psychogenic pseudosyncope

	Vasovagal Syncope	Seizure (tonic-clonic)
Orthostatic/emotional triggers	+	---
Presyncopal symptoms	+	----
Aura/focal seizures	---	+
Number of muscle jerks	<10	>20
The pattern of muscle jerks	Usually asynchronous	Synchronous/rhythmic
Duration of unresponsiveness (min)	<1 min	>5 min
Post recovery disorientation	Significantly less (a few seconds only)	Prolonged (>5 min)
Tongue biting	----	+
Cyanosis	----	+

Why do blackouts or loss of peripheral vision happen before LOC?

Intraocular pressure increases venous pressure in the retina. The driving pressure (Arterial - Venous pressure difference) of the retina is lower than that of the brain

Management
Place the donor on his back if he is in a standing or sitting position
Lower the head end of the couch
Raise the donor's feet above the head level
Provide fluids making sure he is not nauseous
Reassure, reassure, reassure! Talk to him and engage
Instruct him to exercise his limbs
If hyperventilating, encourage relaxation, and provide a paper bag for rebreathing if necessary
Apply a cold cloth to the forehead, back of the neck
Discontinue donation if felt necessary
Support the phlebotomy arm till the removal of the needle
Monitor vitals and seek medical assistance if required

Determinants of Donor Reaction

Not favourable	Favourable
Female gender	Male sex
Younger age (up to 25 years)	>35 yrs
First-time donor	
Lesser Weight, BMI	
Lesser Blood Volume	
Race- white race, Asians	African ancestry
Nervousness, fatigue, and anxiety of the donor	
Abnormal pulse/BP(systolic less than 110)	
Menstruation	
H/O vasovagal symptoms outside blood donation	
Previous reaction to blood donation	
Autologous donation	
Time since Meals (> 4 hrs)	Time since Meals (< 1 hr)
Longer waiting time from screening to the needle in	Better phlebotomy and interpersonal skills of the staff
Prolonged needle in – needle out time	
Afternoons	
Warm, humid spring season	
Antihypertensive medications	Autumn
	Collection in Mobile (Healthy worker effect)

Preventive Strategies
Identify at-risk groups and implement specific preventive measures
Implement stringent donor selection criteria
Ease donor anxiety – distraction, Audio-video, converse during the procedure
Reduce the risk of Injury – move to a safer area, do not leave unattended, allow them to support their back always, squatting, knee-chest
Pre-donation hydration, refreshments, caffeinated beverages
Manoeuvres – leg crossing, fisting,
Resting on the couch after the donation
Post-donation care- education
Training the staff for monitoring and management of reactions

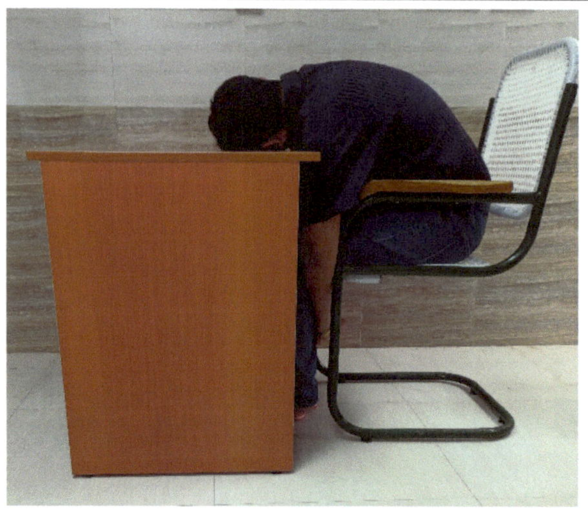
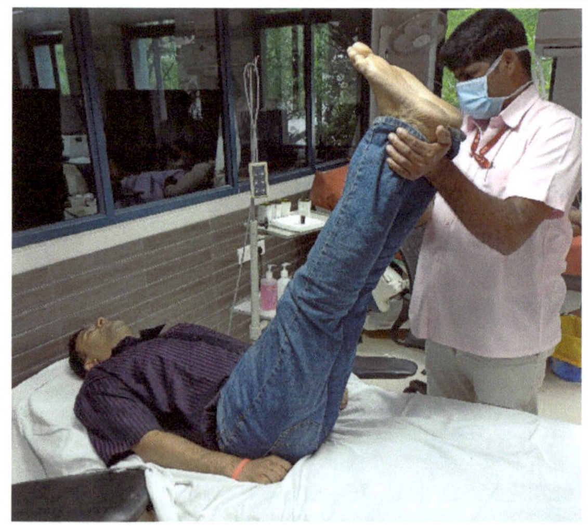
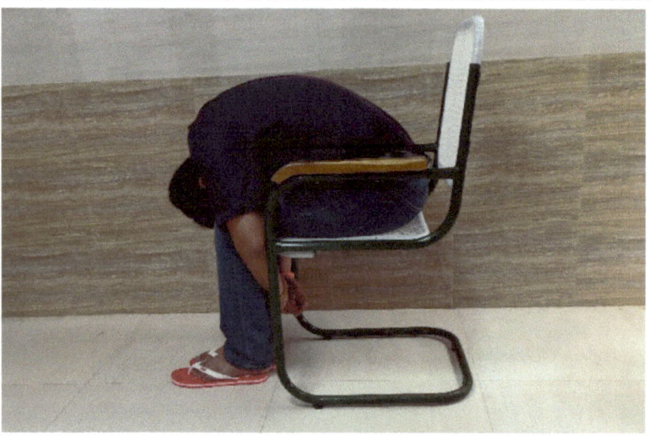
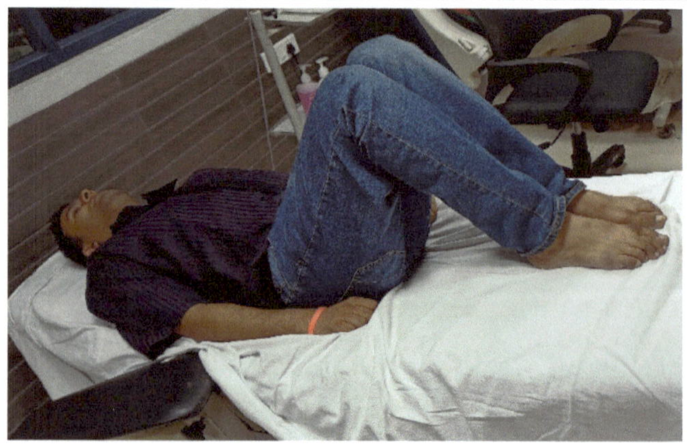

Injury	Description	Management
Nerve Injury (Irritation) CRPS- type II	Sharp, lancinating, burning, or electrical pain radiates to the lower arm Dull, boring, aching chronicity	Symptomatic treatment for pain Analgesics, anti-inflammatory drugs, Tricyclic antidepressants, anticonvulsants, transcutaneous electrical nerve stimulation, nerve blocks, stellate ganglion blockade, and sympathectomy
Arterial Punctures *Pseudoaneurysm* *Arteriovenous fistula* *Compartment syndrome* Contusion and Hematoma Sore Arm		Vascular surgery -"- 4 Ps, as mentioned
Allergic reactions	To- Iodine-based antiseptics, latex gloves, adhesive tapes, gauze, bandage	Use non-Iodine antiseptic-Chlorhexidine Non-latex gloves
Infection and Thrombophlebitis DVTs	Cellulitis, red linear streaks Swelling, increasing pain, and antecubital tenderness	Warm soaks, antibiotics Anticoagulants

15.5 PREPARATION AND CONDUCT OF OUTDOOR BLOOD DONATION CAMP

1. Take account of the details of the organiser, venue, and expected number of donors
2. Make sure the information and sufficient advertisement for the camp have been done
3. Prepare a checklist for all the equipment and materials to be carried to the camp and brought back
4. Reach in time and discuss issues with the organisers; stay till the camp is feasible and agreeable to you and the organisers
5. Deal with the donors in a respectable way and clear their doubts

Human resources requirements for the camp:

Usually, 4-5 donors can be bled per bed in one hour. So accordingly, arrange the number of beds depending on the expected donors. One phlebotomist can manage 2-3 donors at a time

A counsellor can manage about 6-10 donors in an hour.

"To collect blood from 50 to 70 donors in about 3 hours or from 100 to 200 donors in 5 hours, the following requirements shall be fulfilled/complied with: one Medical Officer and two nurses or

phlebotomists for managing 6-8 donor tables; two medico-social workers; three blood bank technicians; two attendants."

Pre-camp Phase	Camp Phase	Post-Camp Phase
Correspondence to the organisers Estimate the requirement Prepare adequately and arrange staff and requirements Information and advertisement for the camps Relevant correspondence should be documented for future reference	Prepare the area/venue Give a small introductory speech Start and execute the camp Make sure blood units are stored properly and reach the blood centre on time **Steps:** Registration→ Examination→ donation→ Refreshments→ Blood storage	Send letters of appreciation to the organiser for arranging the camp. Encouraged to organise similar camps regularly Constant touch with blood donors should be maintained Deficiencies, if any, in the camp should be analysed and improved upon

Equipment	Consumables
BP Apparatus, Stethoscope	Pamphlets, IEC materials
Artery Forceps/Scissors	Donor Questionnaire
Couches, mattresses, bedsheets, blankets, towels	Lancet/swabs/mixing sticks/slides
Test tubes/stand	Hemoglobinometer/copper sulphate
Needle destroyer	Antisera, Glass Slides
Blood Transport boxes	Donor cards/certificates and refreshments
Emergency kit, oxygen cylinder	Blood bags
Infusion stand	Band-Aids/ tape
Donor weighing scale, Blood bag weighing scale	Emergency drugs
Stripper/cutter/sealers	Sodium Hypochlorite, Antiseptic solutions
Dustbins	Ice packs
Banners	Stickers, Marker pens
	Blood collection Monitors/mixers

A typical floor plan arrangement for a camp is shown in the figure. (The path of the donor)

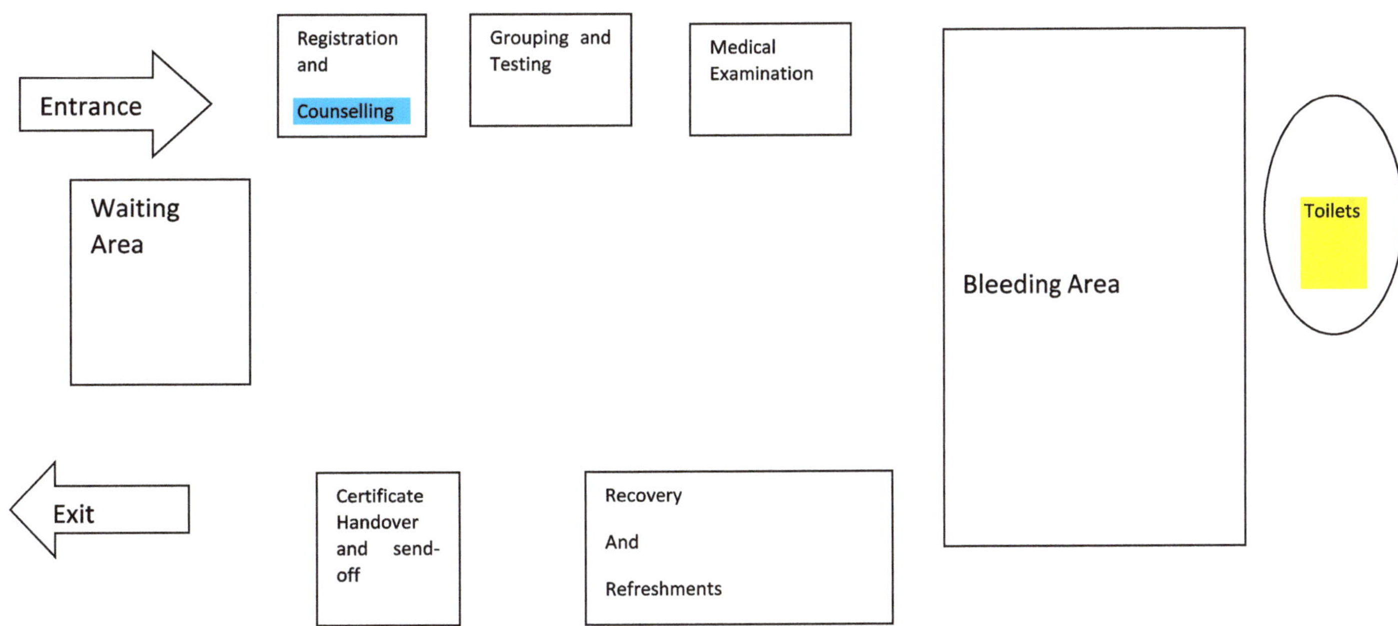

Giving Motivational Speech: Being a resident of Transfusion Medicine, inevitably motivating people to donate in small groups or big gatherings is common. It is an art that all of you must inculcate very early in your residency. Try to connect to the people. Use the local language wherever possible. Do not hesitate to make mistakes. Be assured that a horribly spoken speech in the local language makes a much more significant impact than a fantastically given speech in a language people do not understand. People understand early that this is not your comfortable language and accept it wilfully and appreciatively.

Tips to give a motivational speech on blood donation

- ➢ Introduce yourself
- ➢ Start with catchy poetry or dialogue
- ➢ Connect to the audience
  - • *"Today, I am going to talk with you ......"*
- ➢ Tell real-life stories and scenarios
- ➢ Tell about the ease of donation and bust the popular myths
- ➢ Tell statistics of India or your place and stress the need, shortages
- ➢ Tell about how the blood is utilised
- ➢ Tell about the advantages of donating- for the self and the community
- ➢ Ask questions and address their issues
- ➢ Give the contact of your blood bank and the person they need to get in touch with in case of requirement
- ➢ Leave them wanting more

<table>
<tr><td>Benefits of blood donation</td></tr>
<tr><td>

- The satisfaction of selflessness and "feel good," healthy glow, and positive feeling
- A potential benefit of a health screen. The unexpected clue to the diagnosis of a disorder that may be treatable, infection etc
- Lower the risk of cardiovascular diseases and decreases iron overload, especially in males
- Possible benefits of reducing the risk of cancers
- It helps to keep the body weight in check
- Stimulates blood cell production
- Motivation to imbibe a healthy lifestyle
- Reduces stress and improves emotional well-being
- A better societal acceptance of donors

</td></tr>
</table>

15.6 IRON DEFICIENCY IN BLOOD DONORS:

Each donation leads to a loss of about 25% of the average iron stores in men and 75% in women, as shown in the figure.

Functional iron deficiency is a fall in iron saturation in people with adequate iron stores due to stimulated erythropoiesis either with endogenous EPO–or with therapy. Manifested as reduced Tsat in the presence of normal ferritin levels

Table 15.4. Evolution of Iron Deficiency

	Normal	Stage I Stage of negative iron balance/ pre-latent iron deficiency	Stage II Stage of iron-deficient Erythropoiesis/ latent iron deficiency	Stage III Iron-deficiency Anemia
Marrow iron stores	1+ to 3+	0 – 1+	0	0
Serum ferritin (µg/L)	50-200	<20	<15	<15
TIBC (µg/dL)	300-360	>360	>380	>400
Serum Iron (µg/dL)	50-150	Normal	<50	<30
Transferrin Saturation (Tsat)	30-50(%)	Normal	<20 %	<10 %
Marrow sideroblasts (%)	40-60	Normal	<10	<10
RBC protoporphyrin (µg/dL)	30-50	Normal	>100	>200
RBC Morphology	Normal	Normal	Normal	Microcytic hypochromic

Serum iron (SI) represents the amount of circulating iron bound to transferrin. Sideroblasts are developing erythroblasts having visible ferritin granules in their cytoplasm.

Total Iron-Binding Capacity (TIBC) is an indirect measure of the circulating transferrin

$$\text{Transferrin saturation} = \frac{\text{Serum Iron}}{\text{TIBC}} \times 100$$

$$\text{Body Iron(mg/kg)} = \frac{\log(\text{sTfR/Ferritin}) - 2.8229}{0.1207}$$

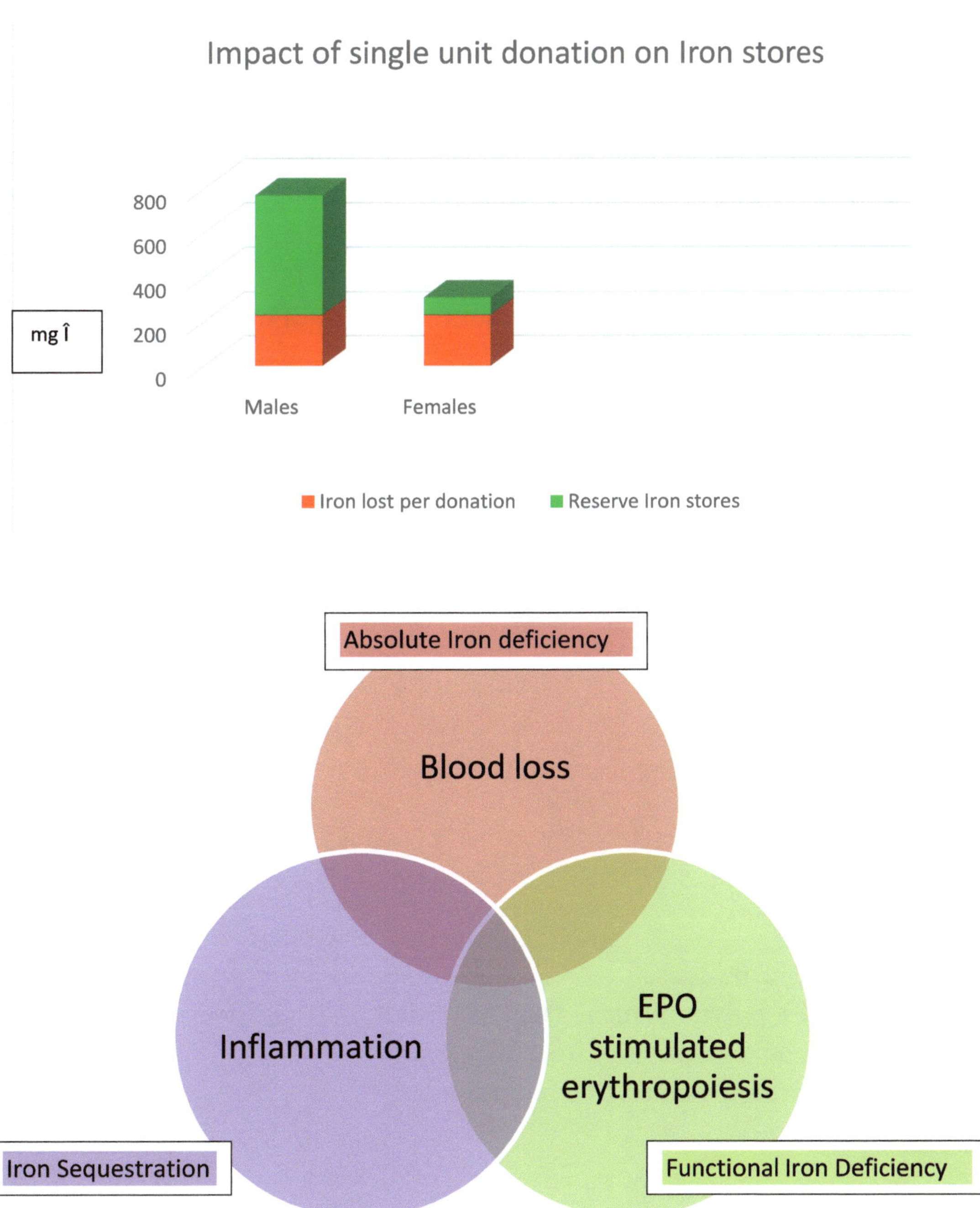

Figure 7. Iron deficiency states

Measurement of Iron status:

a. Hb
b. Red cell indices: MCH decline (hypochromia), MCV decline (microcytosis) and RDW increase (anisocytosis). Warning signals- MCH <28pg, MCV <83fl, RDW >14.6
   CCI: A cut-off of 52·6 for males and 50·6 for female
c. Serum/plasma Ferritin: Depleted body iron store is defined as ferritin <12 µg/L.
   Each ng/ml of ferritin in the blood equals 8-10 gm of storage iron in the storage compartment.
d. Soluble Transferrin Receptor Assay: (normal 4-6 mg/L) Transferrin receptors present on RBCs are synthesised and shed in increased amounts during the reduction of iron availability
e. Ferritin/sTfR ratio:

   - transferrin/log(ferritin) ratio: cut-off value of 1.70
   - LogTfR: Ferritin ratio > 2.55

f. Zinc protoporphyrin (ZnPP), also called free erythrocyte protoporphyrin (FEP): when the iron is deficient, protoporphyrin binds zinc resulting in its increase. (ZnPP>100mmol/mol heme)
g. Percentage of hypochromic mature red blood cells (%HYPOm): a time-averaged indicator of iron that is incorporated within the three-month lifespan of mature RBCs (cut off 0.3%). This is akin to HbA1c for diabetes
h. CHr (cellular haemoglobin content in reticulocytes): incorporating iron into developing reticulocytes that can be detected within their three-day lifespan (cut off 32pg). It is a real-time parameter.
i. Hepcidin levels (normal 8-200 ng/ml). cutoff 18ng/ml has about 80% sensitivity and specificity for predicting Hb decline and correlates with ferritin.

Risk factors:

Age: Younger, the better

Gender: Females >> males

Menstrual status and intensity: Premenopausal is worse

Pregnancy

Weight

Genetic predisposition:

   i. HFE genotype(heterozygous)
   ii. a transferrin (TF) polymorphism (G277S mutation) has been described to predispose individuals to the development of iron deficiency
   iii. Others: DMT1, Ceruloplasmin (CP) mutation

Donation frequency

Donation interval: < 14 weeks

Smoking and diet

Clinical outcomes asserted to be due to iron deficiency even without significant anaemia:
Fatigue: More in women and responds to iron supplements
Lowered exercise tolerance
Altered cognitive function
Pregnancy-related outcomes: Low birth weight
Pica: *the compulsive ingestion of non-nutritious substances like ice(pagophagia), dirt, raw pasta, starch, or chalk*
Restless leg syndrome: *A neurological condition with crawling, aching or burning sensation in legs, the most common feature being an irrepressible urge to move one's legs, particularly in the evening, and the condition can significantly compromise sleep and quality of life. Intense at rest*

Mitigation:

   i.   Increase interdonation interval
  ii.   Raising the minimum haemoglobin level
 iii.   Ferritin testing
 iv.   Iron supplementation:

325 mg oral ferrous sulfate (65 mg elemental iron) once daily for two months

Adverse effects: dark stools, constipation, diarrhoea, nausea, vomiting, and taste disturbance

Table 15.5. Sources of Iron food

	Haem-iron	**Non-haem iron**
Absorption	Better	Poor
Sources	Liver, meat, poultry, fish	Cereals, green leafy vegetables, legumes, nuts, oilseeds, jaggery, dried fruits
Iron bioavailability	Readily	Poor- due to the presence of interference phytates, oxalates, carbonates, phosphates, fibres
Co-absorption	Enhances absorption of non-haem iron	Milk, eggs, and tea can inhibit iron absorption

Etiologic Factors in Iron-Deficiency Anemia (Negative Iron Balance)

❖ Decreased Iron Intake
    • Inadequate diet
    • Impaired absorption: Achlorhydria, Gastric surgery, Celiac disease, Helicobacter pylori infection, Duodenal bypass, Drugs that increase gastric pH, Tannins, phytates, bran, Competing metals, Inflammation, ↑ hepcidin

❖ Increased Iron Loss
- Blood donation
- Iatrogenic: diagnostic phlebotomy for testing
- Gastrointestinal bleeding: Intestinal parasites Anatomic lesions: haemorrhoids, gastritis, diverticulosis, varices, hiatal hernia, Meckel diverticulum, arteriovenous malformation, peptic ulcer, Neoplasm, Inflammatory bowel disease
- Cow's milk protein allergy (infants and children)
- Use of salicylate or nonsteroidal anti-inflammatory agents, Anticoagulant, antiplatelet therapies
- Excessive menstrual flow
- Neoplasm: Gynecologic, Bladder
- Epistaxis, Hemoglobinuria
- Self-induced bleeding (autophlebotomy)
- Pulmonary hemosiderosis
- Tuberculosis, Bronchiectasis
- Hereditary hemorrhagic telangiectasia
- Chronic hemodialysis
- Runner's anaemia

❖ Increased Requirements
- Infancy, Pregnancy, Lactation

❖ Genetic Forms of Iron-Deficiency Anemia
- DMT1
- Glutaredoxin 5: Participates in iron-sulfur cluster biogenesis
- Atransferrinemia
- Aceruloplasminemia
- Matriptase-2: Hepcidin suppressor, acts by cleaving membrane hemojuvelin

15.7 THERAPEUTIC PHLEBOTOMY:

Polycythemia vera is a myeloid neoplastic multi-clonal stem cell disorder classically categorised as BCR-ABL negative.

The rationale for therapy: heightened risk for thrombotic complications

Epidemiology: Male preponderance

Juvenile: less than 20 yrs, Adult: 60-65 yrs (more common)

Transformation: Myelofibrosis and grade 2 bone marrow fibrosis

Acute myeloid Leukemia

Risk factors for leukemic blast crisis include myelofibrosis, abnormal karyotype, TP53 and TET2 and DNMT3A mutations

	Major Criteria	Minor criteria
1	Hb> 16.5 g/dl male, >16 g/dl female (or) Hct >49% male,>48% female, (paediatrics: 53.2) (or) Red cell mass (RCM) above 25% of the predicted value	Subnormal erythropoietin value
2	Positive genetic markers JAK2 V617F point mutation in Exon 14 or various JAK2 mutations in exon 12	
3	Hypercellular bone with the proliferation of erythroid cells, megakaryocytes of different sizes and granulocytosis	
Two major and **one** minor criterion are required to diagnose Polycythemia vera		

Phlebotomy:

Drainage of 300-450 ml (up to 10% of blood volume)

Observe the patient for 20-30 minutes post phlebotomy

About 1 litre of fluids to be consumed divided equally before and after phlebotomy

Frequency: every one to 2 weeks and maintenance monthly to target a Hct of less than 45%

Recalcitrant Hyperviscosity syndrome: target should be about 40-42%

Temporary phlebotomy resistance

High risk	Low risk
≥ 60 yrs	Age <60 yrs
h/o arterial-venous thrombosis	No h/o arterial-venous thrombosis
JAK2 mutation positivity	
Therapy:	Therapy:
Low-dose aspirin: 81 mg once or twice a day	Low-dose aspirin: 81 mg once or twice a day
Hydroxyurea	
Anticoagulation	
Second line: Busulfan, Peg IFN-α2a, Ruxolitinib	

Other indications for therapeutic Phlebotomy: Hemochromatosis, Porphyrias

COMPONENT PREPARATION

16.1 OVERVIEW

Why components?

- Rational use of scarce resources – single donation can benefit several recipients
- The recipient will get only that component that is required
- Reduces the risk of transfusion reactions as the component the patient does not require are not transfused (e.g., PRBC reduces allergic reactions due to plasma in comparison to whole blood)
- Optimisation of storage conditions- correct choice of additive solution, temperature, or bag type to ensure the effectiveness of each component with regard to shelf life

Cells	Specific gravity	Size
Platelets	1.058	1-3µm
Monocyte	1.062	15-20µm
Lymphocyte	1.070	Small 6-9µm Large 10-14µm
Neutrophil	1.082	12-14µm
Red cell	1.100	6-7µm
Eosinophil and Basophil		8-12

	ACD-A	ACD-B	CPD	CPDA-1	CP2D
Citric acid	35	21	14	14	14
Sodium citrate	97	58	116	117	117
Dextrose	136	81	141	142	**284**
Monosodium phosphate	-	-	15.8	16	16
Adenine	-	-	-	2	-
pH	5.0		5.6	5.6	5.6
Coagulant: blood ratio used	1:7	1:4	1:7	1:7	1:7

Relative centrifugal force: It is the force that acts on samples during centrifugation. It is expressed as multiples of the earth's gravitational field (g)

Relative Centrifugal Force (RCF)$= r \times (\text{rpm})^2 \times 118 \times 10^{-7}$

r= radius of centrifuge rotor in cms

rpm= rotations per minute, i.e., speed of rotation

one g is equivalent to the force exerted by gravity at the earth's surface, as applied during the centrifugation

If we know RCF for preparing a product, the required rpm can be calculated either from the formula above or the nomogram below. Or vice versa

The greater the radius of the rotor, the greater will be the force applied to the blood bag for any given rotational speed

To find the relative centrifugal force (RCF) at a radial distance of 30 cm from the centre of rotation for a centrifuge operating at a speed of 5000 rpm, place a straightedge on the chart connecting the 30 cm point on the Rotating Radius Scale (A) with the 3000 rpm. The point on the Speed Scale (B). Read the point at which the straight edge, like a ruler/scale, intersects the Relative Centrifugal Force Scale (C) – in this case, 3000 x gravity

Similarly, suppose the desired RCF is known; the necessary speed for a given rotating radius may be determined by connecting the two known points and reading the intersection of the straightedge with the Speed Scale.

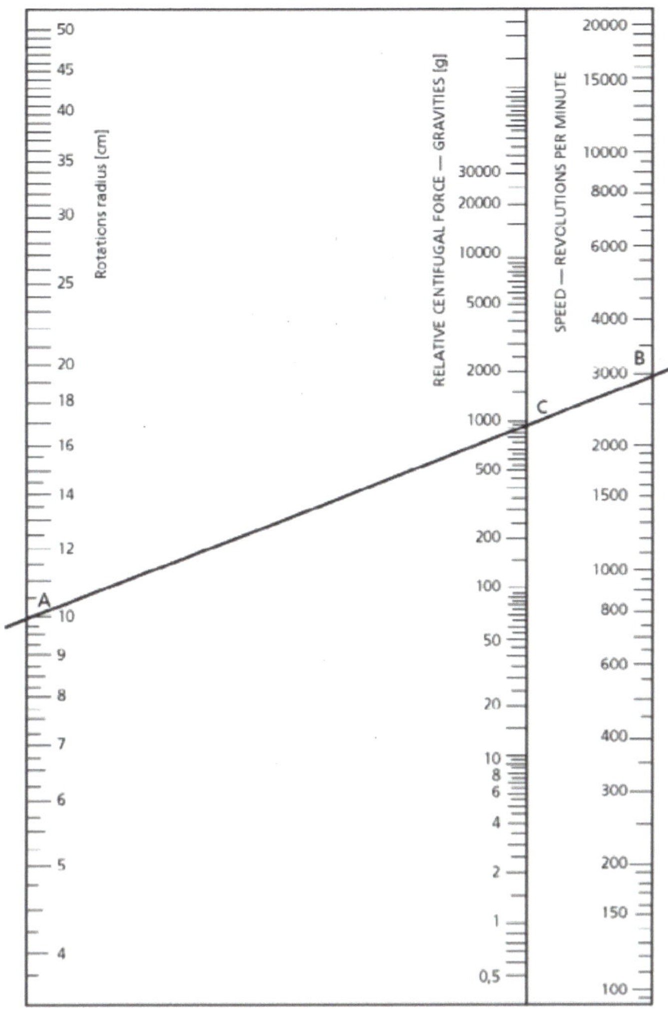

Figure 8. Nomogram to determine RCF or rpm for a given radius of the centrifuge

Components	Specific gravity
Whole blood	1.053
Packed red cells with additive solution	1.06
Packed red cells without an additive solution	1.08
Apheresis platelets	1.03
Plasma	1.02
Extracellular components	**Size**
Fibrinogen	700A°×20A°
IgM	300A°×200A°
IgG, IgA	200A°×50A°
Albumin	100A°
Cholesterol	15A°
Urea, creatinine, glucose	7A°
Na, K, Ca, Cl	1A°

Blood bag systems:

The choice of the bag depends on the following:

- Components needed to be prepared (In turn depends on clinical demand)
- Affordability
- Type of processing: manual, semi-automated or fully automated
- Special consideration, if any: extended storage, pediatric aliquotes, leukoreduction

Types of the blood bag Systems
Single bags
Double bags: primary bag + transfer/satellite bag
Triple bags: platelet by PRP methods
Quadruple bags: platelet by buffy coat method. Top and Top, Top and bottom
Pentabags

What happens if the buckets are not balanced before the operation?

Centrifuge vibrates during spinning, causing damage to itself and the personnel operating it.

The product may not be sufficiently centrifuged (The mismatch allowed is 1 gm)

In the PRP method bag must be left undisturbed for 1-2 hours because immediate attempts to resuspend the platelet button will cause irreversible aggregation

Why should platelets be kept under agitation?

Agitation facilitates gaseous exchange, diffusion of metabolites, and maintenance of platelets in a mobile liquid medium

General QC for all components:

Quantity	To be performed on 1% of the components or 4 units per month (whichever is higher)
TTI	Negative for all mandatory TTI infections
Sterility testing	Negative by culture, both short and extended duration

16.2 INDIVIDUAL BLOOD COMPONENTS

Whole Blood

	Volume(ml) Cut off is ± 10%	PCV(Hct)
450 ml	405-495	30-40
350 ml	315-385	30-40
1% of all units OR at least 4 units per month, whichever is higher, should undergo QC A minimum of 75% of units tested should meet QC. (Except European Council, which requires 90% *COMMENT: 100% of products tested should be sterile.*		

PRBC

		Volume(ml)	PCV(Hct)
From 450 ml WB	With Adsol/SAGM	350±20	55-65
	With CPDA/CPD	280±40	65-75
From 350 ml WB	With Adsol/SAGM	270±15	
	With CPDA/CPD	220±25	

Leukocyte-poor Red Cells

	Leucocytes	Red cells	Plasma
By Centrifugation	<70% of original	>70% of the original	
By washing	<15% of the original	>80% of the original	<1% of the original
By leukoreduction filter	<1% of original	>90% of the original	

Factors affecting PRBC quality:

1. *Donor factors:* Age, gender, Hb, donation status (repeat>first time), diet (Non-veg), smoking status
2. *Collection method:* containers used(DEHP improves quality), the needle size and anticoagulants type and ratio used, sterility, mixing
3. *Preparation method:*
   Centrifugation rpm and type of spin, storage/Additive solutions,
   Temperature and time-lapse during collection and component preparation, time-lapse during storage (metabolism is higher at warmer temperatures)
4. *Modifications performed:* leukoreduction, washing, irradiation, rejuvenation, freezing and pathogen reduction all reduce RBC content and quality

Remember

> ➢ 15-35 ml of blood is lost in the leukofilters depending on their size and content(WB or PRBC)
> ➢ The rejuvenation solution contains: PIPA (Phosphate, Inosine, Pyruvate, Adenine)
> ➢ RBCs expire 28 days after irradiation or original expiry, whichever is earlier

Platelets:

Platelets- Platelet Rich Plasma method	Platelets – Buffy coat method
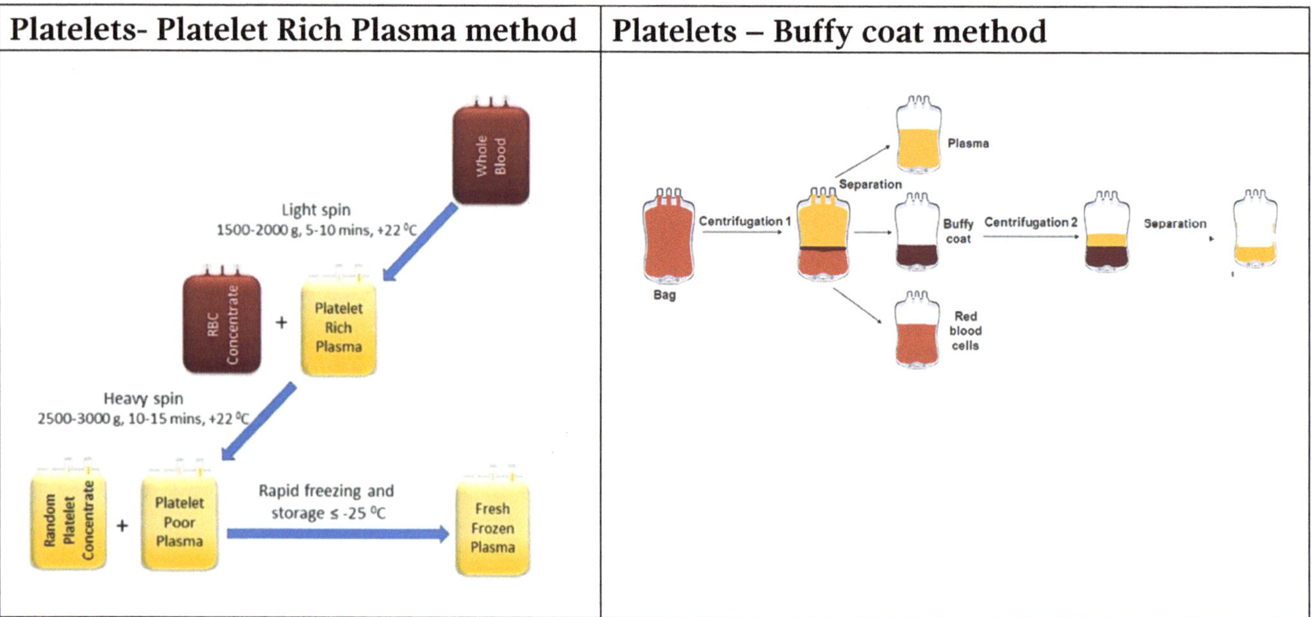	

	PRP Method	Buffy-coat Method(BC)	
First spin	Soft/Light	Hard/Heavy	Platelets are cushioned against RBCs in high spin; hence functionally better platelets in the BC method
Second spin	Hard/Heavy	Soft/Light	RBCs do not undergo hard spin; hence lesser lesions in them in the PRP method

System	Manual/ semi or fully -automated	Semi or fully automated only	
Process control	Inconsistent if done manually	Better	
Interface	Less clear	Clear	Better the interface less the RBC contamination
Plasma yield	Comparatively less	More	
Red cell loss	Minimal or no	30-40 ml	
WBC count	No change	Comparatively less/ reduced	
Viable bacteria	No change	Moderate reduction	
pH	>6.2	Comparatively higher	
Storage lesions		Lesser due to reduced glycolysis, increased oxidative metabolism, better maintenance of bicarbonate levels	
Effect on leukoreduction		More effective	

Indications

1. Hypo proliferative thrombocytopenia
2. Prophylaxis for invasive procedures
3. Inherited qualitative defects in platelets
4. Acquired qualitative defects in platelets: ECMO, cardiac bypass pump, medications
5. Thrombocytopenia due to immune destruction of platelets

Table 16.1. QC parameters for Apheresis platelets

	DGHS	D&C	AABB	NBTC	Council of Europe	WHO
Volume (ml)	200-300	-	-	200-300	>40 per 6×10^{10} platelets	150-300
Platelet count	$3\text{-}7\times10^{11}$	$3\text{-}7\times10^{11}$ (in 75% of units)	3×10^{11}	$3\text{-}7\times10^{11}$	2×10^{11} (For neonates: a minimum of 0.5×10^{11} per unit)	10×10^{11}/L

	DGHS	D&C	AABB	NBTC	Council of Europe	WHO
WBC Contamination (per unit)	$<5\times10^6$	-	-	$<5\times10^6$	$<0.3\times10^9$	$<1\times10^9$
RBC Contamination (per unit)	<0.5 ml	-	-	<0.5 ml	-	$<1\times10^9$
pH	>6	>6	-	>6	>6.4	6.4-7.4
Sterility						Sterile

Table 16.2 QC parameters for RDP by PRP method

	DGHS	D&C	AABB	NBTC	Council of Europe	WHO
Volume (ml)	50-70	-	40-70	50-70	>40 per 6×10^{10} platelets	45-65
Platelet count	$>5.5\times10^{10}$	$>4.5\times10^{10}$	$\geq5.5\times10^{10}$	$\geq4.5\times10^{10}$	$>6\times10^{11}$	$>5.5\times10^{10}/L$
WBC Contamination (per unit)	$<5.5\times10^7$ to 5×10^8	-	-	$<5.5\times10^7$ to 5×10^8	0.2×10^9	$<1\times10^9$
RBC Contamination (per unit)	<0.5 ml	-	-	<0.5 ml 5.5×10^9 RBCs	-	
pH	>6	>6	>6.2	>6	>6.4	6.4-7.4
Sterility						Sterile
Swirling						Present

From 450ml WB, the volume expected is 50-70 ml with a count $>5.5\times10^{10}$

From 350ml WB, the volume expected is 40-50 ml with a count $>3.8\times10^{10}$

Table 16.3 QC parameters for RDP by Buffy method

	DGHS	D&C	NBTC	Council of Europe
Volume (ml)	70-90	-	70-90	>40 per 6×10^{10} platelets
Platelet count	$6-9\times10^{10}$	$\geq4.5\times10^{10}$	$6-9\times10^{10}$	$\geq6\times10^{10}$
WBC Contamination (per unit)	5.5×10^6	-	10^7-10^8	0.05×10^9
RBC Contamination (per unit)	<0.5 ml	-	<0.5 ml	-
pH	>6	>6	>6	>6.4

From 450ml WB, the volume expected is 70-90 ml with a count $>5.5\times10^{10}$

From 350ml WB, the volume expected is 50-65 ml with a count $>3.8\times10^{10}$

Plasma Transfusion

Factor	Plasma levels (mg/L)	Half-life (in-vivo)	% activity Needed for Hemostasis
I	2.5 g/L	3-6 days	12-50
II	150	2-5 days	10-25
V	7	5-36 hrs	10-30
VII	1	2-5 hrs	>10
VIII	0.15	8-12 hrs	30-40
vWF	8	12 hrs	
IX	5	18-24 hrs	15-40
X	10	20-42 hrs	10-40
XI	5	40-80 hrs	20-30
XIII	20	12 days	5
Antithrombin	150	3 days	
Protein C	44	9 hrs	

Component	Collection	Time to Freezing from collection (in Hrs)	Shelf Life	Storage Temperature	Content	Indications
FFP	WB or Apheresis	8	Frozen: 1 yr Thawed: 24 hrs As TP: 4 Days	< -18^{0}C 1-6^{0}C	All clotting factors and plasma proteins	Deficiency of any of the clotting factors or proteins
PF24	WB or Apheresis	8-24 hrs Stored in the refrigerator till frozen	Frozen: 1 yr Thawed: 24 hrs As TP: 4 Days	< -18^{0}C 1-6^{0}C	Reduced Factor VIII, V, protein C	Same as above except for replacing Factor V, VIII or protein C
PF24RT24	WB or Apheresis	Up to 24 hrs Stored at Room Temperature till frozen	Frozen: 1 yr Thawed: 24 hrs As TP: 4 Days	< -18^{0}C 1-6^{0}C	Reduced Factor VIII, V, protein S	Same as above except for replacing Factor V, VIII or protein S
Cryo-poor plasma (CPP)	WB	24 hrs from Cryoprecipitate reduction	Immediate or relabel as thawed Cryopoor plasma5 days)	< -18^{0}C 1-6^{0}C	Absent Factor VIII, XIII, vWF, Fibronectin, Fibrinogen	TTP, Nephrotic syndrome

Thawed plasma (TP)	WB or Apheresis		5 days after thawing	1-6°C	Factor II, Fibrinogen, ADAMTS13	Repletion of stable factors, TTP, massive haemorrhage
Liquid Plasma	WBD	N/A	5 days after the expiration of parent WB	1-6°C	All factors decrease gradually with time	Massive Hemorrhage

WB- Whole Blood, FFP- Fresh Frozen Plasma, PF24- Plasma frozen within 24 hrs after phlebotomy, PF24RT24- Plasma is frozen within 24 hrs after being held at Room Temperature from the time of phlebotomy

Coagulation tests for Plasma Therapy Dosing			
Assay	**Reflection**	**the reference range for adults**	**When to initiate**
PT	Extrinsic pathway (VII) and the common pathway (X, V, II, I)	seconds	>18-24 sec
INR	Same as above	0.9-1.1	> 1.7
aPTT	Intrinsic pathway (VIII, IX, XI, XII) and common pathway (X, V, II, I)		

Clinical situation		Therapeutic options
INR	**Bleeding**	
2.5 -5	Not significant	Lower anticoagulant dosage. Temporarily discontinue drug
5-9	Not significant	Omit 1-2 doses; monitor INR. *If the patient is at increased risk of haemorrhage:* omit a dose and give 1-2.5 mg of vitamin K1 orally. *For rapid reversal before urgent surgery:* 2-4 mg vitamin K1 orally; repeat the dose with 1-2 mg at 24 hours if INR remains elevated
>9	Not significant	Omit warfarin; give 5-10 mg of vitamin K1 orally
Any INR	Serious	Omit warfarin. Give 10 mg of vitamin K1 by slow intravenous infusion. Supplement with plasma or prothrombin complex concentrate depending on the urgency of correction. Vitamin K1 infusions can be repeated every 12 hours.
Any INR	Life-threatening	Omit warfarin. Give prothrombin complex concentrate with 10 mg of vitamin K1 by slow intravenous infusion. Repeat as necessary, depending on INR

QC of Plasma

Parameter	FFP	FP
Volume	200-220 ml	200-220 ml
Stable clotting factors	200 units of each factor	200 units of each factor
Factor VIII	0.7units/ml	
Fibrinogen	200-400 mg	

Thawing plasma

Before transfusion, FFP must be thawed at 30–37°C, which takes 20–30 minutes (termed FFP Thawed). Thawed FFP should be transfused immediately or stored at 1–6°C for up to 24 hours.

QC: Fibrinogen is measured by the dry clot weight method. Fibrinogen level should be 250-300 mg/bag in FFP and 150mg/bag in case of cryoprecipitate.

a. One-stage assay for factor VIII: based on comparing the ability of dilutions of patient's plasma and standard plasma to correct the APTT of substrate plasma lacking F VIII
b. Fibrinogen Assay: based on the precipitation of fibrinogen by ammonium sulphate and measuring the height of the column of the precipitate.

Cryoprecipitate (or) Cryoprecipitated Antihemophilic Factor (or) cryo

1964: Dr. Judith Pool

Preparation:

Centrifugation of cold insoluble proteins after FFP has been thawed either by

a. **Slow-Thaw Method: (overnight thaw)** Bags of frozen plasma are placed directly on wire shelves in a refrigerator (4°C) for 20 h till they are completely thawed. The bags are centrifuged at 4,920g at 0°C for 10min, and the supernatant plasma is allowed to drain from the inverted bags. The cryoprecipitate is then dissolved in the small amount of remaining plasma by warming in a 37 °C water bath
b. **Rapid thaw method:** The plasma units are placed in metal canisters to form the plasma into a uniform layer (approximately 20 mm in thickness), and the canisters are placed on the shelves of the -80°C freezer. After two hrs, the bags of frozen plasma are removed from the canisters and placed in a 4 °C circulating water bath. When all the slushy ice has disappeared, the bags are immediately centrifuged. The conditions of centrifugation, draining of the supernatant and thawing of the cryoprecipitate for the factor VIII assay are as described above for the slow-thaw method.
c. **Thaw-centrifuge method:** The plasma units are frozen in a configuration that fits into a centrifuge cup. The frozen bags of plasma are placed in the centrifuge cups, with each cup at least half-filled with water, and the centrifuge is balanced. They are then centrifuged at 2,000 g and 8 °C for 90 min. The water portion and the plasma concentrate are expressed into the satellite bag leaving behind the cryoprecipitated AHF
d. **Thaw-Siphon Method:** The plasma packs are frozen in metal canisters similar to those used for the rapid-thaw method. The frozen bags of plasma are placed in a 4 °C circulating water

bath, with the satellite bags placed on the bench below the bottom of the bath. After 10 min, two broad rubber bands are stretched around the pack at distances from the bottom equal to one-quarter and three-quarters of the length of the pack. The siphoning is discontinued when the frozen mass remaining in the bag is less than 30ml.

The remaining cryoprecipitate in frozen plasma is thawed in a 37°C water bath.

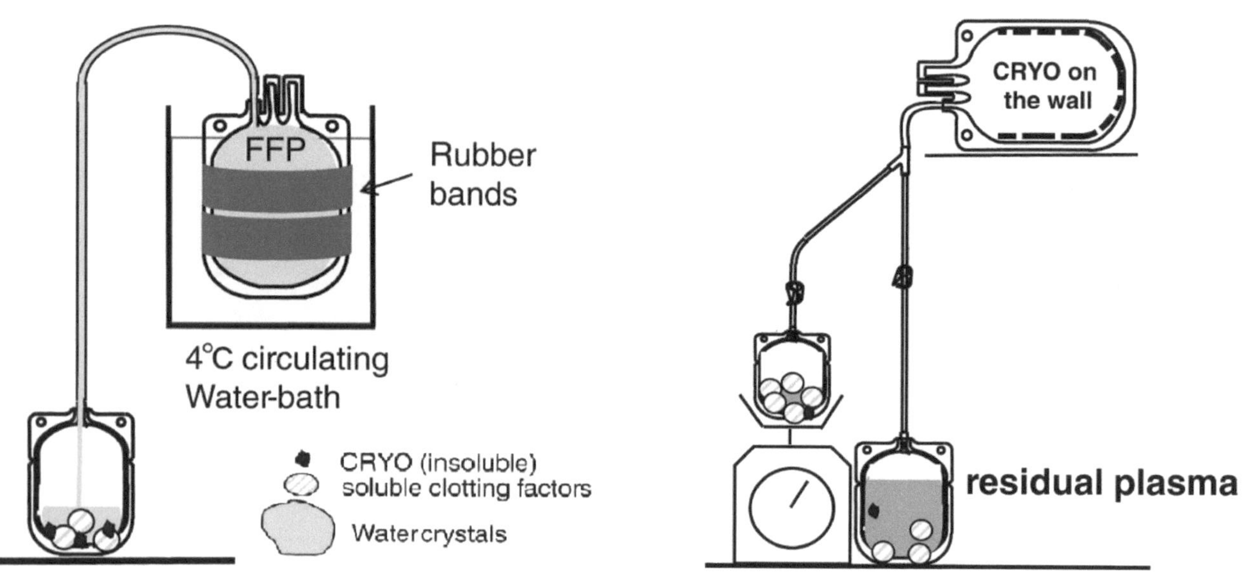

QC of Cryoprecipitate

Volume	10-20 ml
Factor XIII	20-30% of the original
Factor VIII	80-120 units
Fibrinogen	150-250 mg
vWF	40-70% of the original
Fibronectin	55 mg

Thumb rule targets: Non-surgical patients	50-100 mg/dL
(Fibrinogen) Surgical patients	100-200 mg/dL
Thumb rule dosing: Single unit per 5-10 kg (or) Number of units = Desired fibrinogen increment (g/L) × Plasma Volume (L) × 4	Raises fibrinogen by 50-75 mg/dL One dose of cryoprecipitate (1 unit of cryo per 10 Kg) is expected to raise fibrinogen levels in the recipient by 50mg/dL
Rate of transfusion	2-5 ml/min (120-300 ml/hr)

Since factor levels of 5% of factor XIII are hemostatic, the recommended dosage is 1 Unit of cryo per 10-20 kg body weight every 2-3 weeks.

Haemophilia A: second-line treatment for when factor concentrates are unavailable. Loading dose to achieve the desired factor VIII level, followed by maintenance doses every 8 to 12 hours.

Therapeutic indications

	Condition	Remarks
1	Haemorrhage secondary to thrombolytic therapy	Fibrinogen repletion
2	Uremic bleeding	As an adjunct to desmopressin, dialysis and conjugated estrogen
3	L-asparaginase chemotherapy, snake envenomation	Fibrinogen repletion
4	Factor XIII deficiency	
5	Von Willebrand disease	
6	DIC	
7	Blood loss and massive transfusion (Coagulopathy)	Adjunct to FFP
8	Cardiovascular surgery	For non-surgical bleeding

The following formula can be used:

Number of bags of cryo required =

$$\frac{\{Factor\ VIII\ Levels(\%)desired - Factor\ VIII\ levels(\%)\ current\} \times Plasma\ volume}{80}$$

Von Willebrand disease: daily infusions of 1 U of cryoprecipitate per 10 kg body weight

Tip: pregnancy results in increased levels of all clotting factors except factor XI

Complications: Risk of TTI, Hemolysis in children from high-titre antibodies, Respiratory distress, Febrile and allergic reactions, Thrombosis

Granulocytes Concentrates

Granulocyte concentrate can be prepared by:

a. Whole blood (Single donor unit or pooling)
b. Leukapheresis by blood cells separator (from a single donor)

Preparation of Granulocytes from donated whole blood:

1. Collect 450 ml of donor blood in 450 ml of CPDA or Adsol SAGM triple packs system and keep at 20-24°C till separation of buffy coat (in no case MORE THAN 6 HRS AFTER COLLECTION of blood)
2. Keep the bags in the buckets of refrigerated centrifuged and balance them accurately. Centrifuge the blood bags at 20-24°C at light spin for an appropriate time, e.g. 2000x g for 3 minutes.
3. Express the supernatant plasma into the first satellite bag. Leave about 20 ml of plasma above the cellular layer (buffy coat) in the primary bag. Double-seal the tubing between the primary and satellite bag with plasma and separate it.
4. Express 20 ml of plasma and the upper 20-25 ml of the cellular layer, rich in white cells, into another satellite pack. Double-seal the tube and separate it.

Storage: At room temperature (20-24⁰c) for a maximum of 24 hrs

Indication:

If patients with infection and neutropenia (<500 PMN/µL) do not respond quickly and completely to antibiotics alone, the addition of therapeutic GTX should be considered.

The product should be transfused in two to four hours **(NEVER USE LEUKOFILTERS)**

Table 16.4 QC of Granulocytes

	Granulocytes	Other leucocytes	Platelets	RBC	volume	HES (if used)
By Apheresis	10^{10}	$0.1\text{-}0.7 \times 10^9$	$2\text{-}10 \times 10^{11}$	5-50 ml	200-400 ml	6-12%
From Whole Blood	$0.5\text{-}1 \times 10^9$				200-250 ml	

16.3 MODIFICATION OF BLOOD PRODUCTS

Indications for using washed blood products:

Red cells:

1. Intrauterine transfusion, Large-volume or rapid transfusion (to reduce hyperkalemia and arrhythmias)
2. IgA deficient recipients (thorough washing up to 6 times is required)
3. Previous serious allergic reaction without a known attributable cause (Removes allergenic plasma proteins)
4. Patients with T-activated red cells (During ongoing hemolysis, reduces further hemolysis by eliminating lgM anti-T)
5. Paroxysmal Nocturnal Haemoglobinuria patients

Platelets:

NAIT (Removes maternal antibodies from maternal platelet product)

Component	Residual leucocyte count
Fresh whole blood	10^9
Packed Red cell concentrate	$10^8\text{-}10^9$
Buffy coat-depleted red cells	10^8
Washed red cell concentrate	10^7
Frozen deglycerolized red cells	$10^6\text{-}10^7$
Platelet concentrate (RDP)	$10^7\text{-}10^8$
Apheresis platelets (SDP)	$10^6\text{-}10^8$
Fresh frozen plasma	$< 10^4$

Leukoreduction

Established

1. Reduction of HLA alloimmunization risk in patients who require long-term platelet support or for potential organ transplant recipients
2. Reduction of CMV transmission in at-risk patients
3. Reduction of the rate of recurrent febrile non-hemolytic transfusion reactions.

Others:

Prevention of prion or viral reactivation
Prevention of post-operative infections
Reduction of tumour recurrence
Prevention of bacterial infection
Reduction in transfusion-related lung injury
Reduction in transfusion-associated graft versus host disease.

Irradiation

1. Fetal and neonatal recipients of intrauterine transfusions
2. Selected immunocompromised recipients
3. Recipients of cellular components known to be from a blood relative
4. Recipients who have undergone marrow or peripheral blood progenitor cell transplantation
5. Recipients of cellular components whose donor is selected for HLA compatibility

Volume reduction (also known as hyperpacking or hyperconcentrating)

In RBC products:

Methods:

Strauss method (Centrifugation and Aliquoting): whole blood collected in CP2D is centrifuged at 5000 g for 5 minutes, the supernatant platelet-rich plasma is removed, and 100ml of extended storage media, preferably AS-3 (because it does not have mannitol) is added to and mixed with the RBCs/. When an aliquot for transfusion is ordered, the storage bag is centrifuged in an inverted position to pack the RBCs to a hematocrit of approximately 90%. Attached to this primary storage bag, by way of a sterile connecting device, is a cluster of small-volume bags. The volume of RBCs requested flows out into one of the attached small-volume bags, which is disconnected. The remainder of the AS-3 product is mixed and returned to storage. In addition, the AS-3 storage bag is mixed each week thoroughly.

Enables the manufacture of small aliquots of RBCs for neonates with hematocrit 90% using a single RBC product until expiration on day 42

Inverted gravity sedimentation: This method stores RBC products in the refrigerator "upside down," concentrating an additive solution product to a hematocrit of around 70–90% within 72 hours. In addition, this method does not require a refrigerated centrifuge

Indications:

1. To remove the accumulated potassium, which leaks from the RBCs during storage
2. To reduce the Adsol concentration (Or SAGM in neonates)
3. To reduce the volume infused in volume-sensitive patients
4. To reduce antibodies when O whole blood is used out of the group

In platelet products:

Method: The stored platelets may be centrifuged at 20–24°C at 580 g for 20 minutes, **OR** 2000 g for 10 minutes, **OR** 5000 g for 6 minutes

Following centrifugation, the platelets must rest without agitation for 20–60 minutes prior to resuspension and eventual transfusion

Since volume reduction is performed in an open system, the expiration date of the platelet products must be changed to 4 hours, starting from when the product was entered for processing.

Indications:

1. ABO Out-of-group Platelet Transfusion
2. To decrease Febrile Non-hemolytic Transfusion Reactions

Aliquoting: Aliquots can be made from individual products, thus allowing the re-use of a given product for multiple transfusion episodes for a given recipient.

Indications:

- RBC products can be divided into smaller volumes for neonatal transfusions
- Platelet products are often dispensed in small aliquots via syringe for neonatal transfusions; these products are acceptable for 4–6 hours in the syring
- Apheresis platelet products can be divided into smaller volumes for neonatal transfusion
- In splenic or hepatic sequestration in sickle cell disease, RBCs are frequently given in small aliquots (5ml/kg) over 4 hours, as the release of autologous RBCs from the sequestration may occur during the transfusion
- In patients at risk for TACO, It may be necessary to split blood products into two sterile aliquots and infuse each split over 4 hours
- Aliquots of HPC, Apheresis can be separated and frozen individually for future use as DLI

Suggested reading

http://naco.gov.in/sites/default/files/FINAL%20BCSU_HANDBOOK%2014%2010%202015.pdf

PRETRANSFUSION TESTING

17.1 OVERVIEW

Blood Grouping:

False positives	False negatives
Clerical errors, identification errors, mix up	Clerical errors, identification errors, mix up
Suspension too heavy	Suspension too weak
	Failure to add reagents, samples
	Failure to follow the manufacturer's instructions
	Hemolysis
Over centrifugation	Under centrifugation
	Warming during the test/centrifugation
Contaminated reagents	Contaminated reagents

Typing methods:

Slide/tile method:

- Spread the mixture over an area of 2×4 cm
- Before declaring negative, at least 2 min of side-to-side rocking is to be performed
- Weak/doubtful reactions should be retested using a tube test
- Use the Rh view box for Rh grouping only, not for ABO grouping

Disadvantages:

- Risk of exposure to personnel performing the test
- not suitable for reverse or serum grouping
- drying effects, not preservable. Never read beyond 5 minutes

Test tube method:

- Cell grouping; the ratio of the cell is to serum 1:1, Serum grouping; the ratio of the cell is to serum 1:2-3,

- To Enhance weak reactions, a 5-15 min incubation at room temperature is suggested
- Use a lens, magnifying mirrors or even a low-power microscope to confirm the absence of agglutinates

Microplate method:

Procedural steps	IgM antibodies (anti-A, anti-B)	IgG antibodies (anti-D, anti-K)
Enhancement media	None	LISS
Red cell suspension	2-5%	2-5%
Incubation	Room temperature for 30 min	37^{0}c for 1 hr.
Wash	Not required	Minimum of 3 washes with saline
Testing phase	Saline	AHG
Endpoint	Macroscopic agglutination	Macroscopic agglutination

Demonstrate proficiency in preparing cell suspensions of appropriate concentration following cell washing techniques correctly & grade and interpret antibody-antigen reactions according to the established criteria.

Red cell suspension

For the Column agglutination technique	0.8-1%
For tube testing	3-5%
For slide or tile methods	50%

Few points to remember
➢ **Why suspension?** Provides the appropriate serum-to-cell ratio to allow for grading and interpretation of tests results ➢ For best results, red cell suspensions to be used for testing should be prepared on the same day of usage

If the suspension is too highly concentrated: It masks weak agglutination

If the suspension is too weakly concentrated: Challenging to visualize, weak agglutinations are missed

QC: Compare the colour of the suspension or the size of the agglutinate button after centrifugation with the standard commercial suspension available.

A 3% suspension is "tomato red" in colour.

Why washing?

- To avoid clots which can form when RBCs coated with fibrinogen are mixed with a serum that contains residual thrombin
- To avoid Rouleaux, which interferes with the interpretation of agglutination
- Substances in the suspension, like lactose and neomycin, may cause agglutination when corresponding antibodies are present in the patient's plasma

- Secretary blood group substances like ABO, Lewis, Chido/Rodgers, and Ii present in plasma may inhibit the corresponding antibody in the test serum
- Plasma may sometimes contain so-called "albumin autoagglutinins."

Why serum and not plasma?

- Plasma may interfere detection of complement-binding antibodies as it contains the anticoagulant

Grading and scoring agglutination reactions

Observation (macroscopic)	Grade	Score
One solid agglutinate	4+	12
Several large agglutinates	3+	10
Medium-sized agglutinates, clear background	2+	8
Small-sized agglutinates, turbid background	1+	5
Very small agglutinates, turbid background		4
Barely visible agglutinates, turbid background		2
No agglutination	0	0
A mixture of agglutinated and unagglutinated cells	mf	
Hemolysis (complete, no cells remaining)	H	
Hemolysis (Partial, some red cells remain)	PH	

Why scoring?

- Reduces subjective bias
- Numerical scoring permits easy data analysis, and grading needs riders to indicate more delicate degrees of reaction like [w, s]
- It takes into account all the positive reactions in contrast to titres which are based on only the greatest dilution, which gives agglutination
- Allows finer gradations within the existing framework

Grading in Column agglutination techniques

Grade	Description	Illustration
0	All the cells at the bottom of the column	
1+	Most of the cells at the bottom of the column with few tapering from the bottom	
2+	Cells dispersed throughout the column	
3+	Most of the cells at the top of the column with few tapering from the top	
4+	All the cells on the top of the column	

<table>
<tr><td>Donor unit testing

ABO
Rh
Antibody screen
TTI testing
Product labelling</td><td>Patient sample testing

Identification and Consent
Sample collection and labelling
ABO and Rh typing
Antibody screening and identification</td><td>Compatibility testing

Serological crossmatch
Electronic crossmatch
Extended antigen matching
Labelling
Issue</td></tr>
</table>

Why pretransfusion testing?

1. Positive identification of the patient
2. To select suitable units
3. To identify and comply with special requirements, if any
4. To review all transfusion records and history and act upon them.
5. Ensuring the best survival of red blood cell (RBC) units.
6. Minimise harm to the patient concerning ABO compatibility, antibody detection and identification

Essential Elements of a Transfusion requisition form
<ul><li>Patient's complete first and last (family and given) names</li><li>Gender, Age, Weight</li><li>unique identifiers like date of birth (DOB), hospital number, health card number, or AADHAR in India.</li><li>The recipient's location.</li><li>The required blood component or blood product: volume or units.</li><li>Date and time of the order.</li><li>Identity of the person ordering the blood products/ treating physician.</li><li>Date and time of the intended transfusion</li><li>Special requirements: CMV negative, irradiated, washed, leukoreduced</li><li>The patient's transfusion history.</li><li>The patient's history of pregnancy and spontaneous /therapeutic abortions.</li><li>Previous blood group if known.History of an alloantibody, autoimmune hemolytic anaemia or transfusion reactions</li><li>Transplantation recipient</li></ul>

Table 17.1 Timing of pre-transfusion samples

Patient transfused within the last:	Samples to be taken not more than (before pretransfusion)
2 days to 2 weeks	24 hrs
2 to 4 weeks	72 hrs
1-3 months	1 week

Table 17.2 Various Pre-transfusion Schemes

	Scheme	Prerequisites	Tests performed	Advantages	Limitations
1	Hold	Patients who have never been transfused or pregnant previously, and transfusion requirement is unlikely	None	Sample is available	
2	Type and Hold	there is minimal chance of transfusion requirement	ABO and Rh Typing		Antibody screening not done
3	Type and screen	there is a chance of transfusion requirement	ABO, RhD typing, antibody screening and identification	In most situations, compatible blood can be provided	Antibody detection not performed
4	Type and screen with Crossmatch	there is a high chance of transfusion requirement	All in type and screen + Red cell unit phenotyping and crossmatch		Units may not be available for other recipients

Sample: Plasma is preferred. If serum is used, make sure it is completely clotted

Steps	Tests	Remarks
1	ABO and Rh Typing of the recipient	
2	Unexpected antibody screen	
3	Compare results with previous records	Blood group, History of antibodies, adverse reactions, special transfusion requirements or modifications
4	Crossmatching Major	Required for any component containing ≥2 ml of red cells

Compatibility testing:

Methods available: IAT tube test, PEG, LISS, MTS Gel, solid phase, immediate spin (IS), computer or electronic crossmatch (EXM) and the Just In Time (JIT) EXM

JIT method: It electronically issues the blood product at the time of request for transfusion rather than at the time of receipt of the sample in the laboratory. This reduces the amount of inventory assigned to patients and creates a more efficient blood management system

Crossmatch VS Type and screen

Uncertainty on whether a patient will require a transfusion or not and whether there is access to reliable antibody screening

Automation in Blood bank:

Prerequisites for automatising a process:

- Laboratories with high volume workload
- Tests including repetitive works
- Involving a lot of data entry
- Tests whose results are easily interpretable with only positive and negative with no intermediary results
- Tests that have a straightforward unidirectional workflow
- Those that pose a high risk to personnel
- Those that produce highly unreliable results or are challenging to achieve accuracy by manual process
- Tests that take a lot of time and effort
- Others: funding and availability of a standardised technology

Advantages:

- Faster result output or turnaround time
- More reliable as the possibility of human error (e.g., pipetting, sample identification, transcription errors. sample cross-contamination) is reduced.
- Accurate, precise and reproducible reports
- The user remains UpToDate
- Positive sample identification.
- Automatic capture and link to an appropriate computer system.
- Avoidance of human transcription errors.
- Excellent tracking systems for quality control purposes as each step is validated and controlled.
- Uses lesser reagents as they are well titrated
- Reduces the staff's risk of exposure to high risk

Disadvantages:

- Expensive, especially the start-up cost of equipment, also the reagents
- Equipments demand high maintenance and also require regular calibration

- Personnel needs to be trained for usage
- As a result of lack of practice, and when the machine fails, technologists may find difficulty in testing samples manually
- Loss of working time as the equipment cannot be used if calibration fails
- Adequate backup or even duplication is required
- Require uninterrupted power supply

Sample collection:

Labelling the recipient sample for pretransfusion testing
a. Patient's full first and last names
b. Patient's health care record number
c. Date and time of specimen collection
d. Initials (if collected by laboratory personnel) or signature (if collected by nonlaboratory personnel) of a phlebotomist,
e. Possibly a unique blood bank number (found on a special blood bank identification band)

Patient History review:

1. Previous group and screen results. Antibodies identified.
2. Transfusion history
3. History of pregnancies
4. Indication for modification, if any (fresh units, phenotype, CMV-, etc.).
5. Transfusion reactions and their details
6. Testing challenges (autoantibodies, stem cell transplant recipient, multiple alloantibodies).
7. History of bleeding

Choosing the blood product: ABO identical products should always be selected for whole blood products. For other blood components, compatible and alternate selections may be necessary at times

Testing blood products:

Testing the pretransfusion sample:

Typing	
Screening	
Antibody identification	
Compatibility testing	

Compatibility report: Should contain

Two independent patient identifiers (e.g. full name and hospital number).

The donor unit number.

The compatibility test results (e.g. compatible or incompatible). Method used

Recipient's ABO and Rh.

Signature of the person who performed the test and reviewer/approver

Records and specimen retention: Segment samples from RBC units and the patient samples must be retained for at least seven days after transfusion. These samples are essential for retesting/ investigations in case of a delayed transfusion reaction.

Solid phase red cell adherence assays:

Advantage: automation

Limitations: Subjective interpretation

Nonspecific reactivity

	Direct method	Indirect method
Assay type	The antibody is fixed to the well	Red cells/membranes are fixed to the wells
Utility	Grouping	Antibody detection
Indicator cells	Not required	Indicator cells coated with anti-IgG are required to be added

Electronic crossmatch:

Prerequisites:

- Computer system/software validated on site
- The system should recognise, and correlate antibody detection results, compare previous records
- There should be two concordant ABO determinations for patients and blood units
- Logic to alert the user to discrepancies in ABO/Rh confirmatory tests and incompatibility between recipient and donor unit

Advantages:

- Saves technologist time
- Reduced sample handling
- Avoidance of false positive test results (cold agglutinins, rouleaux)
- Decreased turnaround time
- Efficient inventory management

17.2 ABO BLOOD GROUP DISCREPANCY AND ITS RESOLUTION

– Dr. Arun R

Gene	Antigen	Glycosyltransferase	Immunodominant sugar
H(FUT1)	H	α-2-L-fucosyltransferase	L-Fucose
A	A	α-3-N-acetylgalactosaminyltransferase	N-acetyl-D-galactosamine
B	B	α-3-D-galactosyltransferase	D-galactose

ABO Subgroups

Red cell Phenotype	Red cell reactions with Antisera/Lectins				Serum reactions with reagent red cells			Saliva	No of Antigens sites ($\times 10^3$)
	Anti-A	Anti-B	Anti-A, B	Anti-H	A1 cells	B cells	O cells	Secretors	
A1	4+	0	4+	0	0	4+	0	A, H	1000
A2	4+	0	4+	2+	0-2+	4+	0	A, H	250
A3	3+^{mf}	0	3+^{mf}	3+	0-2+	4+	0	A, H	35
AX	0	0	1-2+	4+	0-2+	4+	0	H	5
Ay	0	0	0	4+	0	4+	0	A, H	1
Ael	0	0	0	4+	0-2+	4+	0	H	0.7
Am	0	0	0	4+	0	4+	0	A, H	1
Aend	mf	0	mf	4+	0	4+	0	H	3.5
B	0	4+	4+	0	4+	0	0	B, H	
B3	0	3+^{mf}	3+^{mf}	4+	4+	0	0	B, H	
Bweak	0	+/-	+/-	4+	4+	0	0	H	
Bel	0	0	0	4+	4+	0	0	H	
Bm	0	+/-	+/-	4+	4+	0	0	B, H	
Bx	0	+	+	3+	4+	1+	0	H	

	Cell Grouping		Serum Grouping				Possible causes	Resolution
	Anti-A	Anti-B	A1 cells	B cells	O cells	Auto control		
1	0	0	0	0	0	0	Group O neonates Immunosuppression	Incubate in RT for 30 min At 4⁰ for 15 min
2	4+	0	1+	4+	0	0	A2 with anti-A1	React with A1 lectin
3	4+	4+	2+	2+	2+	2+	Rouleaux Auto-anti I, P, Lea, M	Wash Auto adsorption and panel detection
4	0	0	4+	4+	4+	0	Oh Bombay	Test cells with H Lectin
5	4+	2+	0	4+	0	0	Acquired B	Acidify anti-B and use (at a pH of 6.0)

Landsteiner Law states that "the plasma contains natural antibodies to A or B if these antigens are absent from the red cells of that person". As per the law, the forward grouping, which tests the presence of antigens in the red cells, should correlate with the reverse grouping, which tests the antibodies in the serum. If there is a discrepancy between forward and reverse grouping, it is termed an ABO blood grouping discrepancy and should be resolved before releasing the individual's blood group. Since the ABO blood group system is the most important in transfusions, misinterpreting ABO discrepancies could be life-threatening to patients. Hence it is crucial to recognise discrepant results and resolve them. ABO discrepancy must be resolved in patients before any blood component is transfused and in donors before their blood is labelled with a blood group.

When to expect discrepancy?

1. Forward grouping does not match the reverse grouping
2. If the reactions are weak (<2+ reaction) or negative (expected reaction should be 3+ to 4+)
3. Mixed field reaction
4. If the previous and current blood grouping does not match

Causes of discrepancy:

1. Technical problem
2. The intrinsic problem within the patient sample

Technical issues

Whenever a blood group discrepancy is encountered, the technical problems should be ruled out first, as this is the most common cause of the discrepancy. The technical problem could be due to various reasons like clerical errors, reagent or equipment problems or procedural errors.

Causes of Technical errors:
1. Mislabelled tubes
2. Wrong identification of sample
3. Cell suspension too heavy or too light
4. Contaminated glassware
5. Failure to add sample/reagent
6. Over or under centrifugation
7. Incorrect reagents
8. Contaminated reagents
9. Expired/inactive reagents
10. Incorrect storage temperature
11. Un-calibrated centrifuge
12. Not following manufacturer's instructions
13. Not re-suspending the test tube before the interpretation

Most discrepancies get resolved if the above causes of technical problems are rectified. Either repeat the test with the same sample or get a fresh sample and do the testing.

The inherent problem within the patient sample:

If technical problems are ruled out, we must consider the inherent problem with the patient sample. The following patient information should be obtained before proceeding with resolution.

1. Age
2. Diagnosis
3. Any H/o previous transfusion
4. Any H/o pregnancy or any relevant obstetric history
5. Any H/o medication
6. Any H/o transplantation

If there is no agreement between forward and reverse grouping, repeat ABO typing on the same sample after washing red cells a couple of times with saline. This retest will eliminate many problems due to plasma proteins or autoantibodies. If there is a discrepancy between the current and previous blood groups, ask for a new sample and proceed.

ABO discrepancies are classified into four groups (Group I to group IV) based on either the absence of additional antigens or antibodies.

Group I- Discrepancy due to Missing antibodies (the most common cause)

Group II- Discrepancy due to Missing antigens

Group III- Discrepancy due to protein or plasma abnormalities

Group IV- Discrepancy due to miscellaneous problems

Practically, it will be challenging to determine which group the discrepancy fits, as most of the discrepancies will fit into more than one group.

One clue to discovering the discrepancy is that ABO forward and reverse reactions are typically very strong (3+ to 4+ reactions). So if the reactions are weak (<2+ reaction) or negative, ABO discrepancy should be expected. Since the production of ABO antigens is genetically controlled, they are less prone to problems than ABO antibodies. Hence problems due to serum are more common than in red cells. Most of the time, the strength of the reaction helps to find out whether it is forward grouping discrepancy or reverse grouping discrepancy (Eg. Weaker reaction in forward reaction implies discrepancy in forward grouping)

Case 1: A 90-year-old immunocompromised male patient who is on corticosteroids had the following grading of reaction in the blood grouping test

Anti-A	Anti-B	A cells	B cells	O cells
4+	0	0	1+	0

Here is a weaker reaction (1+) with B cells in reverse grouping (expected is 3+ to 4+). So it is a reverse group discrepancy (Group I discrepancy). This could be due to weaker antibodies because of immunosuppressants or age-related weakened antibody activity.

Resolution:

- Increase the serum-to-cell ratio (from 2:1 to 3:1)
- Incubate the serum being tested for 15 minutes at room temperature to enhance antibody reactions
- If negative, incubate serum testing at 4°C for 15 minutes as IgM antibodies get enhanced at a lower temperature. Include an autocontrol to rule out the enhancement of other cold antibodies at 4°C (**"mini-cold"** panel).

The patient's age and diagnosis should be obtained as weaker reactions are expected in extremes of age (newborn and elderly) and immunocompromised or hypogammaglobulinemia individuals. The reaction could be weak or absent.

There will not be any reaction in the reverse grouping in newborns as ABO antibodies are not present at birth. They develop by 3 to 6 months of age. So reverse grouping is usually not done in newborns. Hence the age of the individual is critical while resolving the discrepancy.

Case 2: A 46 years old male with haemoglobin of 7.2g/dl had an H/o transfusion one year ago. His blood grouping result shows the following

Anti-A	Anti-B	A cells	B cells	O cells
0	4+	4+	1+	1+

Here as per forward grouping blood group is "B". Reverse grouping shows the reaction in all the pooled cells (expected is a reaction in A cells only if the blood group is B). This could be due to cold auto or alloantibodies or rouleaux formation. While A cells showed a 4+ reaction, it is weaker (1+) in B cells and O cells. Note: the reaction strength need not always be weaker; it can range from 1+ to 4+ in the above-said conditions like the following.

Anti-A	Anti-B	A cells	B cells	O cells
0	4+	4+	4+	4+

In the above scenario, if the forward group is O instead of A, B, or AB, then the Bombay phenotype (as mentioned below) is also considered apart from cold auto, alloantibodies, or rouleaux formation.

Anti-A	Anti-B	A cells	B cells	O cells
0	0	4+	4+	4+

Resolution:

Rouleaux formation:

Rouleaux formation is due to abnormal concentrations of serum proteins or altered serum/protein ratios (Multiple myeloma, Waldenstrom's macroglobulinemia) or high-molecular-weight volume expanders (Hydroxyethyl starch, dextran, etc.).It may falsely appear agglutinated due to increased serum proteins (globulins). In the slide, it looks like a stack of coins.

- In such cases, the saline replacement technique is to be performed in the test tube, wherein serum is removed after centrifugation from the cell mixture, leaving the red cell button in the tube.
- Replace the serum with two drops of saline, resuspend the red cell button, and observe for agglutination.
- Rouleaux will get dispersed on saline replacement, whereas true agglutination will be stable in the presence of saline.
- Hence diagnosis and medication history are essential while resolving such cases.
- Sometimes rouleaux affects forward grouping also. In such cases, repeated washing of cells will resolve the discrepancy.

Bombay phenotype (Oh):

Bombay phenotype should be suspected if the forward grouping is O and reverse grouping shows a reaction with all the three pooled cells. This is due to the presence of anti-H in the serum. As anti-H is more potent, the strength of the reaction will usually be 3+ to 4+. Do testing of red cells with H lectin. As the H antigen is absent in the Bombay phenotype, the reaction with H lectin will be negative, whereas, in the O group, the reaction with H lectin will be positive. Salivary testing can be done for ABH antigens (secretor status) as per the standard documented procedure. Bombay phenotype will be non-secretors for ABH antigens.

Anti-A	Anti-B	H lectin	A cells	B cells	O cells	Group
0	0	0	4+	4+	4+	Bombay
0	0	4+	4+	4+	0	O

Another entity termed as Parabombay group will be secretors for ABH antigens. The red cell shows a negative reaction with H lectin. Depending upon the A and B genes present, the forward grouping may show a weak reaction with anti-A, anti-B, or both. Sometimes these antigens will be detected only by the adsorption and elution method. Serum may have anti-A or anti-B depending upon the antigen present. Anti-H present has a broad thermal range (4 to 37°C). Sometimes anti-H may be weak (anti-IH) and reactive at low temperatures. This antibody is nonreactive to cord cells. The reaction options for parabombay are as follows

Anti-A	Anti-B	H lectin	A cells	B cells	O cells	Group
*0/W+	0	0	+ (sometimes due to anti-A1)	+	+/W+ reactive at 37 °C	Ah
0	*0/W+	0	+	W+(anti-B may be detected)	W+ reactive at 37 °C	Bh
*0/W+	*0/W+	0	+/-	+/-	+/W+ (anti-IH reactive at low temperature)	

*sometimes detectable by adsorption and elution only

Cold alloantibodies:

Some alloantibodies are reactive at room temperature (e.g., anti-P1 and anti-M). Antibody identification at room temperature/immediate spin can be made to determine the type of alloantibody. These alloantibodies may react if the pooled red cells have the corresponding antigen. In such cases, use pooled red cells negative for that specific antigen if you know the antigram of the pooled cells (which is usually available if commercially available pooled cells are used). In the in-house prepared pooled cells, select another randomly picked pooled red cell and repeat the test. Autocontrol and DAT will be negative. Another option is to prewarm the serum and pooled red cells at 37 °C separately for 15 minutes to 1 hour and perform reverse grouping.

Cold autoantibody:

Prewarming will help resolve ABO blood grouping discrepancy due to cold autoantibodies. Collect the sample by a 37 °C prewarmed syringe and transport it in a prewarmed vacutainer at 37 °C. Separate the serum at 37 °C. Place the tubes containing pooled red cells, the tube containing the patient's serum, and a pipette at 37 °C for 5-10 minutes. Transfer two drops of prewarmed serum to each tube containing prewarmed pooled red cells using prewarmed tips/pipettes. Incubate at 37 °C for 30-60 minutes. In between, mix without removing tubes from the incubator. At the end of incubation, centrifuge the test tubes and look for agglutination. If extended incubation (60 minutes to 2 hours) is carried out, the settled red cells can be examined for agglutination by resuspending the button alone without centrifuging.

If the cold antibodies are potent even after prewarming, a cold autoadsorption test is to be done by incubating equal amounts of the patient's red cells and serum at 4 °C for 30 to 60 minutes and performing the reverse grouping with the adsorbed serum.

Sometimes these cold autoantibodies may cause autoagglutination and interfere with both forward and reverse grouping by causing false-positive reactions. In this situation, autocontrol and DAT will be positive. In such conditions, the forward grouping will look like AB and reverse, reacting with all the pooled cells like the one mentioned below.

Anti-A	Anti-B	A cells	B cells	O cells
4+	4+	4+	4+	4+

Perform forward grouping by washing red cells with warm saline, which will remove autoantibody to determine ABO and Rh type. Perform testing using 6% albumin as a control. If the control is positive, antibodies can be dispersed using sulfhydryl reagents (0.01M DTT) as per the standard documented procedure. For reverse grouping, the method mentioned under cold autoantibody can be done. Another option is to do heat elution at 45°C for 10 to 15 minutes with constant agitation and to do grouping.

In newborns, another reason for spontaneous agglutination is the presence of Wharton's jelly in a cord blood sample.

Resolution: Wash at least 6 times to remove the gelatinous substance and do the grouping. If not resolved, get a new sample from the heel of the newborn.

Case 3:

A 26-year-old healthy voluntary blood donor donated his blood. He has mentioned A positive in the donor questionnaire. While performing his blood grouping in the laboratory, the blood grouping shows the following

Anti-A	Anti-B	A cells	B cells	O cells
3+	0	1+	4+	0

Forward grouping is A, while in the reverse grouping, there is an extra reaction (1+) with A cells (expected is negative with A cells if the blood group is A). In such conditions, A2 with anti-A1 in the serum is suspected.

Resolution:

Test the red cells with A1 lectin. A2 red cells do not react with A1 lectin. Test the reverse grouping with both A1 and A2 cells separately. The serum will react with A1 cells, not A2 cells, confirming anti-A1 in the serum. (see below)

Anti-A	Anti-B	A1 lectin	A1 cells	A2 cells	B cells	O cells
3+	0	0	1+	0	4+	0

As mentioned below, it can also happen with the AB group (A2B with anti-A1 in the serum).

Anti-A	Anti-B	A cells	B cells	O cells
3+	3+	1+	0	0

Resolution for A2B with anti-A1 in the serum:

Anti-A	Anti-B	A1 lectin	A1 cells	A2 cells	B cells	O cells
3+	3+	0	1+	0	0	0

ABO discrepancy in unique clinical conditions:

Case 4:

A 45-year-old male patient was diagnosed to have a snake bite. Fifty vials of anti-snake venom were given, and his blood sample was sent for blood grouping. His report is as follows

Anti-A	Anti-B	A cells	B cells	O cells
0	4+	0	0	0

Forward grouping shows the "B" group, whereas, in the reverse grouping, there is no reaction with A cells (expected is a positive reaction with A cells if the blood group is B).

Resolution: Obtaining proper clinical history is the resolution as anti-snake venom is reported to neutralise anti-A in the serum. So these kinds of discrepancies can occur in B and O group individuals where anti-A is present in their serum. So have a hospital policy to send a sample for blood grouping before administering anti-snake venom.

Case 5:

A blood sample from 53-year-old male suffering from carcinoma of the pancreas was sent for blood grouping.

Anti-A	Anti-B	A cells	B cells	O cells
0	0	0	4+	0

The forward group is "O", and the reverse group is "A".

Possibility 1: "O" blood group with the absence of reaction with A cells (reverse group discrepancy)

Possibility 2: "A" blood group with the absence of reaction with anti-A antisera (forward group discrepancy)

Resolution:

For possibility 1: If the blood group is considered O, anti-A and anti-B should be present in the serum. As described above, the isolated absence of anti-A alone is unusual unless it occurs in certain exceptional cases like anti-snake venom administration. Hence blood group O can be ruled out. If the O group is still suspected, the reaction with A cells can be enhanced by performing as in case 1.

For possibility 2: If the blood group is considered as A, the expected is a positive reaction with anti-A antisera. The patient is suffering from carcinoma pancreas. It has been reported that blood group-specific soluble (BGSS) substances will be present in certain conditions like carcinoma of the stomach, pancreas etc., which will neutralise anti-A or anti-B antisera, thereby causing a false-negative reaction. In such conditions, wash the red cells several times to remove the BGSS substance and repeat the test. Another possibility to produce such a kind of reaction is subgroups of A.

Other rare conditions:

Case 6:

A 44-year-old male was diagnosed to have Intestinal obstruction with gangrenous ileum. His blood group result came as

Anti-A	Anti-B	A cells	B cells	O cells
4+	1+	0	4+	0

The forward group shows "AB", while the reverse group shows "A".

Possibility 1: "AB" blood group with extra antibody in serum reacting with B cells alone.

Possibility 2: "A" blood group with additional weak reaction with anti-B reagent (weak B antigen)

Resolution:

Possibility 1: If we consider the blood group as AB, there is a weak reaction (1+) with anti-B antisera (expected is 3+to 4+ reaction), and also, there is a reaction with B cells (expected is a negative reaction). So it could be a cold alloantibody that reacts with B cells alone (but there should not be a weaker reaction with anti-B antisera if a cold alloantibody is suspected). Hence AB blood group can be ruled out. If still suspected, the procedure to resolve cold alloantibody can be done.

Possibility 2: If we consider it as an A blood group, there is an additional B antigen that reacts weakly (Pseudo-B antigen). Since the patient has gangrenous ileum, there is a chance of gram-negative bacterial infection (sepsis). Gram-negative bacteria modify the immunodominant sugar of the A group into D-galactosamine, which is similar to B sugar (D-galactose) that cross-reacts with anti-B antisera (Acquired B phenomenon). So this phenomenon occurs in blood group A.

Autocontrol will be negative, i.e., anti-B in serum will not react with the patient's red cells having acquired B antigen. If the pH of the anti-B antisera is greater than 8.5 or less than 6, there will not be any reaction with the acquired B antigen. The secretor test shows only the presence of A antigen in secretions. Adding acetic anhydride decreases the reactivity of the acquired B red cells when tested with anti-B antisera, whereas normal B cells are not affected.

Case 7:

A 46-year-old female was admitted for a hysterectomy. Her blood group shows

Anti-A	Anti-B	A cells	B cells	O cells
0	0	0	4+	0

The forward group is O, and the reverse group is A. This reaction is similar to the reaction described under BGSS, where we have mentioned that subgroups should also be considered. Here the weak reaction is due to the weak expression of the A antigen. It could be due to

1. Inheritance of a weak ABO subgroup
2. Malignancies like Hodgkin's disease, Lymphomas, and Leukemias may result in the loss of ABH transferases
3. Massive transfusion with group O blood to a non-group O blood type, e.g. a group A person receiving lots of group O blood (can produce mixed field reaction).
4. Bone marrow transplant and chemotherapy.

Resolution:

Incubate the antisera and red cells for up to 30 minutes at room temperature, centrifuge, and look for agglutination.

If still negative, incubate at 4 ^{0}C for 15 to 30 minutes. Autocontrol should be tested as a control simultaneously. The reaction can also be enhanced by treating the red cells with enzymes before grouping. Diagnosis and medication history are essential while resolving this type of discrepancy.

Subgroups of A are A3, Ax, Aend, Am, Ay, Ael, and B is B3, Bx, Bm, and Bel. The strength of the reaction varies from negative to weak to mixed field. Anti-AB may be used in addition while resolving subgroups of A and B. There will be weak agglutination with anti-A and anti-AB antisera for A3, Ax, and Aend and no agglutination for Am, Ay, and Ael. Sometimes anti-A1 may be present in A3, Ax and Aend. Adsorption and elution study and secretor status help in resolving such conditions. A molecular study for blood grouping helps in confirming the blood group.

Anti-A	Anti-AB	Unexpected Anti-A1 in serum	Secretor status	Group
Mixed filed (mf)	Mf	+		A3
Very weak mf	Very weak mf	+++		Aend
0/w+	w+	+		Ax
*0/w+	*0/w+	-	A+++	Am
*0	*0	-	A+	Ay
*0	*0	+	Only H	Ael

*detected only by adsorption and elution

There will be weak agglutination with anti-B and anti-AB antisera for B3, Bx and no agglutination for Bm, Bel.

Anti-B	Anti-AB	Extra antibodies in serum	Secretor status	Group
Mixed filed (mf)	Mf	-		B3
W+	W+	Weak anti-B		Bx
*0	*0	-	B+++	Bm
*0	*0	Weak anti-B	Only H	Ael

*detected only by adsorption and elution

Algorithm for ABO discrepancy

Forward grouping

Extra Reaction

Rouleaux formation:- Do saline replacement technique

Wharton's jelly in cord blood:-

- Wash several times and repeat grouping (OR)
- Do grouping with blood collected from heel etc.,

Cold auto Antibody:-

- Wash red cells with warm saline with 6% albumin as control.   (OR)
- If not resolved, treat red cells with sulphydryl reagent (0.01M DTT). (OR)
- Do heat elution at 45° C for 10-15 mins with control.

Acquired B:-

- Occurs in blood group "A" having gram negative bacterial sepsis.
- If the p^H of anti-B reagent is <6, there won't be reaction with acquired B antigen.
- Adding acetic anhydride decreases the reactivity of the red cells when tested with anti-B reagent.
- Auto control will be negative.

Absent /weak reaction

Blood group specific soluble substances (BGSS):-

- It occurs in ca stomach and pancreas etc.,
- BGSS neutralizes anti-A or anti-B reagent.
- Wash red cells several times to remove BGSS and repeat grouping

Sub groups/ chemotherapy/ leukemia patients:-

- Incubate antisera and red cells at RT for 30 mins and centrifuge.
- If not resolved, Incubate at 4^oc for 15-30 mins with Aurocontrol.
- Testing with anti-AB reagent will show agglutination sometimes
- Perform adsorption and elution
- Perform secretor status.

Algorithm for ABO discrepancy

Reverse grouping

Extra Reaction

Rouleaux formation:- Do saline replacement technique.

Cold Allo Antibody:-

- Do antibody identification at RT/IS.
- Use antigen negative pooled cells. (OR)
- Prewarm serum of pooled red cells separately at 37°c for 15 mins to 1hr and repeat grouping.
- Autocontrol and DAT will be negative.

Cold Auto Antibody:-

- Do prewarming technique for sample collection and separation.
- Incubate serum and pooled red cells at 37°c for 30-60 mins and centrifuge.
- If not resolved do grouping with adsorbed serum after cold auto adsorption at 4°c for 30-60 mins.
- Autocontrol and DAT will be positive.

Bombay / parabombay phenotype:-

- Negative reaction with H lectin.
- Perform salivary secretor status

A2 or A2B with anti-A1:-

1. Negative reaction with A1 lectin.
2. Negative reaction with A2 cells and positive reaction with A1 cells in reverse grouping.

Absent /weak reaction

- Increase serum to cell ratio.
- Incubate reaction mixture at RT for 15 mins.
- If not resolved, Incubate at 4°c for 15 mins (include Autocontrol).

Note:

a. Newborn :- No ABO antibody formation till 3-6 months of age.

b. Elderly and immunocompromised:- weak reaction can occur due to weakened antibody

c. H/O anti snake venom administration neutralizes anti-A in B and O group serum.

17.3 RESOLVING RH DISCREPANCIES

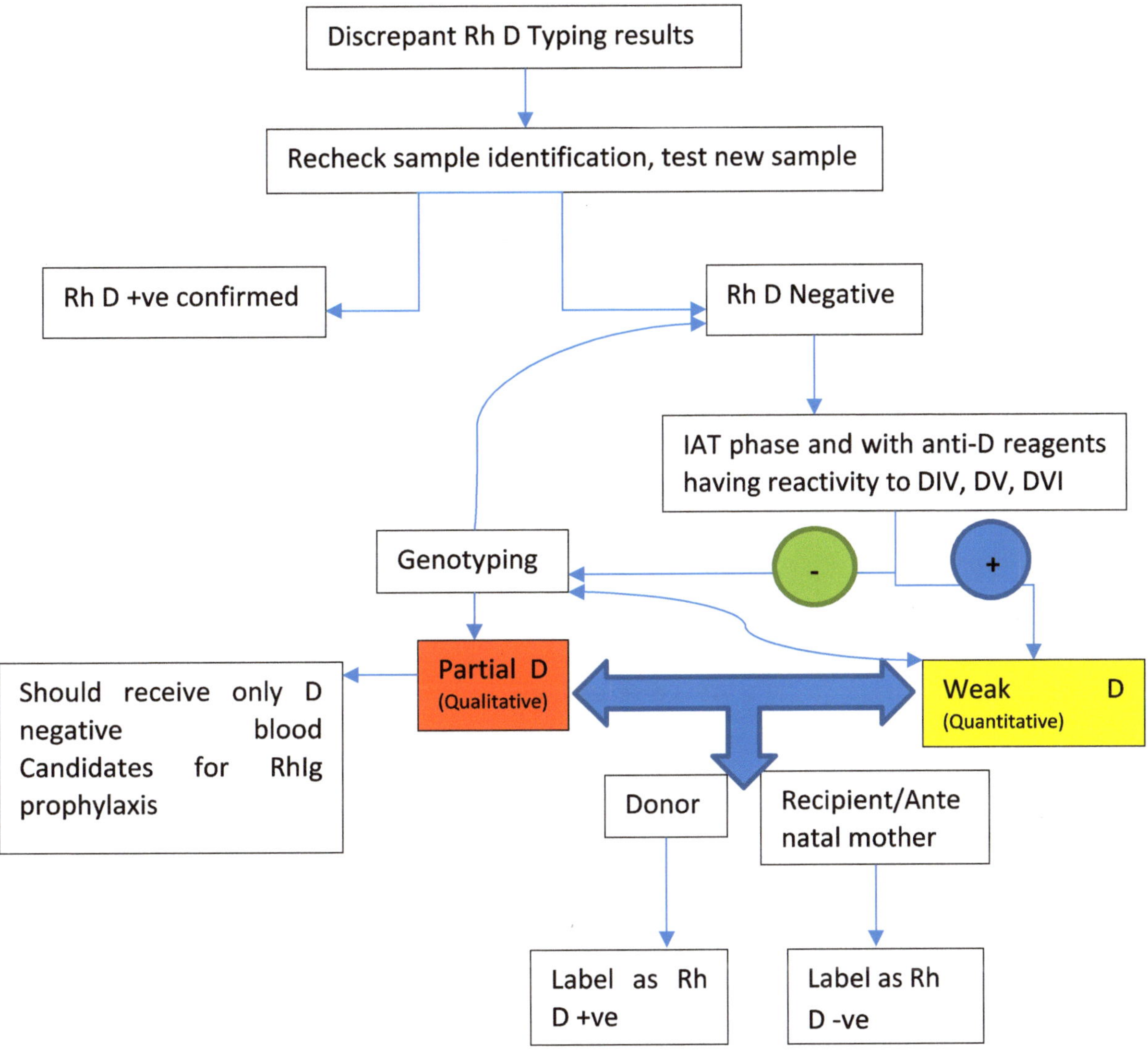

Figure 10. Algorithm to approach Rh D grouping discrepancies

False positive results	False-negative results
Warm/agglutinins coating red cells	**Suspension**: too heavy (for tube test) or
Polyagglutinable red cells	too weak (in slide test)
Reagent factors: preservative, dye, antibiotic, high protein or macromolecular additives	**Non-functioning reagent**: contamination, improper storage, expired
Reagent contamination	Failure to add reagents
Serum factors causing rouleaux	Aggressive resuspension dispersing agglutination
Use of wrong reagents	Use of wrong reagents
Not following manufacturers instructions/SOP	Not following manufacturers instructions/SOP
Reagent reactive with RhCE variant	Weak D/ Partial D, Blocked D

Variables resulting in Rh Typing discrepancies:

1. The method used: slide, tube, microplate, gel, automated analyser
2. The sample used: enzyme treated, suspension(
3. The phase of testing: AHG, LISS
4. Clone of the reagent used (manufacturer)
5. Gene variations: affecting expressions and epitopes

17.4 THE INCOMPATIBLE CROSS-MATCH:

Three significant clinical situations may lead to difficulty in providing crossmatch compatible blood:

1. Difficulty determining the patient's ABO type
2. Presence of Alloantibodies
3. Presence of Autoantibodies

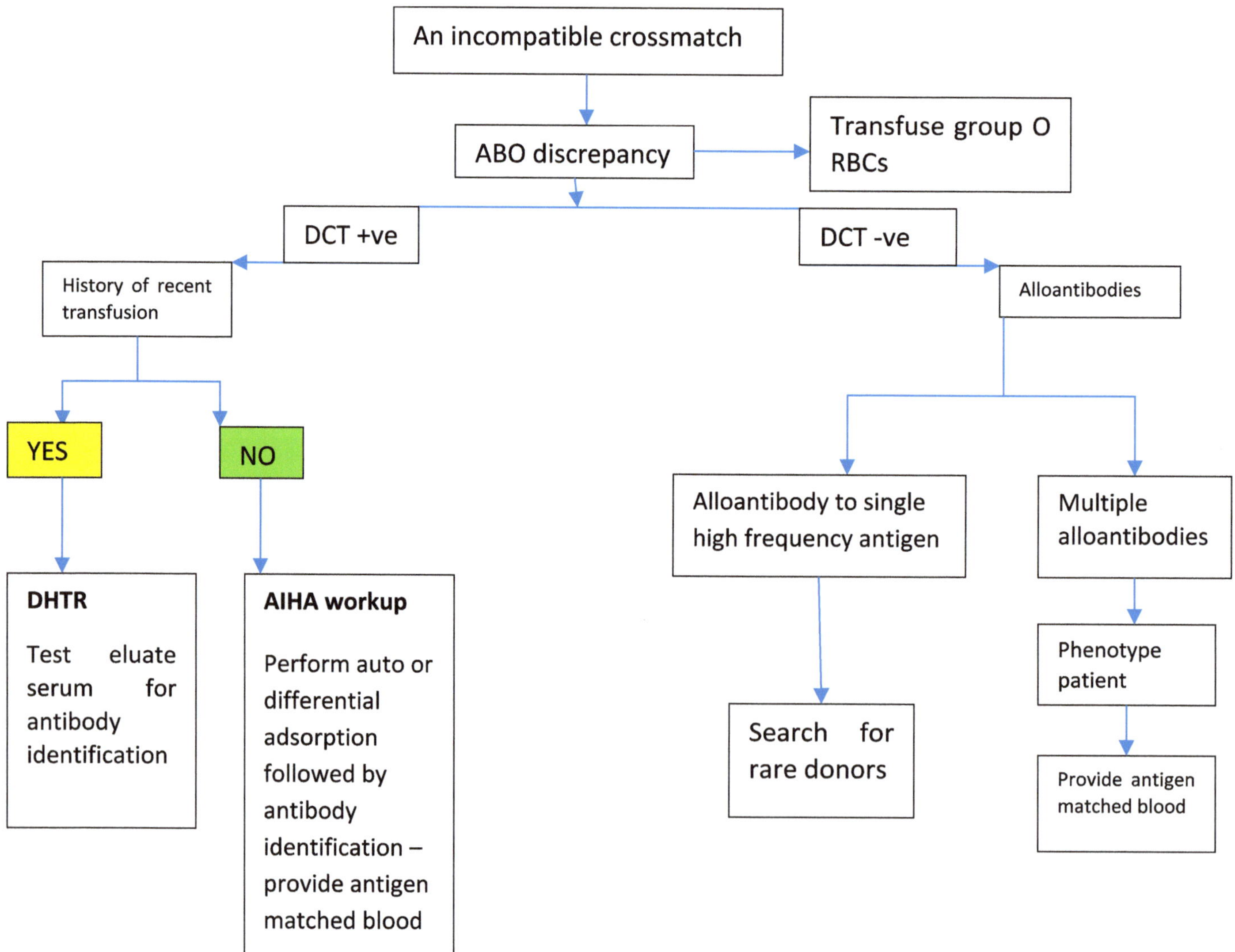

Figure 11. Approach to an incompatible cross-match

In such cases approach includes:

1. **Communication between the clinical team and the transfusion team**

   Laboratory personnel must let the clinician know the complexity of the laboratory testing, the estimated timeframe required to complete the testing, and what kind of patient history would help find possible causes of the incompatibility.

   The clinician must let the laboratory know the clinical urgency of transfusion, detailed pertinent history, and a treatment plan related to managing anaemia and other concurrent medical problems

2. **Patient history**

   A history of use of certain drugs (e.g., methyldopa, procainamide, fludarabine) suggests that the patient may have drug-induced autoimmune hemolytic anaemia (AIHA)

   A history of a lymphoproliferative disorder (particularly chronic lymphocytic leukaemia), autoimmune disease (mainly systemic lupus erythematosus), or immune deficiency disorder (particularly AIDS) suggests secondary AIHA

   A history of pregnancy or prior transfusion raises the possibility of multiple RBC alloantibodies

   A history of difficulties in finding blood for family members suggests the presence of an alloantibody against a high-frequency antigen

   A history of recent transfusion raises the possibility of a delayed hemolytic transfusion reaction

3. **Immediate management**

   Given the time required to perform the appropriate laboratory evaluation, the severity of the patient's condition determines clinical management during the testing. The patient's ability to withstand severe anaemia while awaiting transfusion can be maximised by enforced bed rest to decrease oxygen demand and administer supplemental oxygen. For patients with an urgent need for transfusion, blood can be issued under a nonstandard release approved by a physician as an emergency release. Patients with a confirmed ABO type can receive uncrossmatched, type-specific blood, and patients without an available ABO type can receive type O blood. The best practice for attempting to transfuse these patients is to infuse blood slowly while carefully observing the patient for signs and symptoms of an acute hemolytic transfusion reaction, and in the event of such signs or symptoms, the transfusion should be discontinued immediately.

   If the alloantibody is not clinically significant, multiple random units can be cross-matched with the patient's plasma. The most compatible units can be safely transfused.

   If the alloantibody is clinically significant, the following options are available:

   - A rare donor file may be contacted for compatible blood.
   - The patient's close family members, especially siblings, may be tested to determine if one or more of them also lacks the same RBC antigen and may serve as blood donors.
   - Autologous donations, when the need can be anticipated, such as prior to elective surgery

- **Antibodies that are ALWAYS considered to be potentially clinically significant include:** ABO (A, B), Rh (D, C, c, E, e), Duffy (Fya, Fyb), Kidd (Jka, Jkb), Kell (K, k), SsU (S, s, U), and Lutheran (Lub)
- **Antibodies that are rarely or never considered to be clinically significant include:** Lewis (Lea, Leb), MN, Lutheran (Lua), P1, Xga, Cartwright (Yta), Bg, York (Yka), Chido/Rodgers (Cha/Rga), Sda, and HTLA (high titer low avidity)
- The most significant concern in transfusing patients with AIHA involves the detection of concurrent alloantibodies

Techniques can be used to detect an underlying alloantibody:

auto adsorption method

allogeneic adsorption

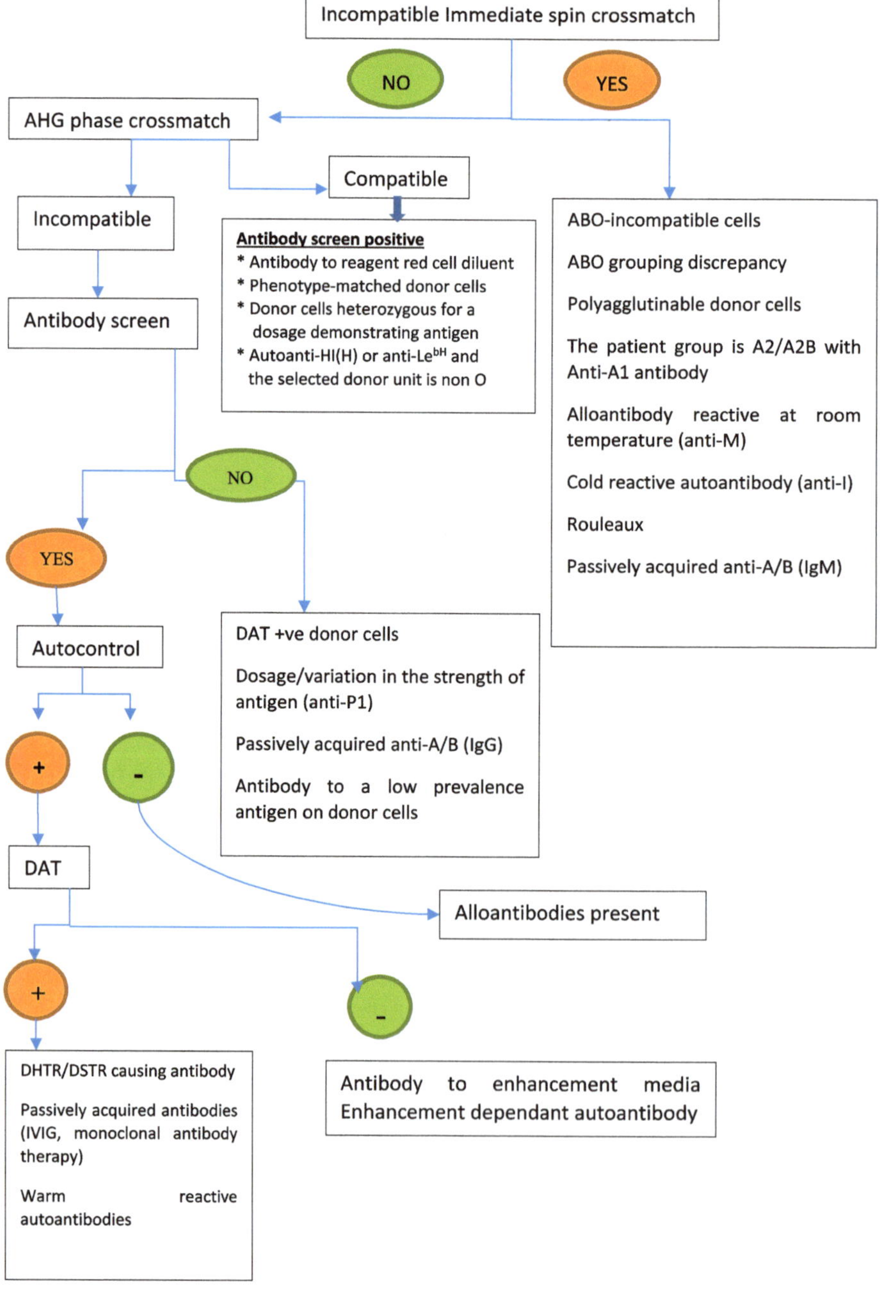

Figure 12. Causes of incompatible cross-match

17.5 TRANSFUSION REACTIONS:

Every undesired event, symptom, diagnosis or worsening of a preexisting medical condition during and/or after a blood transfusion

Hemovigilance: A set of organised surveillance procedures relating to serious adverse or unexpected events or reactions in donors or recipients and donors' epidemiological follow-up.

It helps us to know what is expected, serious, emerging, operational or biological.

Why know/identify transfusion reactions?

Successful patient outcomes depend on early recognition, prompt cessation and clinical intervention

Grade: severity of clinical features observed in the patient

Imputability: likelihood that the reaction can be attributed to the transfusion

Diagnosing transfusion reaction:

Is the symptom new or an exacerbation of an existing condition?

What was the rate of transfusion? Any other premedication?

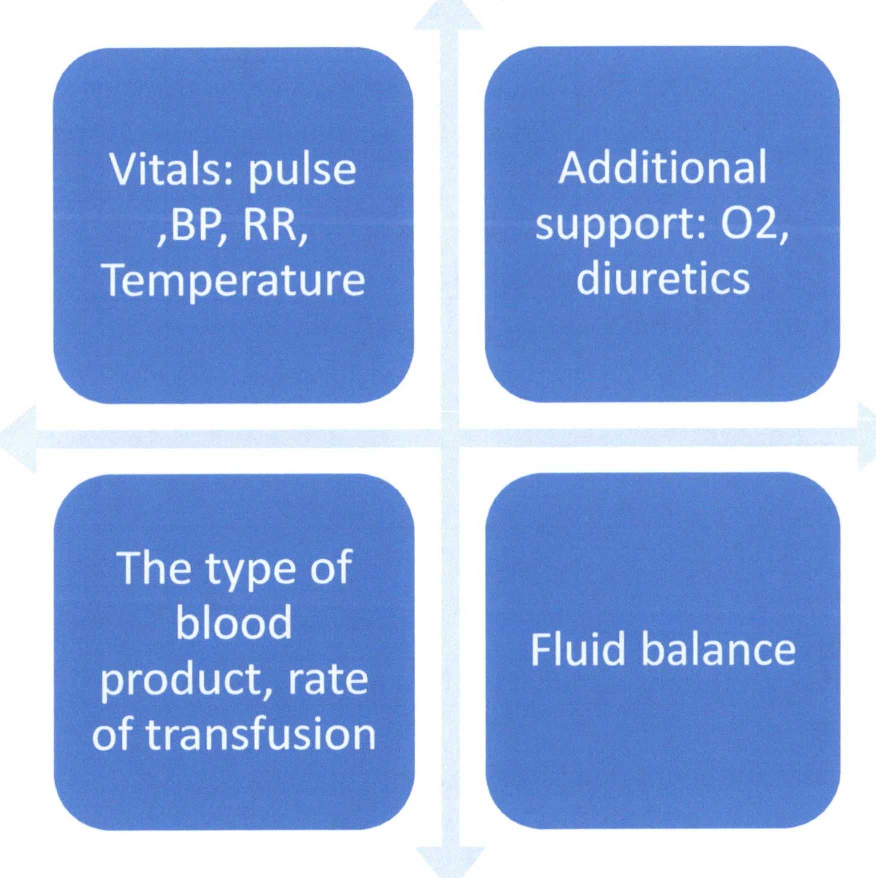

Symptoms	
Fever	≥ 38⁰ C oral or ≥ 1⁰ C raise from pretransfusion value
Chills	With or without rigours Chill is a feeling of coldness accompanied by shivering Rigour is an episode of shaking or exaggerated shivering
Respiratory distress	Wheeze, cough, dyspnoea(difficulty in breathing, sudden and severe shortness of breath
Pain	Local: At the infusion site Remote: Abdominal, chest, flank or back
Skin manifestations	Pruritis
Nausea	Sometimes vomiting
Signs	
Hypoxia	Pao2/FIo2 <300 mmHg, maybe TRALI
Fever	≥ 10 C rise in temperature (or) ≥ 380 C
Altered BP	Hyper or Hypotension
Skin manifestations	Rash, flushing, urticaria, localised oedema, Icterus
Urine changes	Hemoglobinuria Oliguria refers to a 24-h urine output of <400 mL, and Anuria is the complete absence of urine formation (<100 mL).
Lab Findings	
Altered CBC	Anemia, Reticulocytosis, thrombocytopenia, micro spherocytes
Altered RFT	Increased Blood urea, serum creatinine, Hyperkalaemia
Altered LFT	Raised bilirubin, AST, ALT
Hemoglobinemia	Free Hb in plasma
Hemoglobinuria	Free Hb in the urine
Bacterial contamination	Gram staining and blood culture
LDH, Haptoglobin	

Evaluation and Management:

Patient-related steps
<ul><li>Stop the transfusion immediately. Keep the line open with normal saline</li><li>Perform clerical recheck</li><li>Draw fresh samples for testing</li></ul>
<ul><li>Assess vitals, treat symptoms, establish Differential diagnosis</li></ul>
Component related steps
<ul><li>Preserve residual component and infusion set</li><li>Repeat testing</li><li>Quarantine other products from the same unit, if any, till further evaluation</li><li>Perform a visual check for a change in colour or consistency, hemolysis</li></ul>

Is the laboratory investigation necessary?

- **No If:** only urticaria, the temperature rise is less than 1^0c, TACO (transfusion can continue)

Whether to continue the transfusion or not depends on the following:

- Original indication of transfusion
- The present condition of the patient
- Results of the evaluation

Table 9 Transfusion reactions by the time of onset

	Onset during/ within	Type of reactions
Acute transfusion Reactions	0-1 Hr	Transfusion Associated Hypotension
	0-4 Hrs	FNHTR, Allergic reactions
	6-12 Hrs	TRALI/TACO
	24 Hrs	HTR, TAD
Chronic Transfusion Reactions	1-28 days	DHTR, DSTR
	5-12 days	Post Transfusion Purpura
	7-12 days	TA-GVHD

Allergic Transfusion reactions-

Urticaria/Hives- is an intensely itchy rash (sometimes burn or sting) consisting of a raised, irregularly shaped wheal with a blanched centre surrounded by a red flare

Angioedema - is an area of well-circumscribed swelling that may involve any part of the body, more commonly the lips and eyelids

Anaphylaxis is an acute immunologic reaction that presents mucocutaneous signs of urticaria and Angioedema with Multiple organ systems involved, including the pulmonary, cardiovascular, gastrointestinal, and neurologic systems.

Anaphylactoid reactions -are acute hypersensitivity reactions that are clinically identical to anaphylaxis but are not mediated by IgE antibodies, or IgE involvement cannot be established

Differential Diagnosis for **Anaphylactic Reaction**
Vasovagal syncope
Hypotensive reactions - especially in patients on ACE inhibitors
TRALI
Asthma exacerbations
Septic shock

Scope of hemovigilance

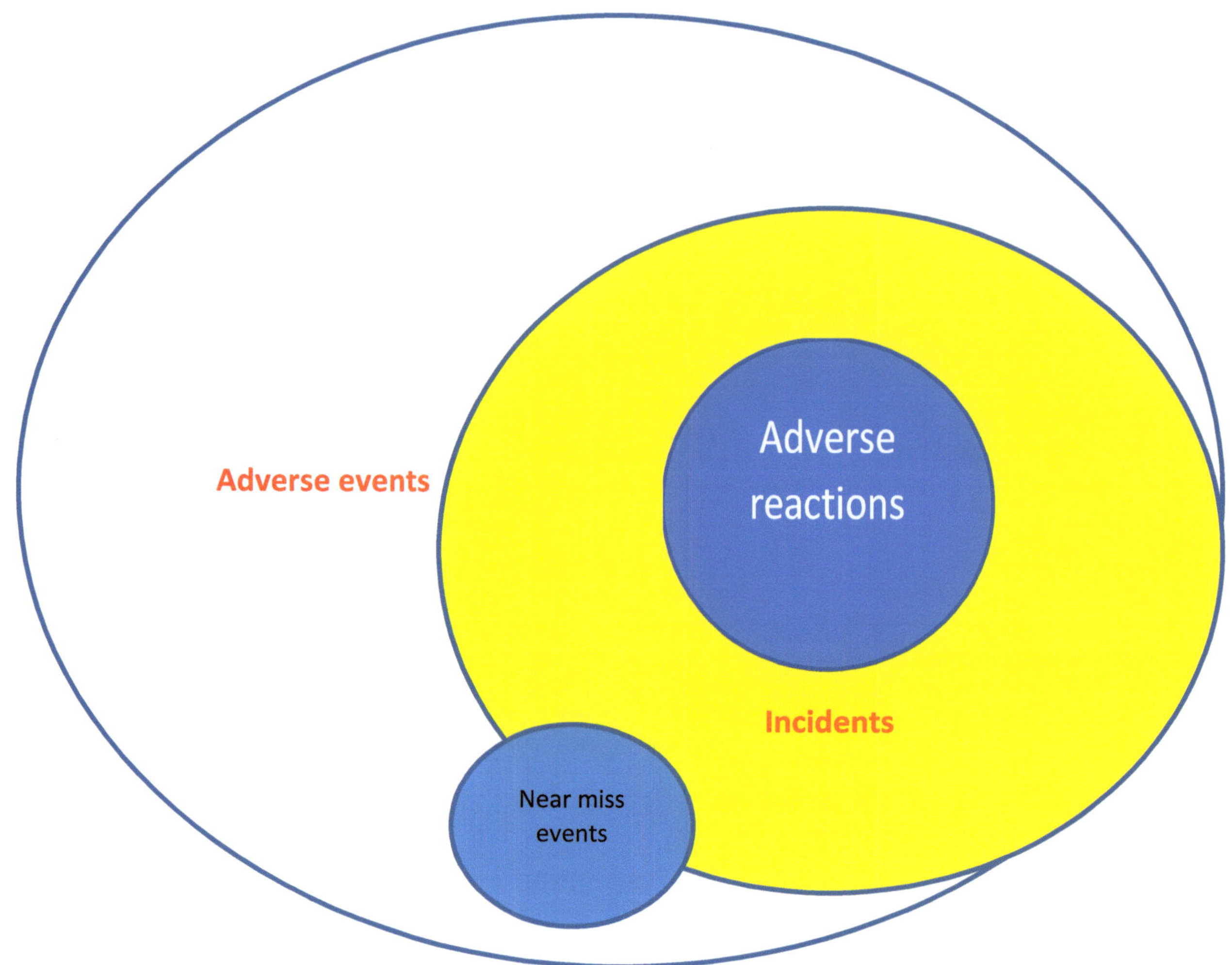

Adverse event: an undesirable and unintended occurrence before, during, or after transfusion of blood or blood components. It may be the result of an error or an incident, which may or may not result in an adverse reaction in the recipient

Incident: when the patient receives a blood component that did not meet all the requirements for a suitable transfusion or was intended for another patient. It thus includes transfusion errors and deviations from standard operating procedures or hospital policies. It may or may not result in an adverse reaction.

E.g., Transfusion of O blood group unit to A group recipient unintentionally

Near Misses: error or deviation from standard procedure or policy that is discovered before the start of the transfusion

E.g., a pretransfusion blood sample taken from the wrong patient or labelled with the wrong patient's details

Adverse reaction: undesirable response or effect in a patient temporally associated with the administration of blood or blood components

Product transfused	Fever	Chills	Hypotension	Respiratory Distress	In presence of	Diagnosis
Plasma> platelets> RBC's					Urticaria pruritis angioedema	**Allergic or anaphylactoid**
RBC's				---	Hemolysis or renal failure	**HTR**
Platelets> Plasma> RBCs				---	Gram stain and Culture positivity	**Septic transfusion Reaction**
Plasma> Platelets					Leukopenia and chest infiltrates	**TRALI**
Platelets>RBCs> Plasma			---	---	Non-leukoreduced products	**FNHTR**

Transfusion-related sepsis:

DDs:

1. AHTR
2. FNHTR

FNHTR:

DDs:

1. HTR
2. Sepsis
3. TRALI
4. Transfusion transmitted malaria

TA-GVHD:

Differential Diagnosis for **TAGVHD**	Drug reactions
	Viral illness

Suspected transfusion reaction

<table>
<tr>
<td>

Patient-Focused steps

- **STOP** transfusion
- Establish/maintain patent IV
- **CONTACT** transfusion services and clinical team for the plan of care
- Check for clerical errors, correct components and patient
- Assess the patient for signs and symptoms
- Collect fresh samples for lab investigations and transfusion services
- Imaging: Chest X-ray if required

</td>
<td>

Component -Focused steps

- **CONTACT** transfusion services for directions on further steps
- Check for clerical errors, correct components and patient
- Return any remaining component, the bag, administration set, fluids
- Repeat testing as appropriate
- Donor management if any

</td>
</tr>
</table>

AHTR: (DDs)

1. TRALI
2. Transfusion-related sepsis
3. Patient's disease itself: G6PD deficiency, AIHA, SCD, membrane defects, Hemoglobinopathies
4. Microangiopathic Hemolytic anaemia:

    a. TTP
    b. HUS
    c. HELLP Syndrome

5. Non-immune mediated hemolysis:

    a. improper shipping
    b. improper storage
    c. incomplete deglycerolization
    d. pressure devices, warmers, infusion pumps
    e. improper bore size
    f. incompatible fluids, drugs
    g. bacterial contamination
    h. mechanical thrombectomy

6. Immune-mediated:

    a. alloantibody-induced hemolysis
    b. AIHA
    c. DSTR
    d. cold Hemagglutination disease
    e. drug Induced hemolysis
    f. PNH

7. Bleeding
8. Artificial Heart valve disinfection
9. Polyaggultination
10. Infections: Malaria, Babesiosis, Clostridia

Allergic reactions:

DDs:

1. Vasovagal reactions
2. Urticaria

With ARDS

- Circulatory overload- Hypertension, CCF

TRALI

- Underlying disease: Acute asthmatic effect, acute exacerbations
- Pulmonary embolism

Hypotension and Shock

- HTR
- Sepsis
- Underlying diseases

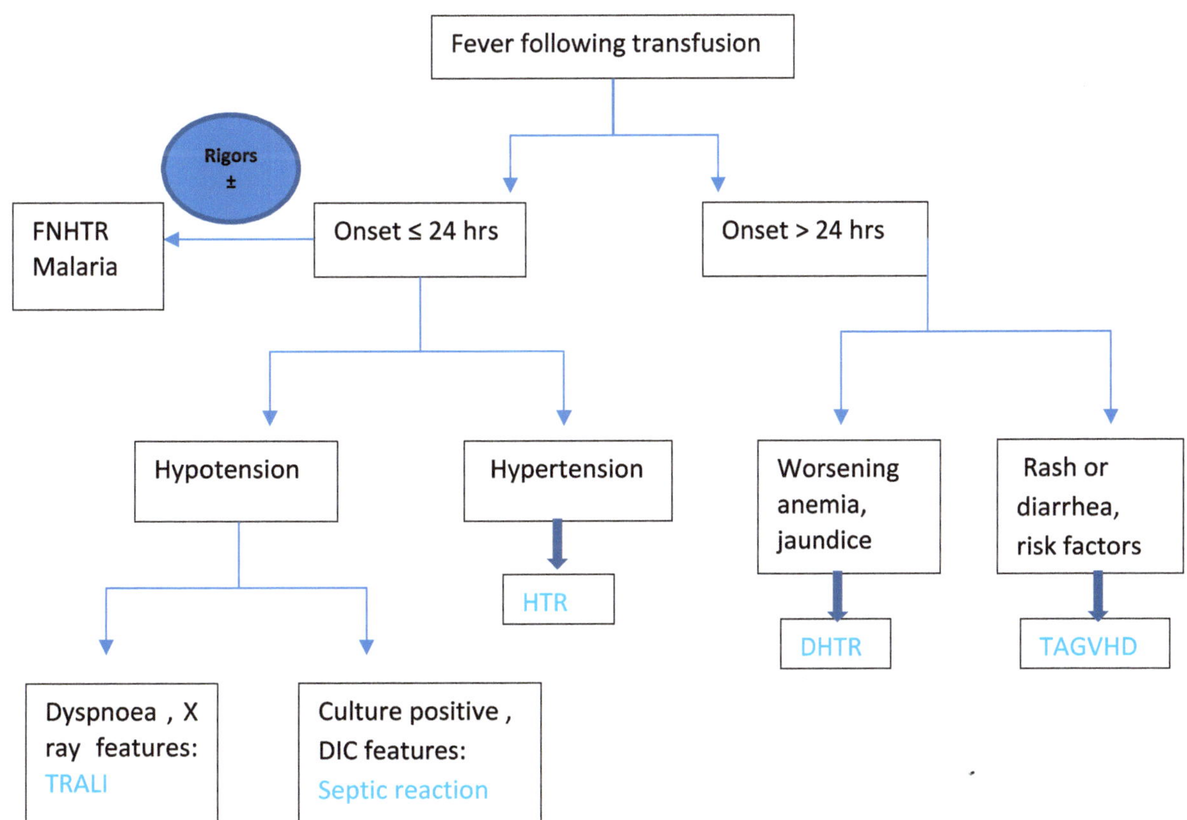

Figure 13. Approach to a patient with transfusion-associated pyrexia

TRALI:

DDs:

1. Anaphylactic reactions
2. TACO
3. Transfusion-related sepsis
4. Coincident MI
5. Pulmonary embolus
6. TAD (Transfusion-associated Dyspnea)

Differential Diagnosis for Post Transfusion Purpura
Idiopathic Thrombocytopenic Purpura
Alloimmune thrombocytopenia
Thrombotic Thrombocytopenic Purpura
Heparin-Induced Thrombocytopenia
Disseminated Intravascular Coagulation
Drug-induced Thrombocytopenia

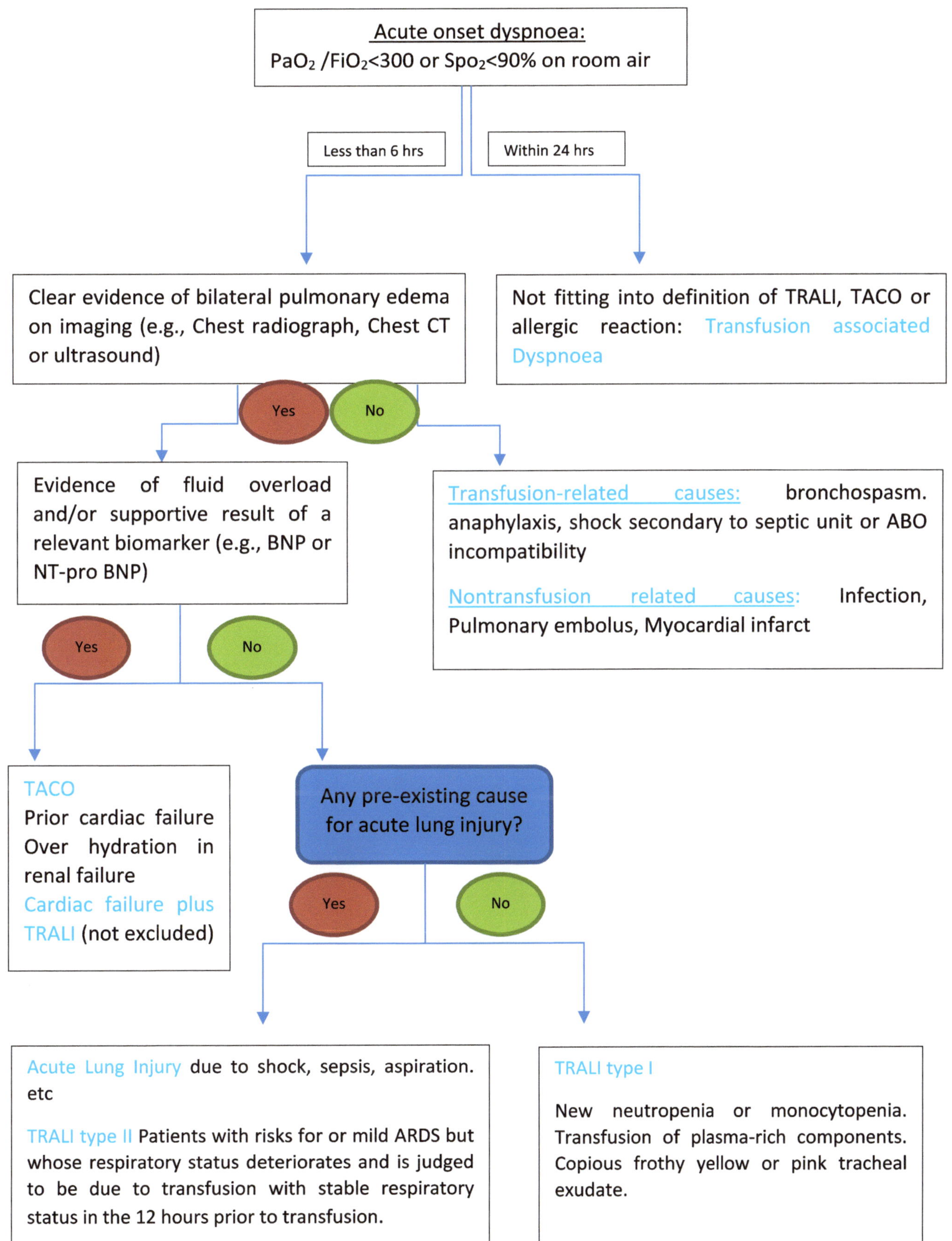

Figure 14. The differential diagnosis for respiratory problems in transfusion reactions

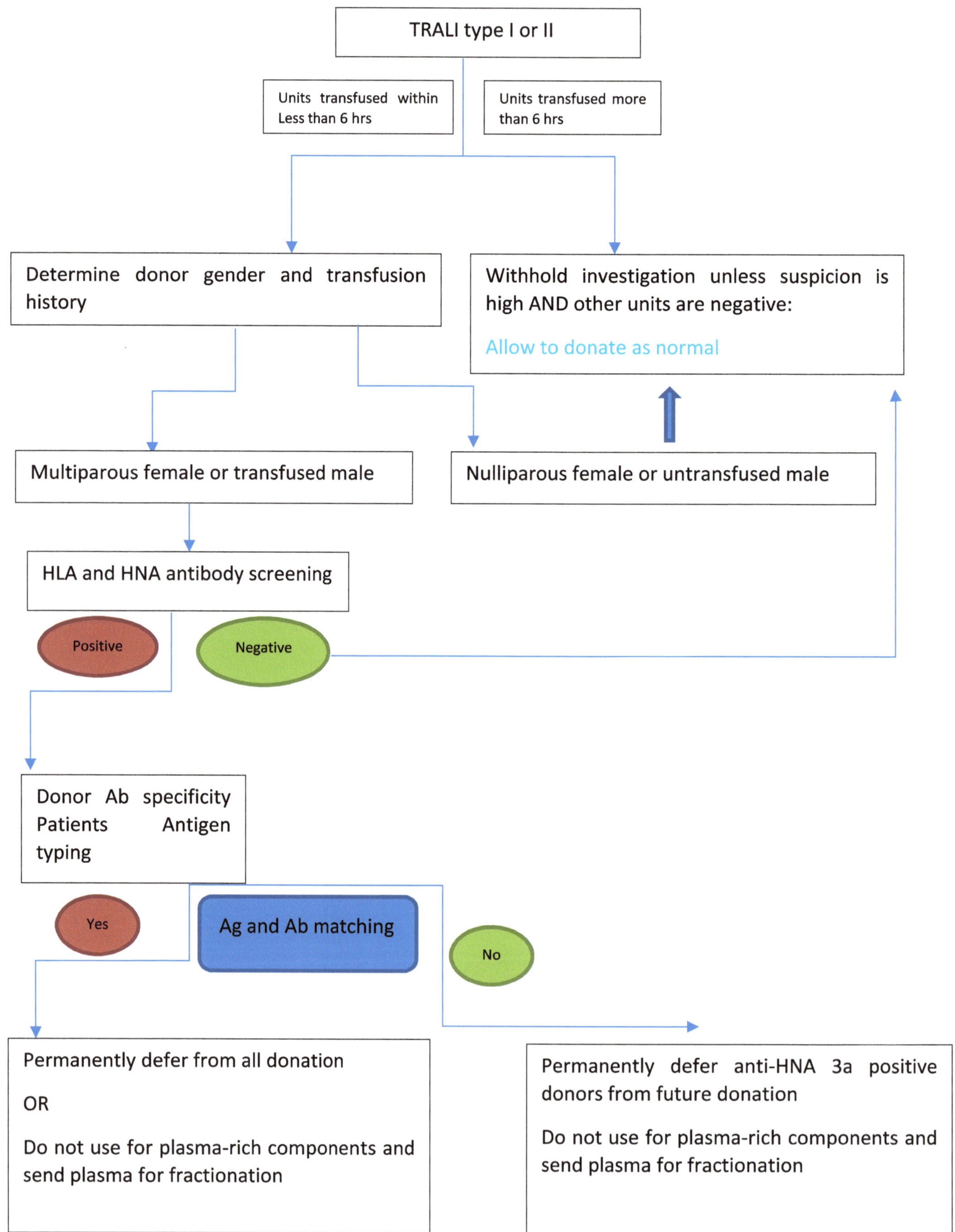

Figure 15. Management of donors whose blood products are implicated in TRALI

Differential Diagnosis for Delayed Hemolytic Transfusion Reaction
Infections- Malaria, Babesiosis, CMV, TTI
TAGVHD
Passenger Lymphocyte Syndrome
Disseminated Intravascular Coagulation
Drug-induced Thrombocytopenia

Time Line of DHTR

Time(Days)	Events	Explanation
0	Negative Pretransfusion tests	Antibody titre below detectable levels
1	Red cells transfused	-
3-10	Clinical signs of hemolysis	The accelerated destruction of transfused red cells
11-21	Positive DAT, Positive Antibody screen	Antibody titre increases
> 21 days (or)	DAT becomes negative	Removal of antibody-bound cells from circulation
21-300 days	DAT may persist as positive; eluates may demonstrate alloantibody specificity or pan agglutination	Nonspecific binding of alloantibody to autologous red cells or development of warm autoantibodies

Laboratory investigations for suspected DHTR- outline
1. **Initial serologic investigation:** Post-transfusion sample tests. Antibody identification tests. DAT profile- IgG, anti-c3 Eluate studies- on DAT-positive cells 2. **Supplemental serologic tests:** *From pretransfusion samples:* DAT and repeat Antibody screen *From retained segments of transfused unit:* Phenotype for antigen corresponding to identified antibody 3. **Review serologic findings and Transfusion History** 4. **Assess the patient for clinical signs and symptoms**

- ➤ Approximately 5% of transfusion recipients develop antibodies against transfused RBC antigens.
- ➤ The development of one alloantibody predisposes an individual to the subsequent production of additional alloantibody

➢ Can adversely impact the outcome of solid organ transplantation
➢ 25% of all antibodies become undetectable over time (median follow-up of 7 months). Antibodies detected with a more sensitive screening technique are less persistent.
➢ Up to 13% of individuals are transfusion immune responders (risk of forming alloantibody). There is a 30% chance of alloantibody after each transfusion episode.

Kidd antibodies are the common culprits. Mortality and morbidity can be much more than AHTR.

Incidence: 1 in 2000 patients or 1 in 11000 transfused units

Typical presentation: 7-10 days post-transfusion (range 5-21 days)

Signs and symptoms: unexplained anaemia, low-grade fever, jaundice, worsening renal function.

Painful crisis in sickle cell patients

Lab findings: raised bilirubin, LDH, retic count, positive DAT, spherocytes in smear

Management: serial monitoring of blood counts and renal functions, adequate hydration, transfusion of antigen-negative blood subsequently and not merely crossmatch compatible blood.

Mitigation strategies:

1. Identify patients at higher risk

Transfusion responder phenotype (transfusion recipients who are at higher-than-average risk of RBC Antigen alloimmunization		
	Factor	**Examples of higher risk**
Patient factors	Genetic predisposition:	
	HLA	HLA DRB1 (04 and 15 alleles)
	Other immune modifiers	Treg
	Age at first transfusion	More the age higher the risk
	Gender	Women>men
	Number of transfusions	More the transfusion higher the risk(exponentially)
	Type of transfusion	Lesser chance if transfused emergently or massively
Donor factors	Racial disparity	
Disease factors	Sickle cell disease	HLA-B35
	WAIHA	
	Inflammatory bowel disease	Inflammation increases risk
Testing factors	Frequency of testing	More the frequency, the better the identification
	Enhancement techniques used	
	Unavailable/irregular previous records	PEG/LISS
	Antibody specificity	Kidd, Duffy

2. Address the problem of antibody evanescence

    a. Routine Surveillance antibody screening at 7-10 days after transfusion (for secondary immune response)
    b. Repeat screening at 3-6 months after transfusion (to detect primary immune response)
    c. Adoption of highly sensitive antibody screening techniques (PEG)

Delayed Serologic Transfusion reaction (DSTR): Much more common (2.5%)

Defined as positive DAT or antibody screen without biochemical evidence of hemolysis

Hypotensive Reactions:

Definition: a drop in systolic blood pressure of more than or equal to 30 mm Hg occurring during or within one hour of completing transfusion and a systolic BP≤ 80 mm Hg after all the other causes, including underlying recipient condition, have been excluded.

Risk factors:

- patients receiving bedside leukofiltration
- patients on ACE inhibitors
- high MELD Score/ liver dysfunction
- filtration during intraoperative recovery
- in the setting of apheresis- hypocalcemia, air embolism or intravascular volume depletion
- few surgeries- Cardiopulmonary bypass, radical prostatectomy

DDs:

1. Anaphylaxis
2. Septic reaction
3. AHTR
4. TRALI
5. Medications

Management:

Trendelenberg position

Isotonic fluids

vasopressor therapy

Experimental drugs: Nafamostat Mesylate (synthetic serine protease inhibitor)

Icatibant (Selective specific Bradykinin B2 receptor antagonist)

Classification	Mechanism / mediators	Examples	Remarks	Time taken
Type I: Immediate	Preformed IgE antibodies, Th2 cells	Allergic or anaphylactic transfusion reactions, IgA deficient patients	Fast and Furious reactions,	Minutes
Type II: Antibody-mediated	IgM, IgG	Acute hemolytic transfusion reaction, HDFN	Cy-2-toxic, Ag+Ab	Hours-days
Type III: Immune complex-mediated	Immune complexes of circulating antigens and IgM/IgG antibodies	Drugs can cause all 4 types, Hep B infection RhIg mediated hemolysis	III: Ag+Ab+Complement	Hours-days
Type IV: Delayed hypersensitivity	CD4+ Cells (Th1 & Th17) CD8+ Cells	Graft rejection, TA-GVHD	T cells, Transplant rejection, Terminal(delayed), Touch (contact related)	Days to Yrs

Mnemonic: ACID, Allergic(I), Cytotoxic (II), Immune complex (III), Delayed (IV)

Transfusion Associated Circulatory Overload:

Acute or worsening respiratory compromise during or up to 12 hrs after transfusion and ≥2 of the following criteria

- Acute or worsening pulmonary oedema evidenced by
- Changes in CVS like tachycardia, hypertension, distended JVP,
- Evidence of fluid overload
- Elevated BNP (>1.5 times the pretransfusion value)
  - ➢ Clinical physical examination (crackles on lung auscultation, orthopnea and cough, cyanosis and decreased O2 saturation)
  - ➢ Radiological imaging (new or worsening pleural effusions, progressive lobar vessel enlargement, peribronchial cuffing, b/l Kerley lines, alveolar oedema with nodular areas of increased opacity and/or cardiac silhouette enlargement
  - ➢ BP monitoring (raised arterial BP, widened pulse pressure, sometimes hypotension)
  - ➢ Change in weight: increases usually but may decrease following diuretic therapy

Table 6. Comparison of features of TRALI and TACO

Feature	TRALI	TACO
Body Temperature	Fever may be present	Unchanged
Blood Pressure	Hypotension	Hypertension
Dyspnoea	Present	Present
Neck veins	Unchanged	Can be distended
Auscultation	Rales	Rales ± S3
X-Ray Chest	Diffuse bilateral infiltrates	Diffuse bilateral infiltrates
Ejection Fraction	Normal or decreased	Decreased
Pulmonary artery occlusion pressure	≤ 18 mm Hg	> 18 mm Hg
Pulmonary oedema fluid	Exudate	Transudate
Fluid balance	Variable	Positive
Response to diuretics	±	+++
WBC Count	Decreased	Unchanged
BNP (pg/ml)	<200	>1200
Leucocyte Antibodies	Present	Usually not

BNP- Brain Natriuretic Peptide

IMMUNOHEMATOLOGY

18.1. IMMUNOGENETICS

Immunogenetics, as a scientific field, deals with the genetic and molecular polymorphisms of blood and tissue antigens as well as of receptor and effector molecules involved in the immune and alloimmune response. Concerned with certain aspects of biodiversity, it is supported by population genetics.

Immunogenetics can be said to have had its start with the discovery of the ABO blood groups. Blood groups provided some of the clearest examples of the role of Mendelism in humans and some of the most important examples of the application of genetic principles in human health and disease, particularly blood transfusion and maternofetal Rh incompatibility.

So in that line, we have Red cell immunogenetics dealing with blood groups, Immunohistogenetics for HLA, Human neutrophil antigens and the Human Platelet Antigen system.

An understanding of immunogenetics is required for understanding concepts in transfusion medicine, including,

- Blood group genetics and antigen systems for other blood cells, WBCs, platelets etc.
- Understanding rejection and tolerance: tissue and blood
- Immune and alloimmune response
- Immunological modulations and reactions to blood transfusion
- HDFN
- Monoclonal antibody development
- Serology, molecular typing and cellular assays
- Cytokine and cytokine receptor gene polymorphism

Terms in genetics:

Pedigree chart: demonstrates the inheritance patterns of each family member

Punnett square: square used to illustrate the probabilities of phenotypes in the offspring from known or inferred genotypes, E.g.:

Parents	A	B
O	AO	BO
A	AA	AB

Gene: the basic functional unit of inheritance on a chromosome

Genetic loci: sites/position of a gene on a chromosome

Alleles: alternate forms of a gene at a given locus

Antithetical: opposite allele

Genome: all the genetic information of a cell

Genomics: the study of the entire genome of an organism

Marker: detectable characteristics to recognise a gene's presence and allelic forms

Trait: genetically determined characteristic or condition

Haplotype: a group of alleles that tend to be inherited together

Independent assortment: each daughter cell randomly receives either maternally or paternally derived homologous chromosomes, resulting in a mixture of genetic material in the offspring.

Crossover: exchange of genetic material between homologous chromosome pairs

Polymorphism: occurrence of allelic variations(two or more alleles at one locus) in the population of genomes

Dosage effect: the observable difference in the strength of reaction, based on the zygosity of an allele(homo/hetero)

Genotype: the set of alleles at a single gene locus comprising the complement of genes inherited from parents

Phenotype: the observable expression of the genes inherited by a person reflecting their biological activities

Linkage: physical association between two genes located on the same chromosome and inherited together. E.g., RHD and RHCE on chromosome 1

Syntenic: gene loci that are not closely linked but carried by the same chromosome, e.g., RH and FY on chromosome 1

Linkage disequilibrium: the tendency of a specific combination of alleles at two or more linked loci to be inherited together more frequently than would be expected by chance.

Inheritance	Examples	Remarks
Autosomal dominant	A or B allele over O	Antigen appears in every generation
Autosomal codominant	S+s+ phenotype	Products of both alleles are expressed
Autosomal recessive	Lu(a-b-), Rhnull, O	More common in consanguineous mating
Sex-linked dominant	Xg^a	If the female is homozygous, then all her children are affected irrespective of sex
Sex-linked recessive	XK gene encoding Kx protein	Prevalence more in males than females

Structural variation	Examples	Remarks
Linkage	RHD and RHCE on chromosome 1	Physical association between two genes that are inherited together
Crossing over	FY and KN on the long arm of the chromosome cross over such that gene coding Fyb travels with the gene that encodes SI(a-)	Exchange of genetic material between homologous chromosome pairs
Linkage disequilibrium	MNSs	Linked genes do not assort independently, and hence the actual prevalence is less than observed

18.2. BASICS OF IMMUNOLOGY

Reaction	IgG	Ig M	IgA
Agglutination	Weak	Strong	Moderate
Precipitation	Strong	Weak	Variable
Complement fixation	Strong	Weak	Nil
Lysis	Weak	Strong	Nil

Properties	Ig M	Ig G	Ig A	IgE	IgD
Subtypes	-	IgG1, G2, G3, G4	IgA1, A2	-	-
Secreted form	Pentamer	Monomer	Dimer	Monomer	Monomer
Molecular Wt.	9,00,000	1,50,000	1,60,000	1,90,000	1,80,000
Serum concentration (mg/ml)	1.5	13.5	3.5	0.05	0.00004
Half-life (days)	5	23	6	2	3
Daily production (mg/kg)	3.3	34	24	0.0023	0.4
Intravascular distribution (%)	80	45	42	50	75
Complement fixation	Classical	Classical	Alternative	-	-
Placental transport	-	+	-	-	-
Secretion in milk	-	+	+	-	-
Secretion by seromucous	-	-	+	-	-
Heat stability(56^{0}C)	+	+	+	-	+
Carbohydrate (%)	12	3	8	12	13
Sedimentation Coefficient(S)	19	7	7	8	7

	Isotype	Allotype	Idiotype
Genetic variations or differences in	Fc portion of the heavy chain of Ig classes and subclasses	Multiple alleles that exist for some of the genes leading to subtle amino acid differences	The variable region of the heavy and light chain
Seen in	Within a species	Occurs in only some populations of the species	Resemble epitopes of an antigen
The stimulus for Antibody formation	IVIG of nonhuman origin	pregnancy, blood transfusion	immunisation/ vaccines
Eg:	IgG: IgG1, IgG2, IgG3, IgG4 IgA: IgA1, IgA2	H chains of IgG1 can carry either G1m(z) or G1m(f); a single amino acid substitution determines the difference	G4m(a) is an allotype in subclass IgG4 but is an isotype in IgG2

Proforma for Case taking in Immunohematology:

Patient Demographics	Name	
	Age	
	Sex	
	Ethnicity	
	Diagnosis	
	Transfusion history	
	Pregnancy history	
	Drugs	
	IV fluids	
	Immunoglobulins	
	Infections	
	Malignancies	
	Hemoglobinopathies	
	Transplantation	

Sample characteristics	Site and technique of collection	
	Age of sample	
	Anticoagulant	
	Hemolysis or Lipemia	
	Colour of serum/plasma	
	Agglutinates/aggregates	

Laboratory values	CBC: Hb, Hct, Retic, RBC morphology	
	Bilirubin, LDH	
	Haptoglobin, Hemoglobinuria	
	Albumin/Globulin	

Immunohematology basic	ABO	
	Rh	
	DAT	
	Phenotype	
	Antibodies detected	
	Autologous control	
	Compatibility testing	

	Direct Antiglobulin test	Indirect antiglobulin test
Components detected	Antibodies and complements attached to RBCs	Antibodies (allo)
Specimen required	Washed red cells/EDTA blood	Serum or plasma
Procedure	No incubation Wash red cells and add coomb's antisera and centrifuge	Incubation of serum with red cells Wash the red cells and add coomb's antisera, and centrifuge
Detection	In vivo antigen-antibody binding	In vitro antigen-antibody binding

DIRECT ANTIGLOBULIN TEST

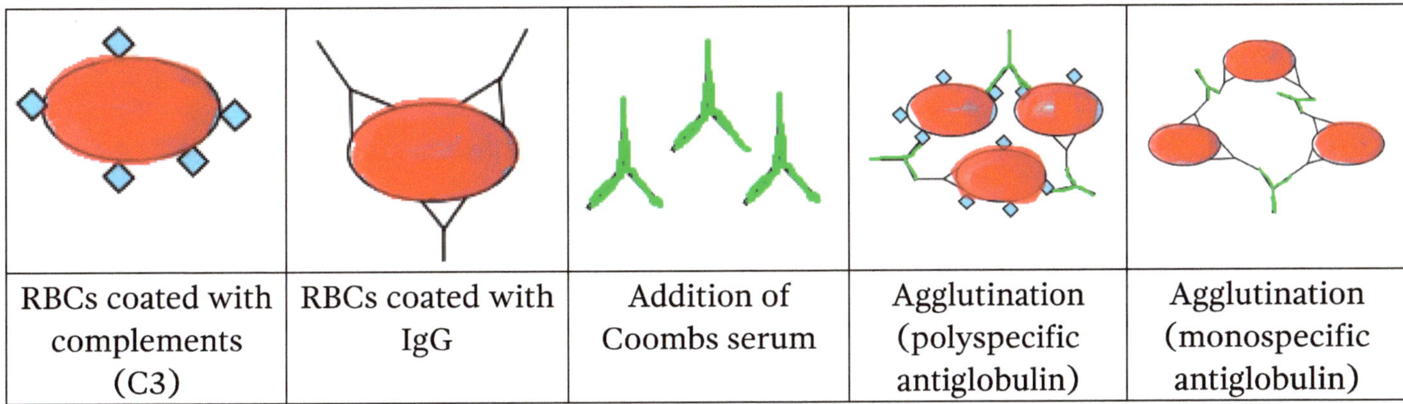

RBCs coated with complements (C3)	RBCs coated with IgG	Addition of Coombs serum	Agglutination (polyspecific antiglobulin)	Agglutination (monospecific antiglobulin)

INDIRECT ANTIGLOBULIN TEST

1. Patient's serum with suspected antibodies	2. Incubate with pooled or reagent red cells (with antigens to the antibody in question)	3. Sensitisation	4. Wash and incubate with antiglobulin (coombs) serum	5. Agglutination

Modalities/methods:

1. Test tube
2. Capillary tube

   The passage of red cells through a column of serum provides multiple opportunities for antibody molecules to come in contact with its antigens and hence are exquisitely sensitive and use significantly fewer volumes of reagents.

3. Column agglutination
4. Flow cytometry

Modifications:

1. Albumin additive IAT

   Albumin creates a low-ionic environment as its osmolarity is lower than that of normal saline, thereby accelerating the antibody coating

2. LISS additive IAT or IAT on LISS-suspended cells
3. PEG IAT
4. Enzyme IAT

Proteolytic enzymes cleave extracellular glycoproteins like sialic acid N-acetylneuraminic acid(NeuAc). NeuAc contains a carboxyl group that imparts a negative charge to RBCs.

5. LIP IAT (Low ionic Polybrene)

   Polybrene is a positively charged polymer which can neutralise negative charge on the red cell surface

6. EDTA IAT

   Complement binding antibodies (anti-Jka, Le) may become undetectable/less detectable on storage due to the formation of anti-complement activity due to the denaturation of complement components(conversion of C3b to C3c and C3d). EDTA destroys the anti-complement properties of stored sera.

Applications:

1. Blood group phenotyping.
2. To ascertain the clinical significance of the antibody. It tells about the capability to fix complement at 37^0C. E.g., Anti-P1
3. Detection weak D
4. Compatibility testing
5. Antibody detection and identification in prenatal testing or pretransfusion testing
6. For confirming weak A or B subgroups by adsorption and elution.

Some weak ABO subgroups are too weak to be detected by direct agglutination, even after cold temperature and antibody enhancement, which requires adsorbing anti-A or anti-B to red cells, followed by elution of bound antibodies. The eluate is then evaluated for the presence of anti-A/B antibodies by testing against A1 or B reagent red cells.

False positive reactions	False negative reactions
Over centrifugation	Failure to wash
Microscopic examination	Interrupted testing
Bacterial contamination	Usage of wrong reagents
Improperly clotted sample	Loss of activity in AHG reagents
Antibody to reagent constituent	Too heavy/light suspension
DAT-positive or polyagglutinating donor cells	Omission/failure to add reagents/plasma

QC: Intralaboratory competency testing:

IAT reading and grading procedure (Titrate with 2% R1r red cells)

Important Notes: Do not read enhanced tests like albumin IAT microscopically, as unwanted positive reactions may occur

18.3 ALLOANTIBODY SCREENING AND IDENTIFICATION

Indications for red cell antibody screening:

- As a part of pre-transfusion testing.
- Antenatal cases.
- Screening of the blood donor.
- As a part of transfusion reaction investigation.
- To investigate a case of HDFN

Antibody screening proforma:

History – (for prior red cell antigen exposure) pregnancy, transfusion, transplantation, needle sharing, immunogenic material injection

Ethnic Origin – In(b-) and Oh in Indians, Yt(a-) in Arabs

Disease- sickle cell, thalassemia, Cold agglutinin syndrome, Raynaud Phenomenon, M Pneumonia, Infectious mononucleosis, PCH, AIHA, SLE, Multiple Myeloma, CLL, Lymphoma

Infection- environmental, bacterial, viral

Passive transfer- IVIG, RhIG, Donor plasma, passenger lymphocytes, HPSC

Medication and therapies- Daratumumab(anti-CD38), Isatuximab(anti-CD38), Magrolimab (anti-CD47)

Clinical Significance

Only HDFN	Sc, RHAG
Only HTR	P1PK, Lua, Lub
Both HTR and HDFN	D, K, Fy
None	LW, Ch/Rg, Cr, Kn

A Clinically significant Red Cell Antibody is defined as an antibody that is associated with Hemolytic transfusion reactions, Hemolytic disease of the fetus and newborn or a notable decrease in the in vivo survival of transfused red cells

Unexpected/Irregular Antibody- All the antibodies other than the naturally occurring Anti-A and Anti-B.

An Alloantibody is an antibody to an antigen that an individual lacks.

An autoantibody is an antibody to an antigen that an individual possesses.

VARIABLES ASSOCIATED WITH ALLOIMMUNISATION

- **Route** - subcutaneous > intramuscular>> intravenous>> intraperitoneal.
- Presence of an infection.
- The dose of the antigen.

Characterising an Antibody

- **Type** - Auto or Allo
- Specificity and Clinical Significance

Condition	Frequency
Sickle cell anaemia	29% (18-45%)
Thalassemia	26%
AIHA	32% (12-40%)
MDS	21-58%
Aplastic Anemia	11%
Renal Failure	14%
Myelogenous Leukemia	16%
Lymphoblastic Leukemia	< 1%
GI Bleed	11%
Overall, in Hospitalised patients	2-6%
General population	0.5-1.5%

Sources of Active Alloimmunisation	Passive acquisition of Antibodies
Pregnancy	IVIG
Transfusion	RhIG
Transplantation	Plasma Transfusion
Injection of Immunogenic materials	HPSCs
Needle and hospital equipment sharing	Passenger Lymphocytes

Methods available: Tube testing, Column agglutination, Solid-phase

Capillary tubes, microplates, ELISAs

Immunofluorescence, Flow Cytometry, Immunoblotting

Panel cells

Detection Panel	Should have 19 Antigens (5 of Rh, 4 of MNSs, two each of Le, K, Fy, Jk)
	Double dose expression of Rh, Fy, MNS, Jk
	A set of 2-3 cell samples of group O
Identification Panel	Usually provided as 2-5% suspension with preservatives
	Should identify with confidence all the clinically significant antibodies
	Patterns should not overlap (e.g., every red cell which is K+ cannot also be E+)
	Expired cell panels can be used as long as they are functioning or used for confirming or excluding uncommon specificities

Abbreviated Identification panel	Used when the patient is already known to have antibodies or has been phenotyped
	Skip the cells which are known to be positive for the antibodies that the patient has or the ones for which he is phenotypically positive
	Exception: when the phenotype is predicted by genotyping and not serologically

Factors that influence the antigen expression:

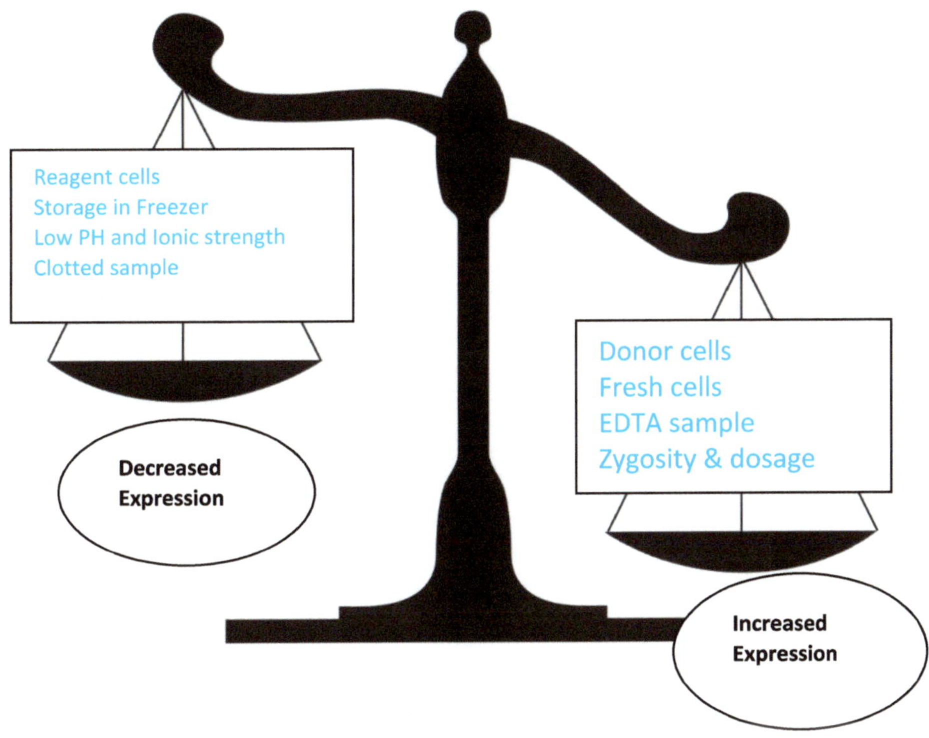

Zygosity and dosage:

Zygosity is the degree of similarity of alleles present at a given locus. (Homo or heterozygous)

Dosage is the degree of expression of an antigen on red cells. (Single or double dose)

Double-dose expression(dosage) is seen for the following common antigens:

Dumb	Kidds	R	Never Dozed
Fya, Fyb	Jka, Jkb	D, C, E, c, e	M, N, S, s

Variation in expression unrelated to zygosity is seen in P, A, I, Le, S

Variation in antigen expression on red blood cells of Neonates and adults:

Antigens that are Negative on Cord blood red cells: Le[a], Le[b], Sd[a], Ch, Rg, and AnWj

ChildRen	Lack	Sd	Antigens
Ch, Rg	Le[a], Le[b]	Sd[a]	AnWj

Antigens that are weakly expressed on Cord Blood cells compared to adults: I, P1, Lu

Antigens that are strongly expressed on Cord Blood cells compared to adults: i, LWa, LWb

The presence of some antigens may suppress the expression of other antigens
In(Lu) is known to suppress the expression of LU Antigens, P1, In^b and AnWj
Kp^a is known to weaken the expression of KEL Antigens

Changes with storage

Blood group antibodies may be weakly reactive with stored red cells than fresh red cells, especially regarding these antigens.

Blood group	Phenotype	MiniMise on	Freezing in	Kelvinator
Bg	P1	M, McCa	Fya, Fyb	Kna

Approaches to Identification

Approach	Basis	Criteria (P- Positive cells, N- Negative cells)
Standard	Fisher Exact method	3P + 3N
Liberal	Harris and Hochman	2P+3N (or) 1P+7N or the Reciprocal
Other		2P+2N

Assess these:

- ✓ Is the agglutination direct (saline) or in IAT only?
- ✓ Are all panel cells positive? (Pan agglutination)
- ✓ Is the auto control reactive? Is the grade similar to that with panel cells?

Steps of Antibody identification:

Step	Principle	Remarks
1	Examine the reaction with own cells (Auto control). Observe the DCT.	Autoantibody, Drug intake or alloantibodies to recently transfused red cells that are still circulating in the recipient are the possibilities
2	Examine the strength of reactions	Dosage effect or presence of multiple antibodies
3	"Ruling out": antibodies against antigens present on non-reactive cells are likely to be absent	Keep in mind that the low-frequency antigens and antigens are not represented in any of the panels
4	Examine the phase of reactivity	IgM reacts as direct agglutinins at Room Temperature, whereas IgG preferentially reacts by IAT. In the early stages of the immune response, predominantly IgG antibodies can have IgM specificities

5	Examine the results with enzyme-treated cells	
6	Apply the reactivity rule	Standard or Liberal
7	Phenotype the patient cells for corresponding antigens of the suspected/identified antibodies	Exceptions for antibodies being present when corresponding antigens appear to be positive are usually in the Rh system, where partial antigens are seen

❖ A single common alloantibody usually produces a clear pattern of agglutination with positive cells and no agglutination with negative cells

❖ **When to suspect multiple Antibodies?**

The observed pattern of reactive and non-reactive do not fit a single antibody

Reactivity at different test phases and different grades in the same phase

Unexpected reaction when attempted to confirm the specificity

The phenotypically similar red cell is non-reactive

❖ **Reactivity without apparent specificity**

- Alternate test method:

  Use a more sensitive method: PEG, enzymes, increased incubation time or serum-to-cell ratio

  Use a less sensitive method: to avoid the detection of unwanted and clinically insignificant reactivity

- Inherent variability: as in anti-Bg[a], -Kn[a], McC[a], -Sl[a], -JMH, Yka, Cs[a]
- Unlisted specificity: Do[a], Do[b], Yt[b]
- Some reactions are stronger with reagent cells but not with their own ABO group cells because reagent cells are usually O cells. E.g., anti-H, anti-IH, anti- Le[bH]
- Sometimes the reagent red cells are incorrect concerning provided antigram or are themselves DAT positive

Methods to resolve Complex antibody identification Problems		
1	Alteration of temperature	**Common IgM antibodies that react at room temperature or lower(22⁰C)** Allo antibodies - Le, MNS, A, Lu Autoantibodies- I, H, HI, Pr,
2	Increase Serum: cell ratio	Increase to 4:1(Serum: cell), 60 min at 37⁰C. Contraindicated when PEG/LISS is used
3	Increase incubation time	Increase it to 30-60 minutes in case of saline/albumin tests Contraindicated when PEG/LISS is used

4	Alteration of pH	If unbuffered saline with a pH <6.0 is used to prepare red cell suspensions or for washing in an IAT, Rh, Duffy, Kidd, and MNS blood groups may lose reactivity

Kidd loses	**Reactivity**	**if**	**Mixed with Acid**
Kidd	Rh	Fya, Fyb	MNS

5	Modification by enzymes	**Ficin and papain destroy or weaken antigens, such as**

ChRonje	**Jointly**	**Fixed**	**Match**	**with X**
Ch Rg	JMH	Fya, Fyb	M, N	Xga

Ficin-treated and Papain-treated red cells show enhanced reactivity with other antibodies

PICKLED - P, I, Kidd, Le, D(Rh)

6	Chemical modification		

Agent	**Destroys**
DTT (0.2M),2AET (6%), 2ME	K, YT, LW, DO, KN
DTT (0.002M)	Js^a, Js^b
Glycine-Hcl/EDTA	Bg, KEL, Er^a
Chloroquine	Bg and Rh

7	Inhibition techniques		

Substance	**Source**
Le^a, Le^b	The saliva of individuals with the LE gene (FUT3) and Le(a-b+) usually have both substances
P1	Hydatid fluid cyst, ovalbumin of pigeon eggs, Earthworms
Sd^a	Urine of Sd(a+) individuals
Ch/Rg	C4 Complement in Plasma
I	Human milk

8	Denaturation of Immunoglobulins	*Using Sulfhydryl compounds such as DTT and 2-ME in the following situations:* Antenatal cases, as we are interested in IgG only When IgM is masking IgG in a mixture of alloantibodies and/or autoantibodies
9	Adsorption and/or Elution	Auto or Allo adsorption as per the situation Elution alone for concentrating and purifying antibodies, especially of weakly expressed antigens or those showing multiple antibody specificities
10	Dilution/Titration	When dealing with multiple antibodies, if one of the antibodies is reactive at a higher dilution than the other, then dilution effectively removes the lower-titred one and thereby allowing the other to be identified

Situations wherein the genotype of a person may not predict the red cell phenotype:

➢ Mutations that inactivate gene expression
➢ Rare new alleles not included in the assay performed
➢ In patients with a Transplantation history, when genotyping is done by blood samples

High titre, Low avidity antibodies: The antibodies that weakly agglutinate in undiluted/ neat concentration continue to react weakly in dilutions as high as 1 in 2048 compared to other antibodies that generally weaken progressively with serial dilutions.

E.g., anti-Ch/Rg, Cs^a, Yk^a, Kn^a, McC^a and JMH – not clinically significant

Anti-Lub, -Hy, Yt^a – can shorten red cell survival

Selecting Blood for Transfusion

1. Antigen-negative blood: should be chosen even when the antibodies are no longer detectable
2. Crossmatch for compatibility:

Typing the donor units may not be necessary. The patient's serum can be used to select a serologically compatible RBC unit for antibodies that characteristically are reactive below 370C and do not ordinarily produce a secondary immune response following the transfusion of antigen-positive RBC units. Anti-M, -N, -P1,-Lea, -Leb, and -A1

$$\boxed{\text{LMNAP}}$$

3. Phenotype matched blood:

   – prophylactic in the case of, say, Rh antigens
   – the patient has warm autoantibody
   – patients on monoclonal antibody therapy
   – the antibody has not been demonstrated, but decreased survival of red cells is observed

Anti-Ch, anti-Rg, and many Knops and Cost antibodies have little or no clinical significance despite their reactivity in an IAT.

Knowing the Clinical Significance of **C**hido **R**ogers **C**osts Nothing

Antibodies that are reactive only at cold temperatures yet may cause red cell destruction in vivo: anti-Vel, -P, $PP1P^k(Tj^a)$

Tests for predicting the clinical significance of antibodies		
Test	**Principle**	**Remarks**
Monocyte Monolayer assay	Quantifies phagocytosis, adherence of antibody-coated red cells	
Antibody-dependent cellular cytotoxicity	Measures lysis of antibody-coated red cells	
Chemiluminescence assay	Measures respiratory release of Oxygen radicals after phagocytosis	Particularly for predicting the severity of HDFN
In vivo thermal amplitude studies		For cold reactive antibodies
Radiolabelled red cell survival study(^{51}Cr)		Can measure survival of as less as 1 ml
Flow cytometry		10 ml of transfusion is required

Rare Blood unit/donor: units that are negative for high prevalence antigens (>1 in 1000 units) or negative for a combination of many common antigens (<1 in 100 each)

Scenario 1: (Perfect Fit)

All the positive cells for the antigen gave a positive test, and all those negative gave a negative test. The variation in the grade of reaction here is the zygosity.

	Cell ID	D	C	E	c	e	P1	M	N	S	s	Le^a	Le^b	K	k	Fy^a	Fy^b	Jk^a	JK^b	IS	LISS	IAT
1	R1R1	+	+	0	0	+	0	+	0	+	0	0	+	0	+	+	0	+	+			0
2	R1R1	+	+	0	0	+	+	+	+	0	+	0	+	0	+	+	0	+	+			0
3	R2R2	+	0	+	+	0	+	0	+	0	+	0	+	0	+	0	+	+	0			0
4	R2r	+	0	+	+	+	+	+	+	+	+	0	0	+	0	+	+	0	+			3+
5	rr	0	0	0	+	+	+	+	0	+	+	+	0	0	+	+	+	0	+			0
6	rr	0	0	0	+	+	+	+	0	+	+	0	0	+	+	+	0	+	+			2+
7	r'r	0	+	0	+	+	0	0	+	+	0	0	+	0	+	+	+	+	0			0
8	r''r	0	0	+	+	+	+	+	+	0	+	0	+	0	+	0	+	+	0			0
9	R1r	+	+	0	+	+	+	0	+	0	+	+	0	0	+	+	0	0	+			0
10	R1R2	+	+	+	+	+	0	+	0	+	+	0	+	0	+	0	+	+	0			0
11	Ror	+	0	0	+	+	+	+	+	0	+	0	0	0	+	0	0	+	+			0
12	Auto control																					

Scenario 2: (3 plus 3 rule)

A minimum of 3 antigen-positive cells test positive with the antibody being tested, and a minimum of 3 antigen-negative cells do not react

	Cell ID	D	C	E	c	e	P1	M	N	S	s	Le^a	Le^b	K	k	Fy^a	Fy^b	Jk^a	JK^b	IS	LISS	IAT
1	R1R1	+	+	0	0	+	0	+	0	+	0	0	+	0	+	+	0	+	+			3+
2	R1R1	+	+	0	0	+	+	+	+	0	+	0	+	0	+	+	0	+	+			3+
3	R2R2	+	0	+	+	0	+	0	+	0	+	0	+	0	+	0	+	+	0			3+
4	R2r	+	0	+	+	+	+	+	+	+	+	0	0	+	0	+	+	0	+			3+
5	rr	0	0	0	+	+	+	+	0	+	+	+	0	0	+	+	+	0	+			0
6	rr	0	0	0	+	+	+	+	0	+	+	0	0	+	+	+	0	+	+			0
7	r'r	0	+	0	+	+	0	0	+	+	0	0	+	0	+	+	+	+	0			0
8	r''r	0	0	+	+	+	+	+	+	0	+	0	+	0	+	0	+	+	0			0
9	R1r	+	+	0	+	+	+	0	+	0	+	+	0	0	+	+	0	0	+			3+
10	R1R2	+	+	+	+	+	0	+	0	+	+	0	+	0	+	0	+	+	0			3+
11	Ror	+	0	0	+	+	+	+	+	0	+	0	0	0	+	0	0	+	+			2+
12	Auto control																					

Scenario 3 (Multiple antibodies)

	Cell ID	D	C	E	c	e	P1	M	N	S	s	Le^a	Le^b	K	k	Fy^a	Fy^b	Jk^a	JK^b	LISS IgG	Ficin IgG	DTT IgG
1	R1R1	+	+	0	0	+	0	+	0	+	0	0	+	0	+	+	0	+	+	3+	3+	0
2	R1R1	+	+	0	0	+	+	+	+	0	+	0	+	0	+	+	0	+	+	3+	3+	0
3	R2R2	+	0	+	+	0	+	0	+	0	+	0	+	0	+	0	+	+	0	3+	3+	2+
4	R2r	+	0	+	+	+	+	+	+	+	+	0	0	+	0	+	+	0	+	1+	3+	1+
5	rr	0	0	0	+	+	+	+	0	+	0	+	0	0	+	+	+	0	+	3+	3+	0
6	rr	0	0	0	+	+	+	+	0	+	+	0	0	+	+	+	0	+	+	3+	3+	0
7	r'r	0	+	0	+	+	0	0	+	+	0	0	+	0	+	+	+	+	0	3+	3+	0
8	r''r	0	0	+	+	+	+	+	+	0	+	0	+	0	+	0	+	+	0	3+	3+	1+
9	R1r	+	+	0	+	+	+	0	+	0	+	+	0	0	+	+	0	0	+	3+	3+	0
10	R1R2	+	+	+	+	+	0	+	0	+	+	0	+	0	+	0	+	+	0	3+	3+	1+
11	Ror	+	0	0	+	+	+	+	+	0	+	0	0	0	+	0	0	+	+	3+	3+	0
12	Auto control																			0	0	0

Scenario 4 (Warm autoantibody, alloantibody anti-S)

	Cell ID	D	C	E	c	e	P1	M	N	S	s	Le^a	Le^b	K	k	Fy^a	Fy^b	Jk^a	JK^b	Anti IgG	Autoadsorbed serum LISS 37^{0}C	DTT IgG
1	R1R1	+	+	0	0	+	0	+	0	+	0	0	+	0	+	+	0	+	+	3+	0	2+
2	R1R1	+	+	0	0	+	+	+	+	0	+	0	+	0	+	+	0	+	+	3+	0	0
3	R2R2	+	0	+	+	0	+	0	+	0	+	0	+	0	+	0	+	+	0	3+	0	0
4	R2r	+	0	+	+	+	+	+	+	+	+	0	0	+	0	+	+	0	+	3+	0	1+
5	rr	0	0	0	+	+	+	+	0	+	+	+	0	0	+	+	+	0	+	3+	0	1+
6	rr	0	0	0	+	+	+	+	0	+	+	0	0	+	+	+	0	+	+	3+	0	1+
7	r'r	0	+	0	+	+	0	0	+	+	0	0	+	0	+	+	+	+	0	3+	0	2+
8	r''r	0	0	+	+	+	+	+	+	0	+	0	+	0	+	0	+	+	0	3+	0	0
9	R1r	+	+	0	+	+	+	0	+	0	+	+	0	0	+	+	0	0	+	3+	0	0
10	R1R2	+	+	+	+	+	0	+	0	+	+	0	+	0	+	0	+	+	0	3+	0	1+
11	Ror	+	0	0	+	+	+	+	+	0	+	0	0	0	+	0	0	+	+	3+	0	0
12	Auto control																			3+		

Factors aiding Antibody identification	Autologous control	
	Phase of reactivity	
	Potentiator	Saline, albumin, LISS, PEG
	Strength of reaction	
	Effect of chemicals on Ag	Proteases, Thiol
	Pattern of reactivity	Single/Multiple
	Reaction characteristic	Mixed field/Rouleaux
	Hemolysis	
	Preservatives /antibiotics in reagents	
	Use of washed RBCs	

Table 10. Mechanisms of autoimmunity

Mechanism	Remarks	Examples
Antigenic alterations	Neoantigens	Drug-induced AIHA, T-Antigen
Sequestered antigens	Crypt Antigens	Polyagglutination
Cross-reacting foreign antigens		GBS, Alloantibody with auto specificity
Molecular mimicry		HUS
Polyclonal B cell activation		PCH, Mycoplasma pneumonia infection and Cold AIHA
Forbidden clones	Breakdown of immunological homeostasis	Adjuvant usage for immunisation
Altered B or T cells function		Lymphomas

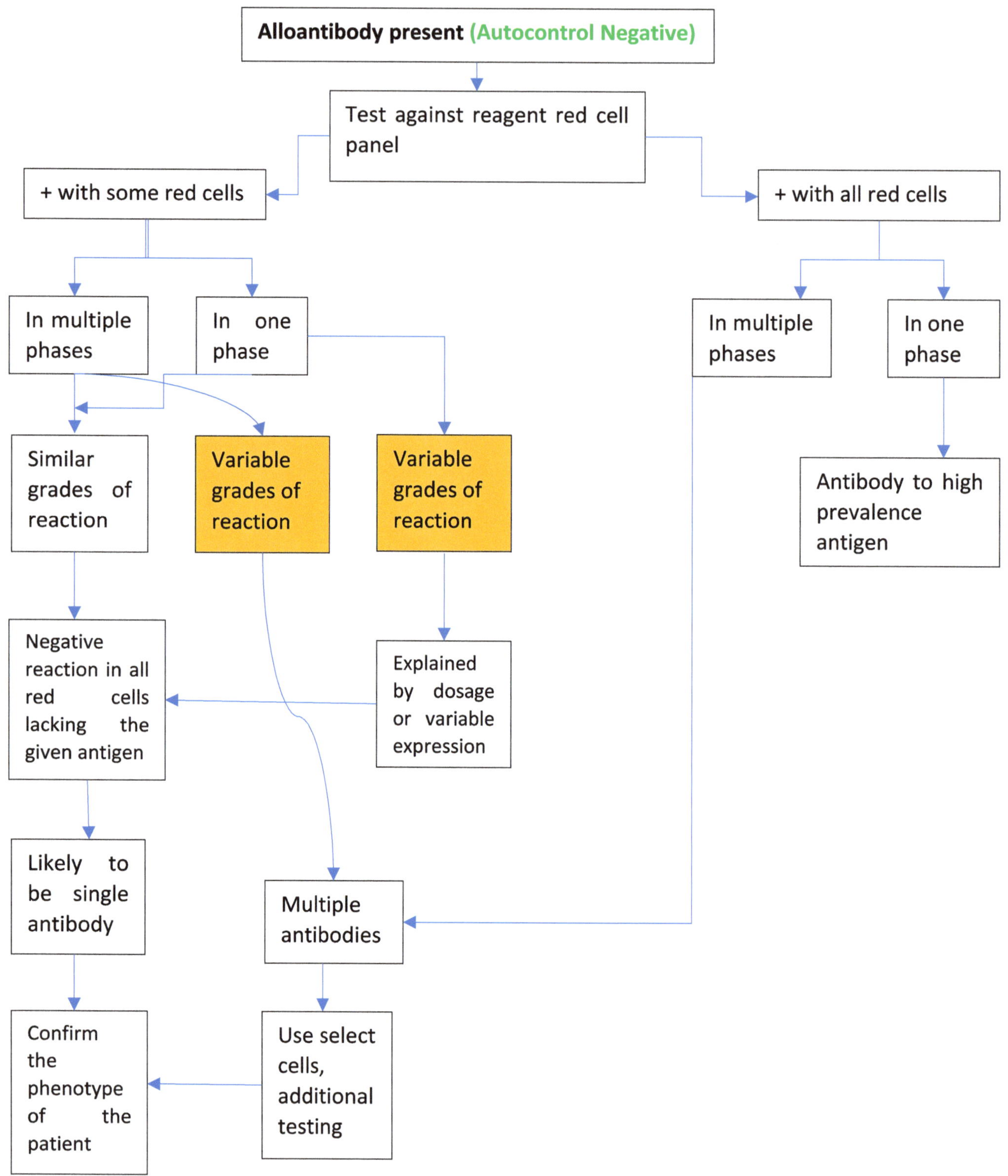

Figure 16. Algorithm for unexpected antibody in the presence of negative autocontrol

Figure 16. Algorithm for unexpected antibody in the presence of negative autocontrol

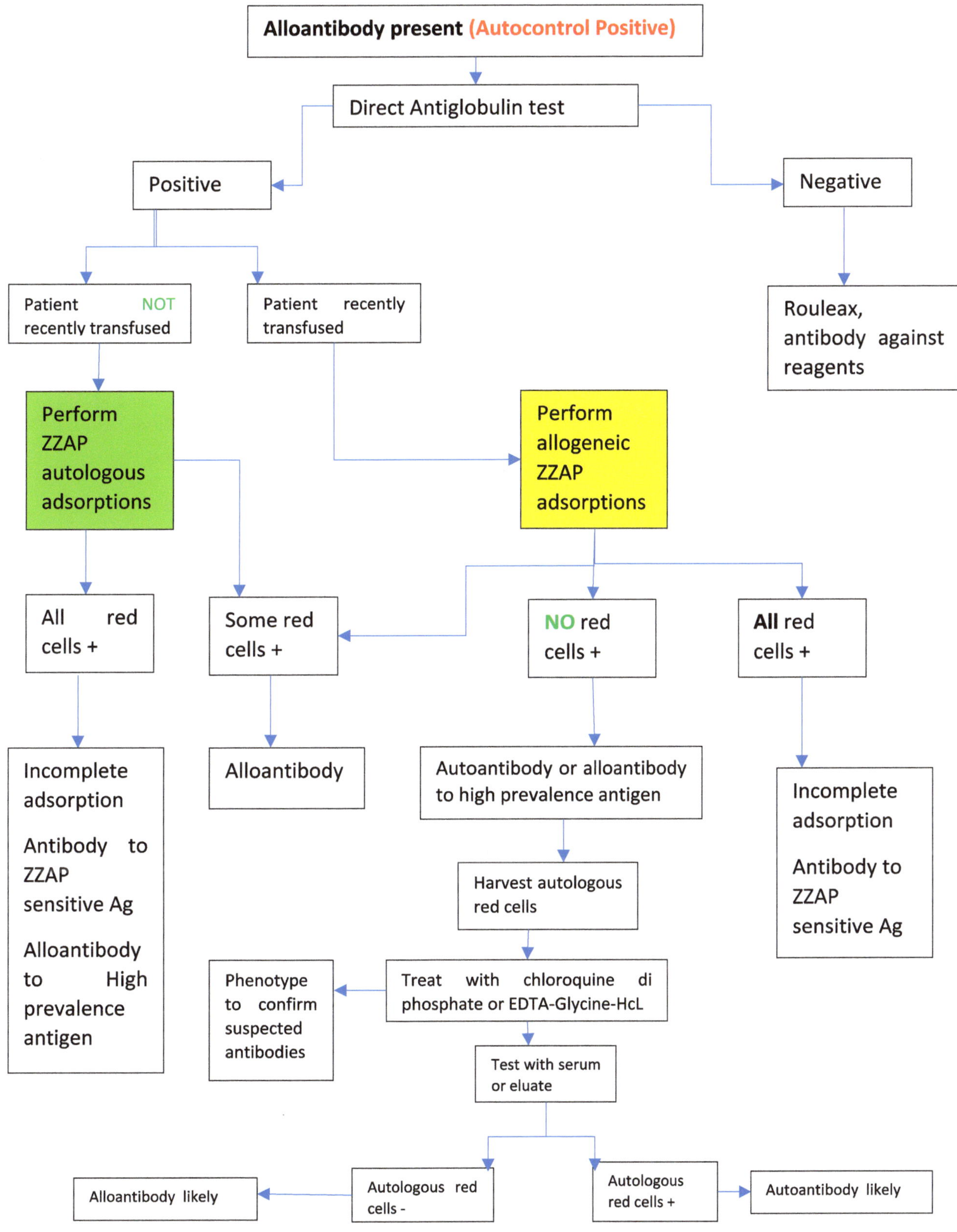

Figure 17. Algorithm for antibody identification when autocontrol is positive

Figure 17. Algorithm for antibody identification when autocontrol is positive

18.4 APPROACH TO A DAT POSITIVE CASE

Classification of Immune Hemolytic Anemias			
Cold-active antibodies	Cold agglutinin disease	*Primary or idiopathic*	
		Secondary	*Lymphoproliferative diseases*
			Autoimmune disorders
			Infections- Mycoplasma pneumoniae, Infectious mononucleosis, Other viruses
	Paroxysmal cold Hemoglobinuria		*Syphilis*
			Measles, mumps, other viruses
Mixed cold- and warm-active antibodies			
Warm-active antibodies (70-80%)	Idiopathic autoimmune hemolytic anaemia		
	Secondary autoimmune hemolytic anaemia	*Lymphoproliferative disorders* *Autoimmune – SLE, Inflammatory Bowel diseases* *Immunodeficiency disorders – CVID, Wiskott Aldrich* *Malignancy- ovarian dermoid cyst, lung, renal cell ca* *Viral infections- HIV, adenovirus, measles* *Others- Chlamydia pneumoniae, Mycobacterium, Leishmaniasis*	
Drug-induced immune hemolytic anaemia	Drug adsorption type	*Penicillin*	
	Neoantigen type	*Quinidine, stibophen*	
	Autoimmune type	α-methyldopa	
	Nonimmune type	*first-generation cephalosporins*	
Transplant-associated hemolytic anaemia	Hematopoietic stem cell transplant	*Minor ABO group mismatch*	
		Major ABO group mismatch	
		Passive antibody transfer	
	Solid-organ transplant	*Passenger lymphocyte syndrome*	
		Passive antibody transfer	

Questions before investigating a positive DAT for patients other than neonates

1. Is there evidence of in-vivo hemolysis?
2. Has the patient been transfused recently?
3. Does the patient's serum contain unexpected antibodies?
4. Is the patient receiving any drugs?
5. Has the patient received blood products or components containing ABO-incompatible plasma?
6. Is the patient receiving antilymphocyte globulin or anti-thymocyte globulin?
7. Is the patient receiving IVIG or IV RhIG?
8. Has the patient received a Haematopoietic or organ transplant?

Serological Investigations:

(i) Characterise the DAT with anti-IgG and anti-C3d reagents
(ii) Detect alloantibodies, if any
(iii) Test the eluate for specificity

Causes of DAT Positivity	
Specific:	**Nonspecific:**
Autoantibodies to red cell antigens	Sickle cell disease
Hemolytic Transfusion Reactions	Beta- thalassemia
HDFN	renal diseases
Drug-induced antibodies	multiple myeloma
Passively acquired alloantibodies	autoimmune disorders
Non-specifically adsorbed proteins	AIDS
Complement activation	elevated BUN
Passenger Lymphocyte syndrome	Elevated serum globulin

Method	Sensitivity (IgG molecules/red cell)	Sensitivity (C3d molecules/red cell)	Remarks
Conventional tube technique	300-500	1100	Gold standard
CAT/Microplate/SPRCA	120-180		
ELISA	80-120	400	
Flow cytometry	30-40		Most sensitive

Warm reactive autoantibodies:

- Apparent Rh Specificity: anti-D, -C, -c, -E or -e

  Against common RhD and RhCE determinants except for Rh-deletion types

- Non-Rh specificities: rarely anti-Jk^a/Jk^b

  against high prevalence antigens like anti-En^a, -U, -Wr^b, -Ge, -I, -Kp^b, -K13, -LW

Cold reactive autoantibodies:

- Anti- I/i, P1, Pr, Sd^x, Gd

	WAIHA	CAD	Mixed AIHA	PCH	DIAIHA
DAT	IgG- 20% C3 - 13% IgG+C3 - 67%	C3 only	IgG+C3 C3	C3 only	IgG+/-C3
Ig type	G	M	G, M	G	G
Eluate	IgG	-	IgG	-	IgG
Serum	35% agglutinate untreated red cells at 20 C	60% titer >/= 1000 at 4C reactive at 30 C	IgG IAT reactive antibody plus IgM agglutinating antibody reactive at 30 C	Negative routine IAT, IgG biphasic hemolysin in Donath Landsteiner test	
Specificity	Pan reactive	I > i >Pr	Pan reactive	anti-P	Rh related

Pentad of Establishing hemolytic Anemia:

1. Normocytic or macrocytic anaemia
2. Reticulocytosis (corrected reticulocyte count >2% or absolute reticulocyte count >100,000/ µL)
3. Low haptoglobin
4. Elevated lactate dehydrogenase (LDH), and
5. Elevated unconjugated (indirect) bilirubin

Predictive value of a positive DAT In a patient with hemolytic anaemia In a patient without hemolytic anaemia	 83% 1.4%
Prevalence: Blood donors Hospitalised patients	0.1- .01% 1-5%
Risk of future development of malignancy in DAT-positive patients	1:8 hematopoietic 1:2 others
Percentage of AIHA patients who are DAT Negative	2-11%

Adsorption with autologous red cells:

Prerequisite: Patient NOT transfused in the recent past (<3 months)

Additional modifications: Gentle heat elution at 56^0 C for 3-5 minutes

Proteolytic enzyme treatment

Treatment with ZZAP

Multiple sequential autologous adsorptions with new aliquots of red cells (generally, three times)

Adsorption with Allogeneic Red Cells:

Indications:

- The patient recently transfused (<3 months)
- Insufficient availability of autologous red cells (severe anaemia)

Prerequisite:

- Allogenic cells used should not contain antigens against which alloantibodies are reactive

Goal:

- To remove autoantibody and leave the alloantibody in the adsorbed serum

Drawbacks:

- Antibodies to high-frequency antigens cannot be excluded
- Selecting the cells is very cumbersome

Adsorption with allogeneic red cells:

1. Autoadsorb serum with the patient's red cells treated with

   a. ZZAP
   b. Chloroquine diphosphate
   c. Variable pH/gradient centrifugation
   d. Partial heat elution at 56^0C

Cell selection: Clinically significant alloantibodies need to be ruled out – Rh antigens, K, Duffy, Kidd, S, s

If the patient's phenotype is not known, use O red cells of R1R1, R2R2, and rr with at least one lacking Jk^a and the other lacking Jk^b.

If the patient's phenotype is known choose cells that match the patient's phenotype

Enzyme treatment can be used to remove Fy

DTT removes K. ZZAP can remove both Fy and K (ZZAP is DTT+ Enzyme)

Enhancement using PEG or LISS may be used.

If adsorption fails to remove reactivity, the possibility of autoantibody or alloantibody to high prevalence antigen is to be considered.

Identify alloantibodies in the patient's serum in tests with serum diluted to a point where the autoantibody reacts only weakly

Testing adsorbed serum: With cells that either lack or carry antigens for Rh, Kell, Duffy, Jk

Selection of Blood for Transfusion

- Exclude the presence of potentially clinically significant alloantibodies.
- Select a unit of appropriate ABO, Rh type
- If a significant antibody is present, transfused cells should lack the corresponding antigens
- For long-term transfusion, obtain extended phenotype. Try to match the Rh phenotype, Kell, Duffy, Kidd, and Ss antigen type.
- If autoantibody has a specificity (e.g. anti-e), blood lacking the corresponding antigen should be sought.

DAT negative AIHA (5%)

- quantity of bound IgG is too low to be detected by a DAT
- the bound autoantibody is not of the IgG immunoglobulin class (IgA in <1%)
- some other immune mechanisms mediate the hemolysis (e.g., cell-based cytotoxicity)
- the patient possesses very low-affinity autoantibodies
- antibody-coated cells get rapidly destroyed and cleared

Further testing: Test the eluate

Polybrene or PEG-modified direct RBCassays.

Flow cytometry

Indications for antibody adsorption:

- Removal of autoantibody activity to permit detection of coexisting alloantibodies.
- Reagent preparation.
- Separation of multiple antibodies to aid in identification.
- Confirmation of the presence of a weak antigen on red cells.
- Confirmation of antibody specificity

Adsorption and elution combined:

- Separating suspected mixtures of antibodies in a patient's serum/plasma.
- Detection of weak red cell antigen variants. E.g. Group O sample with missing anti-A isoagglutinin

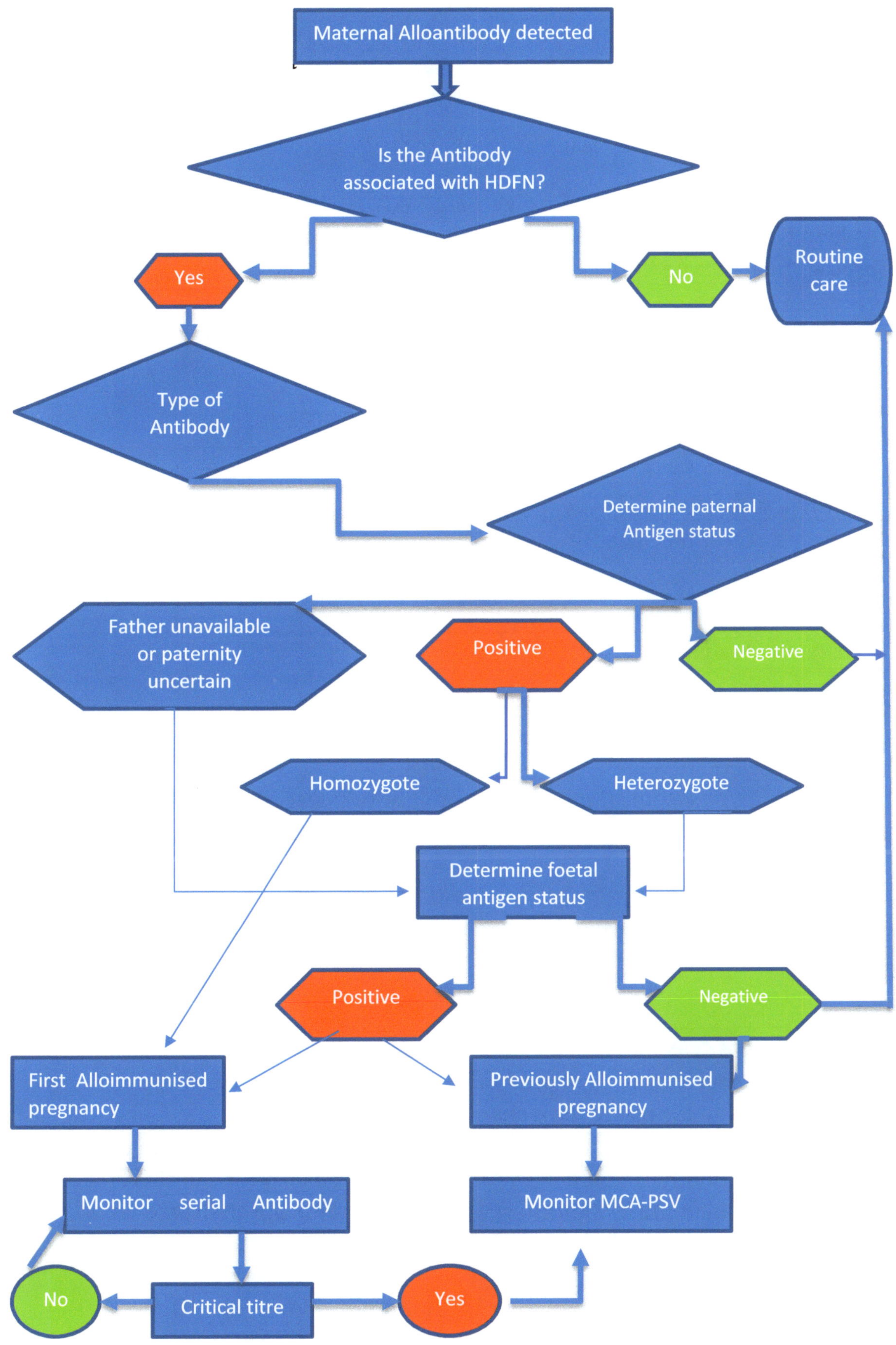

Algorithm for fetal alloimmunisation management

18.5 ELUTION

Elution is a procedure of dissociating antibodies from sensitized red cells, the primary objective being to recover bound antibodies for study by routine serologic techniques.

How does elution work?

- changing the thermodynamics of antigen-antibody reactions
- neutralizing/reversing the forces of attraction that hold antigen-antibody complexes together
- disturbing the structure of the antigen-antibody binding site

Why elution?

- To recover the bound antibody in a usable form

Table 18.1 Factors that influence the outcome of the elution procedure

Technical factors	
	Washing efficiency
	The type of test tube used
	Incorrect pH
	Tonicity of suspension medium
	Purity and Stability of reagents used
	Contaminant cells
	Temperature
	The time delay from elution to separation
	The medium of suspension (Albumin or antibody-free plasma is better than saline)
Antibody factors	
	Affinity
	Type/class of antibody
	Titre

Applications

1. Investigating a positive antiglobulin test: HDN, HTR, AIHA
2. Purification and concentration of antibodies
3. Detection of weakly expressed antigens
4. Identification/resolving if multiple antibody specificities present in a single serum
5. Preparation of antibody-free red cells for autologous adsorption studies (rendering red cells negative by the direct antiglobulin test and thereby allowing the red cells to be tested with antisera reactive by the indirect antiglobulin test)
6. Preparation of typing reagents
7. Separation of antibodies from a mixture of antibodies

Freeze-Thaw (Wiener):   Uses alcohol and the action of Freezing and Thawing.

Useful for weaker A and B antibodies, ABO-incompatible Transplant recipients, Passive AB antibodies

Microwaves or Ultrasound: Useful for ABO antibodies, cold-reactive IgM antibodies

Eluting Antibodies from Placental Tissue: Use Digitonin and Glycine

Eluting Antibodies with Xylene/D-Limonene: For AIHA, drug-induced and alloantibodies

necessary safety precautions are needed to use chemicals like xylene/ether, along with unique storage and disposal requirements, make them difficult, if not impossible, to use in today's laboratories

Table 18.2 Commonly used elution techniques

Method	Application	Advantages	Disadvantages
Lui freeze-thaw	ABO HDFN	Quick A small volume of RBCs required	Poor recovery of other antibodies
Heat Elution(56^0C)	ABO HDFN IgM agglutinating antibodies	Easy to perform It can be done in basic laboratories, also	Poor recovery of IgG allo and antibodies Difficult to standardize Lacks consistency
Acid elution (Citric acid, Glycine	Warm auto and alloantibodies	Easy to perform	Possible false results when high titer antibody is present
Chemical/organic solvent elution (Chloroform, Trichloroethylene, Ether)	Warm auto and alloantibodies		Chemical hazards: inflammable, carcinogenicity, chemical toxicity
Others Chloroquine Phosphate	Usage of anti-S and anti-Fya on DAT-positive cells		Can give a negative reaction in Rh Typing

Matuhasi-Ogata phenomenon: unwanted positive reaction in the elution procedures, i.e., presence of antibody specificity in the eluate for which the eluted red cells are antigen-negative. It has been attributed to the non-specific binding of IgG in the presence of a specific antibody. For example, when group B, D-negative red cells are incubated with anti-B and anti-D, an eluate prepared from the cells was also found to contain anti-D. The finding of unexpected antibodies in eluates might be due to the non-specific uptake of IgG rather than the adherence of antibodies to antigen-antibody. The amount of unexpected antibodies in the eluate is usually small and gives only weak reactions

Technical tips:

Washing: To ensure that the antibody recovered in eluates is red cell membrane-derived and does not represent a "free" unbound antibody, red cell samples must be adequately washed before performing the elution procedure. Normal or buffered saline, or low-ionic-strength saline (LISS), may be used to wash red cells before elution. Using ice-cold saline or LISS may help prevent the dissociation of low-affinity antibodies during the washing process

False-positive Eluates	False negative eluates
Incomplete washing	Antibody dissociation during washing

Determining ABH Secretor Status:

The presence of water-soluble A, B, and H antigens is determined by ABO and Se genes in saliva and other body fluids. If Se is present, those ABH antigens will also be found in the secretions. The presence of these secreted antigens is ascertained using a hemagglutination-inhibition assay. Polyclonal antisera or high-titre plasma should be used for the test.

False Positive test: If monoclonal antisera used

False Negative test: Improperly prepared saliva

Principle:

Dilution of the antisera/plasma with PBS (0.1ml + 0.9ml)

Addition of saliva(0.1ml), mixing and Incubation (30 minutes at Room Temperature)

Addition of indicator cells mixing and incubation (15 minutes at Room Temperature)

Centrifuge and interpret. If agglutination is absent(inhibited), the test is positive for secretor status.

18.6 CRYOPRESERVATION OF RED REAGENT CELLS

Freezing and thawing of red cells are used for the long-term preservation of red cells of rare phenotypes for use in antibody identification.

If possible, freeze red cells within one week of collection.

1. Glycerol preservation

   Red cells are diluted with glycerol to prevent membrane damage by ice crystals and may be preserved frozen for many years. Hemolysis during the thawing process is minimized by washing in solutions of decreasing salt content.

   Use brief centrifugation during washing for recovery as over-centrifugation results in aggregation of red cells that is difficult to disperse.

   Red cells frozen in this manner may acquire a positive DAT because of C3 coating; if so, perform indirect antiglobulin tests (IATs) with anti-IgG.

2. Liquid-Nitrogen Preservation

   To prevent membrane damage by ice crystals, red cells in sucrose may be frozen in liquid nitrogen for many years.

Indications for antibody titration:

- To determine the strength of clinically significant antibodies in antenatal cases.
- Resolution of high titre low avidity antibodies.
- To Distinguish between the strengths of multiple antibodies in a single sample.
- ABO isohemagglutinins titrations on apheresis platelet units.
- ABO isohaemagglutinin titrations on recipients due for receiving organs that are to be transplanted across the ABO barrier

Table 18.3 Preparation of check cells

Type of cells	Method	Remarks
C3b/C4b-Coated RBCs	Mix 1 mL of whole blood with 10 mL of sucrose	
IgM/C3b-Coated RBCs	anti-Le^a or anti-Le^{a+b} antisera with packed group O, Le(a+b−) RBCs	
C3b-Coated RBCs (Fruitstone Method)	C3b-coated RBCs may be converted to C3d-coated RBCs either by extended incubation (2 hours) in 20 volumes of freshly collected normal human serum Or by treatment of the RBCs with crude trypsin	Under low-ionic conditions, the complement components C3b and C4b are bound to RBCs without prior attachment of antibody molecules (i.e., via the alternative pathway)
C4b-Coated RBCs	Under low-ionic conditions, C3b and C4b are bound to RBCs without prior attachment of antibody molecules (i.e., via the alternative pathway). The addition of EDTA to the sucrose prevents the uptake of C3b, leaving RBCs coated only with C4b.	used for identifying anti-Ch/Rg
Immunoglobulin-Coated RBCs	Immunoglobulins are coupled to RBCs using chromic chloride	

18.7 POLYAGGLUTINATION

Definition: Polyagglutinability is the state of red cells wherein they are altered by microbial (bacterial or viral) activity, certain forms of aberrant erythropoiesis, or inherited alterations in the RBC membrane, and they are agglutinated by almost all samples of normal ABO compatible adult human serum although not by the patient's own serum.

Category	Type	Causes
Microbial associated	Th	Corynebacterium aquaticum, especially in pregnancy
	Tk	Bacteroides Fragilis, Escherichia Freundii, Flavobacterium keratolyticus, Serratia Marcescens, Candida Albicans
	Tx and Tr	Pneumococcal
	Acquired B	Usually, in colorectal cancer with Gram-negative sepsis
	Passive bacterial product adsorption	Bacillus cereus, Hemophilus Influenza, Bacillus Anthracis, Streptococcus
Non-Microbial associated	Tn	Mutation in the hematopoietic tissue that gives rise to a clone of cells that lack β-3-D-galactosyltransferase: MDS, Leukemias Deficiency of β-3-D -galactosyltransferase in children
Inherited Forms	Cad	an autosomal dominant condition that gives rise to a permanent polyagglutinable state due to Cad antigen
	Haemoglobin M-Hyde Park	heterogeneity in the molecular size of SGPs and a mild reduction in the sialylation of O-linked oligosaccharide chains
	HEMPAS (Hereditary erythroblastic multinuclearity with positive acidified serum lysis test)	Increased amounts of i-antigen and decreased amounts of H antigen and sialic acid
	NOR	Possible related to the P blood group system
Miscellaneous	VA (only up to a temperature of 18^0c)	Reduction in sialic acid and depression of H receptors
	Antibodies against usually hidden antigens	On enzyme-treated red cells, e.g. Trypsin, papain, bromelain, periodate, neuraminidase
	Cold agglutinin reacting with only stored cells	After 4-7 days of storage, probably because of the gradual expression of galactose or mannose-containing epitopes or low-density lipoproteins
	Agglutinin reacting with freshly washed cells	Washing in saline

T-activation is a complicating factor in infants with the following conditions:

- Necrotizing Enterocolitis (NEC)
- Non-NEC Bowel related surgical complications, Sepsis

Organisms causing T-antigen exposure (neuraminidase producing):

- Clostridium Perfringens
- Streptococcus pneumoniae (associated with HUS and Hemolytic anaemia)
- Bacteroides
- E Coli
- Actinomyces
- Influenza virus

Overexpression of T-Antigens:

- Epithelial carcinomas: breast, colon, bladder, prostate

Incidence:

- 0.6% of all patients admitted to NICU
- Up to 30% of infants with NEC

Anti-T:

- Predominantly IgM {react strongly at colder temperatures($<37^0$C)}
- Do not fix the complement
- All have by six months and reach adult levels by 2 yrs

DDs for Hemolysis in T-antigen activation:

- Clostridium Perfringens bacteremia induced (due to phospholipase enzyme)
- DIC
- Sepsis
- MAHA
- Inherited hemolytic disorders
- Lecithinase-producing bacterial infections: Clostridium perfringens, Staphylococcus aureus, Pseudomonas aeruginosa or Listeria monocytogenes

Diagnosis:

- Reverse grouping and minor crossmatch in the at-risk group
- DAT: usually negative except in Strep. Pneumoniae infection

Pathogenesis:

The major RBC membrane glycoproteins, glycophorin A, B and C, carry O-linked oligosaccharides that are disialylated tetrasaccharides.

Removal of Sialic acid(N-Acetylneuraminic acid) from these tetrasaccharides by the enzymatic action of bacterial neuraminidases exposes the hidden β-linked galactosyl residue

(Galactose-β(1-3)-N-acetylgalactosamine) termed T-antigen (Thomsen-Friedenreich cryptantigen)

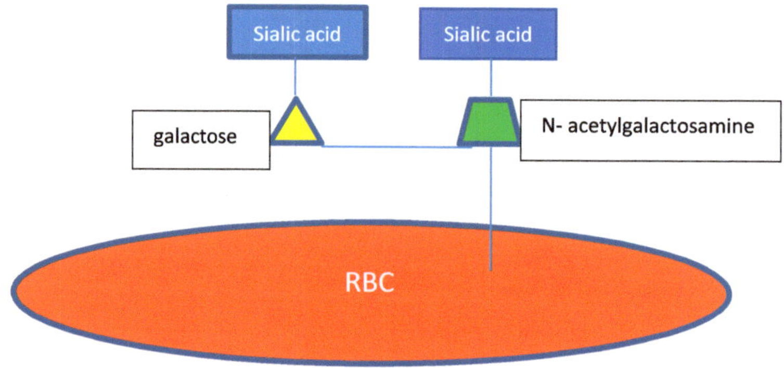

Table 18.4 Lectin panel classification of T-antigen activation variants

Lectin	Common name	T	Th	Tk	Tx	Tn
Arachis Hypogaea	Peanut, groundnut	+	+	+	+	-
Glycine Soja	Soybean	+	-	-	-	+
Salvia sclarea		-	-	-	-	+
Salvia horminum		-	-	-	-	+
Vicia cretica		+	+	-	-	-
Medicago disciformis		+	+	-	-	-

Griffonia Simplicifolia	Ajwain 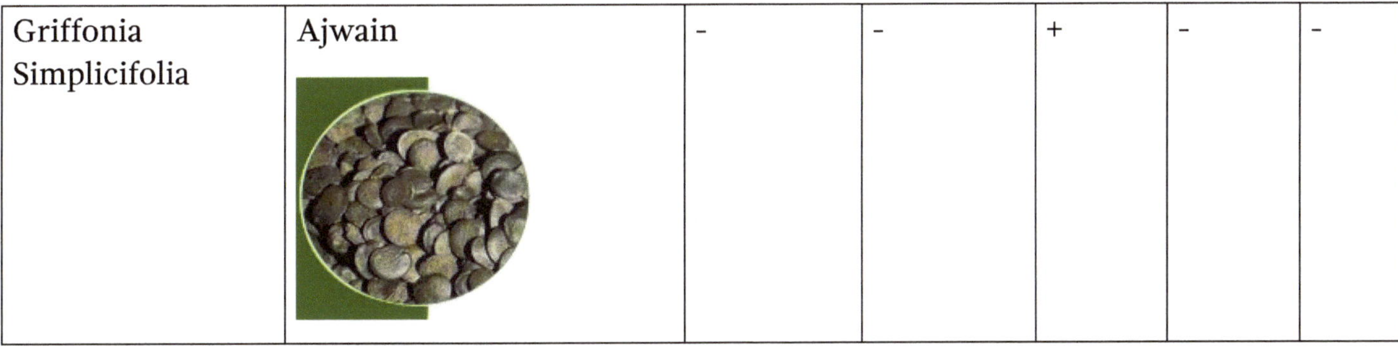	-	-	+	-	-

Anti-T antibodies are usually present in virtually all individuals after six months. The unmasked T-antigen binds with anti-T antibodies in the plasma of individuals leading to polyagglutination and potential hemolysis in vivo.

Transfusion in Polyagglutination:

- Use plasma-reduced or washed RBC and platelet components.
- Plasma, if used, should be low anti-T titred
- If low anti-T titred plasma is not available, monitor closely for hemolysis.
- Exchange transfusion using washed RBCs suspended in albumin may be required in infants with brisk ongoing hemolysis and hemoglobinuria.
- Plasmapheresis can be performed in children with SpHUS(Strep Pneumoniae), avoiding plasma as a replacement fluid to remove autologous anti-D and prevent the passive transfer of anti-T in normal plasma.

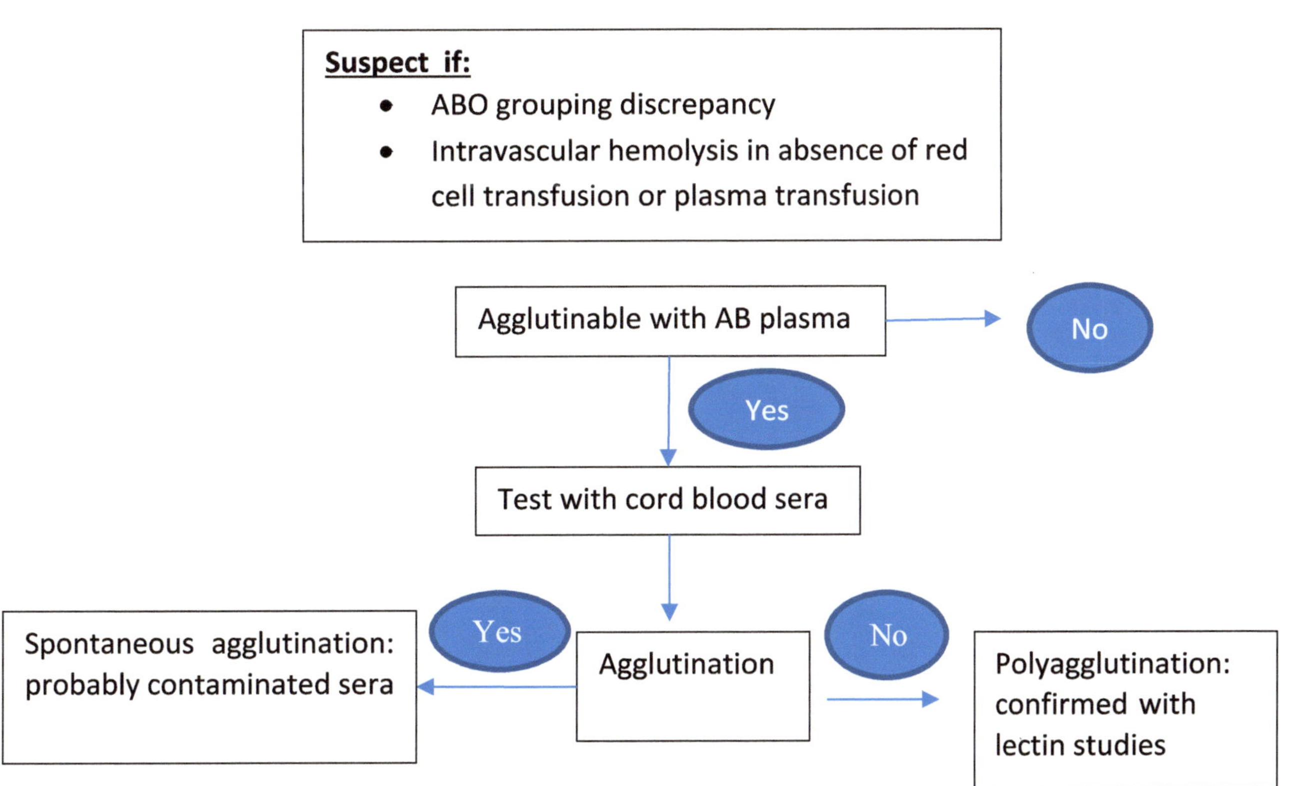

Figure 18. Approach to testing for polyagglutination

Acquired B antigens

- can be changed back to normal A1 determinants by reacetylating with acetic anhydride (CH3CO)2O.
- Readily detected by certain monoclonal anti-B (ES4) at a neutral or alkaline Ph but not in acidic pH.
- The addition of GalNH2-HCl can inhibit the acquired B reactivity but not the normal B antigen.

TTI TESTING

19.1 INFECTION SCREENING AND METHODS

	Screening Tests	Diagnostic Tests
Target Population	Apparently healthy (Blood Donors)	Sick or suspected people only
Application	Mass/Groups	Case-to-case basis
Results	Arbitrary and final	Modified and repeated as the disease progresses
Inclusion	Usually one criterion (like all donations)	Based on symptoms, signs and other lab findings
Accuracy	Less	More
Expense	Low	High
Further action	Always confirmed with another test or modality for evaluation	Used as a basis for treatment
Initiative	As a policy or investigation	Usually, patient/physician initiated based on complaints

In order to be transmissible by blood, the infectious agent or infection usually has the following characteristics:

- ✓ Disease transmitted should be an essential health problem
- ✓ Presence in the blood for long periods and generally in high dosage
- ✓ Stability in blood stored at 4^0 C or lower
- ✓ The long incubation period before the appearance of clinical signs
- ✓ Asymptomatic phase or only mild symptoms in the blood donor, hence not identifiable during the blood donor selection process
- ✓ There should be a screening test available
- ✓ The expected benefits of detection should exceed the costs

Features of a good screening test:

1. Acceptability: technical requisites, infrastructure requirement, trained workforce, cost
2. Repeatability: (Reliability, precision or reproducibility)
3. Validity: (Accuracy)
4. Yield: the amount of previously unrecognised disease that is diagnosed as a result of the screening test

Evaluation of a screening test:

a. Sensitivity
b. Specificity
c. Percentage false negatives
d. Percentage false positives
e. Predictive value

Essential quality elements in the TTI laboratory:

- Quality of the kits used for testing.
- Quality and calibration of equipment used in testing.
- High-quality controls (internal kit controls and external controls).
- Interpretation of results, proper calculation of cut-off.
- Documentation.
- Standard Operating Procedures.
- Establishment and implementation of protocols for troubleshooting and corrective action.
- Application of statistical process.
- Staff Training.

Rapid Immunochromatography:

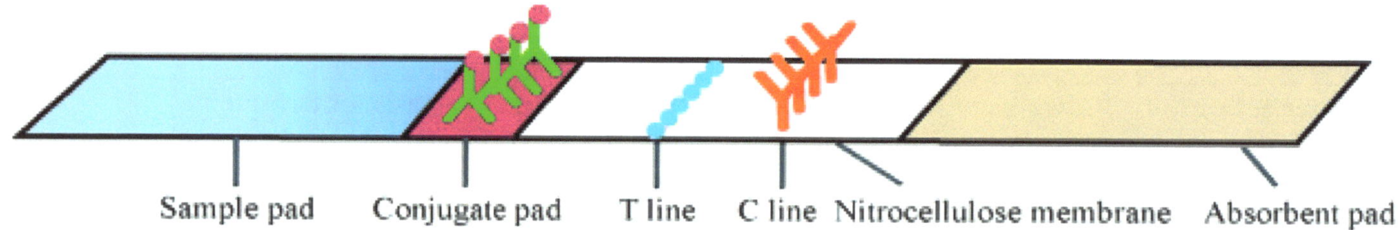

They are 3 main types:

1. Immuno-chromatographic method.
2. Immuno-filtration method (e.g. dot blot assay for HCV).
3. Conventional enzyme immunoassay (EIA

Advantages:

- Almost as sensitive and specific as ELISA
- Very fast and can be performed in the field (Ideal for Emergencies)
- It does not need electric power or other infrastructure or equipment
- Not much sample preparation is required
- It does not require much training, is easy to perform, and can be read visually

Disadvantages

- Lack of permanent records and traceability
- Useful only in low throughput laboratories

ELISA

Microwell plate-based technique. Antigen/Antibody may be fixed to the plate and then captures the corresponding Antibody/antigen if present in the test sample, which is added

Enzymes	Indicators
Alkaline Phosphatase	Coloured latex particles
Horseradish Peroxidase	Colloidal gold sol particles
Acetylcholinesterase	Dyes
Carbonic Anhydrase	Enzymes
Glucose Oxidase	Carbon particles
Glucamylase	
Glucose-6 Phosphate dehydrogenase	
Lysozyme	
Malate Dehydrogenase	
Substrates		**Stop solutions**
TMB	Tetramethyl Benzidine	1 N HCl
OPD	o- Phenlyenediamine	4N H2SO4
DAB	Diaminobenzidine	NaOH
BCIP	5-Bromo 4-chloro 3-indolyl phosphate	
NBT	Nitroblue tetrazolium	

Types of ELISA

The difference between a direct and indirect ELISA is in the detection method of the immobilised antigen on an ELISA plate. Direct ELISAs use a conjugated primary antibody, while indirect ELISAs, an unconjugated primary antibody binds to the antigen, and then a labelled secondary antibody directed against the host species of the primary antibody binds to the primary antibody

Direct ELISA:

Advantages

1. Rapid
2. No cross-reactivity

Disadvantages

1. Low sensitivity
2. Time-consuming and expensive to get specific antibodies for each ELISA

Indirect ELISA

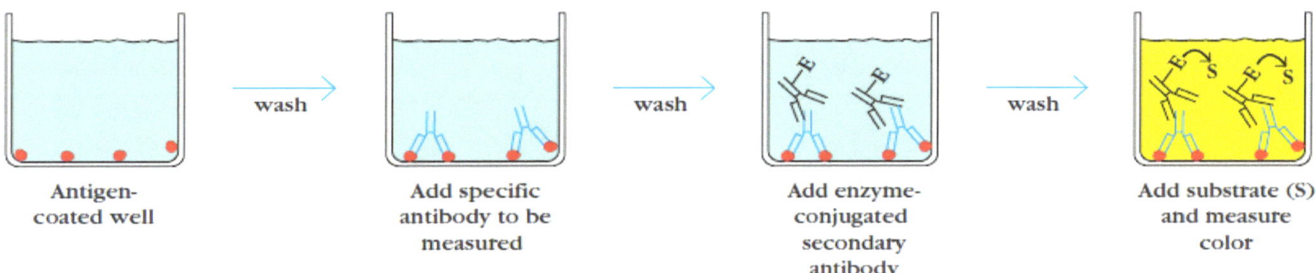

Advantages

1. Labelled secondary antibodies are available commercially in a wide variety. Hence cheaper.
2. It is versatile because many primary antibodies can be made in one species, and the labelled secondary antibody used for detection can be the same.
3. Since the primary antibody is not labelled, maximum immunoreactivity is retained.
4. Every primary antibody contains several epitopes bound by the labelled secondary antibody, which allows for signal amplification, increasing sensitivity.

Disadvantages

1. The secondary antibody can exhibit cross-reactivity, thereby eliciting a nonspecific signal.
2. An extra incubation step is required.

Sandwich ELISA

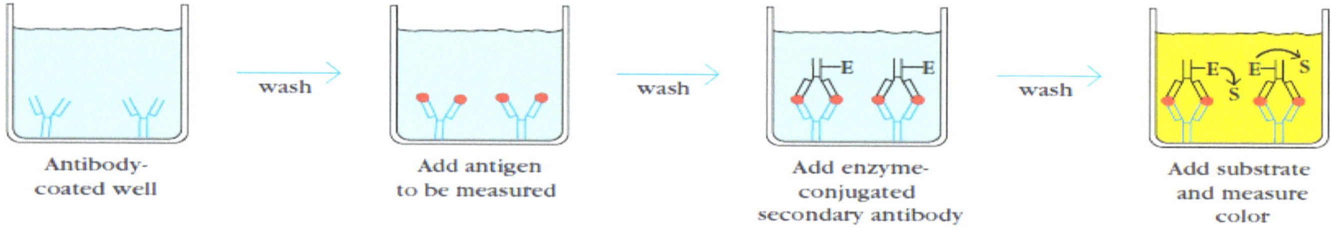

Advantages

1. High specificity because the antigen/analyte is specifically captured and detected.
2. Suitable for complex (or crude/impure) samples as the antigen does not require purification before measurement.
3. Flexible and sensitive, both direct and indirect detection methods can be used.

Disadvantages

1. Requires match paired primary and secondary antibodies
2. Time-consuming and expensive

Competitive ELISA

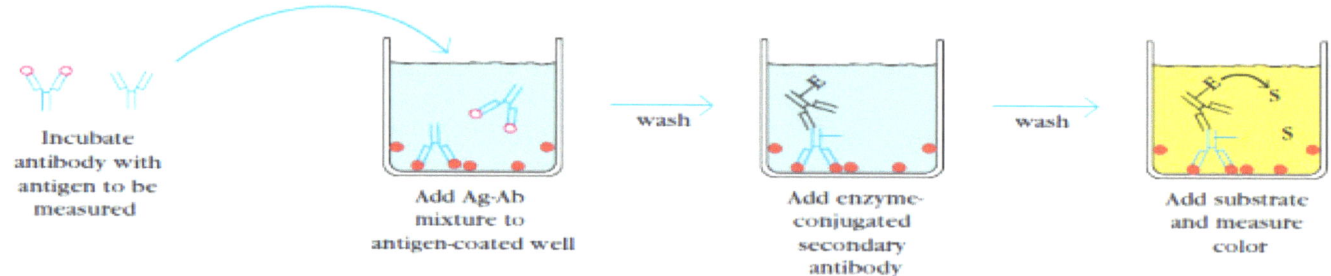

Advantages

1. It is highly sensitive even when the specific detecting antibody is present in relatively small amounts or smaller antigens.
2. Low variability
3. A broad range of antigens in a sample can be tested

Disadvantages

1. Low specificity
2. It cannot be used with diluted samples

- **Hook Effect**- when there are very high antigen levels in the sample, the specific binding of the antigen is insufficient to match analyte levels, and the signal is lower than expected. Rectification: test several dilutions of each sample
- **Edge Effect**- outer wells behave differently with unexpected values out of line with neighbouring wells. Rectification: using duplicates or triplicates for all samples and noting any significant variations in the results for a given sample.

Troubleshooting in ELISA		
Issue	**Cause**	**Resolution/Remarks**
Reactive negative control	Sample contamination	
	Inadequate washing	
	Detection Ab reacting with coating Ab	
High background	Background wells contaminated	
	Inadequate washing	
High signal	Antigen content more than the assay range	
	Oversaturated samples	decrease incubation time/ temperature
	Inadequate washing	
High variation	Bubbles in wells	
	Inconsistent pipetting	
	Edge effect	Ensure wells have the same temperature and humidity, use plate sealers and shaking
	Non-homogenous samples	
	Stacked plates	

The normalised OD value is calculated as follows:

1. Non-competitive EIAs: divide the sample OD value by the cut-off OD value
2. Competitive assays: divide the cut-off OD value by the sample OD value.

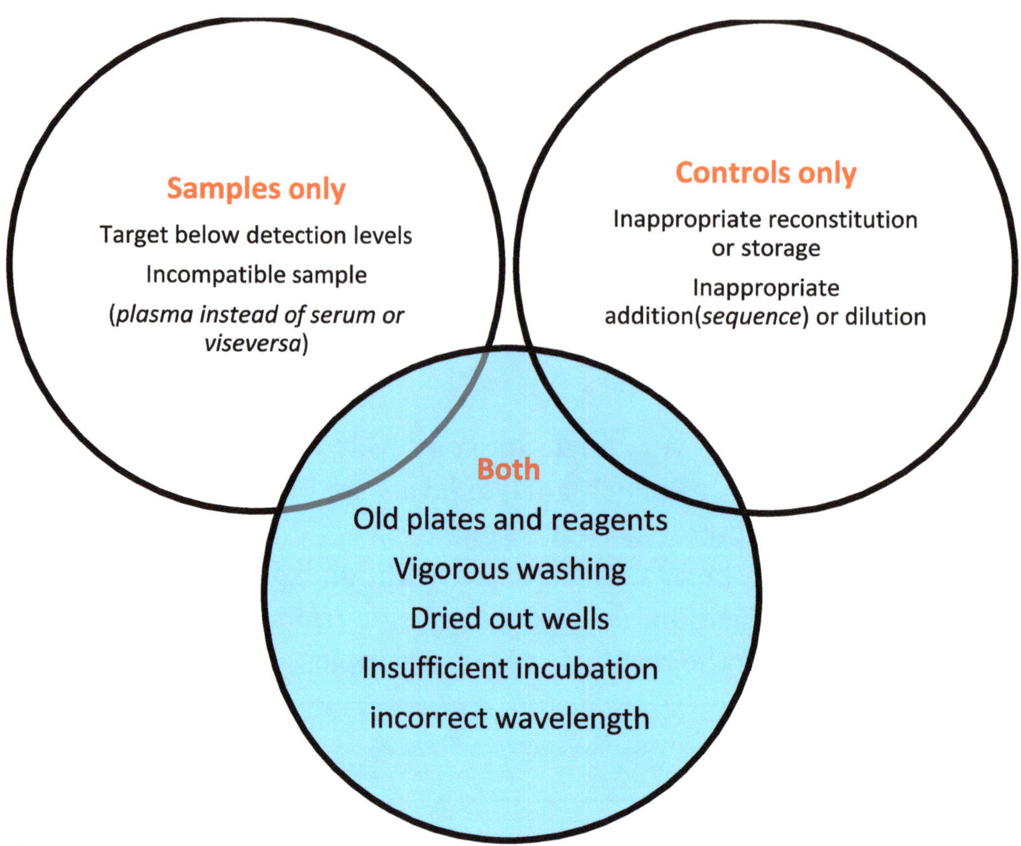

Figure 1. Possible sources of low signals in ELISA

Chemiluminescent immunoassay (CLIA): an immunoassay technique where the label, i.e. the actual "indicator" of the analytic reaction, is a luminescent molecule.

Principle: Luminescence is the emission of visible or near-visible (λ = 300–800 nm) radiation generated when electron transitions from an excited state to a ground state. The resultant potential energy in the atom gets released in the form of light.

Luminescence has an advantage over absorbance in Spectrophotometry because it is an absolute measure, whereas the latter is relative. We reference chemiluminescence because the type of luminescence applied to immunoassay techniques generally identifies exergonic chemical reactions as the most suitable energy source for producing the electronically excited state.

   i. Direct—uses luminophore markers; competitive or non-competitive
  ii. Indirect—uses enzyme markers; competitive or non-competitive

Luminophore markers	Enzymatic markers		Enhancers
Acridinium and Ruthenium esters	**Substrate**	**Enzyme**	Ferrocyanide Metallic ions
	Adamantyl 1, 2-dioxetane aryl phosphate (AMPPD)	Alkaline phosphatase	
	Luminol or its derivatives	Horseradish peroxidase	

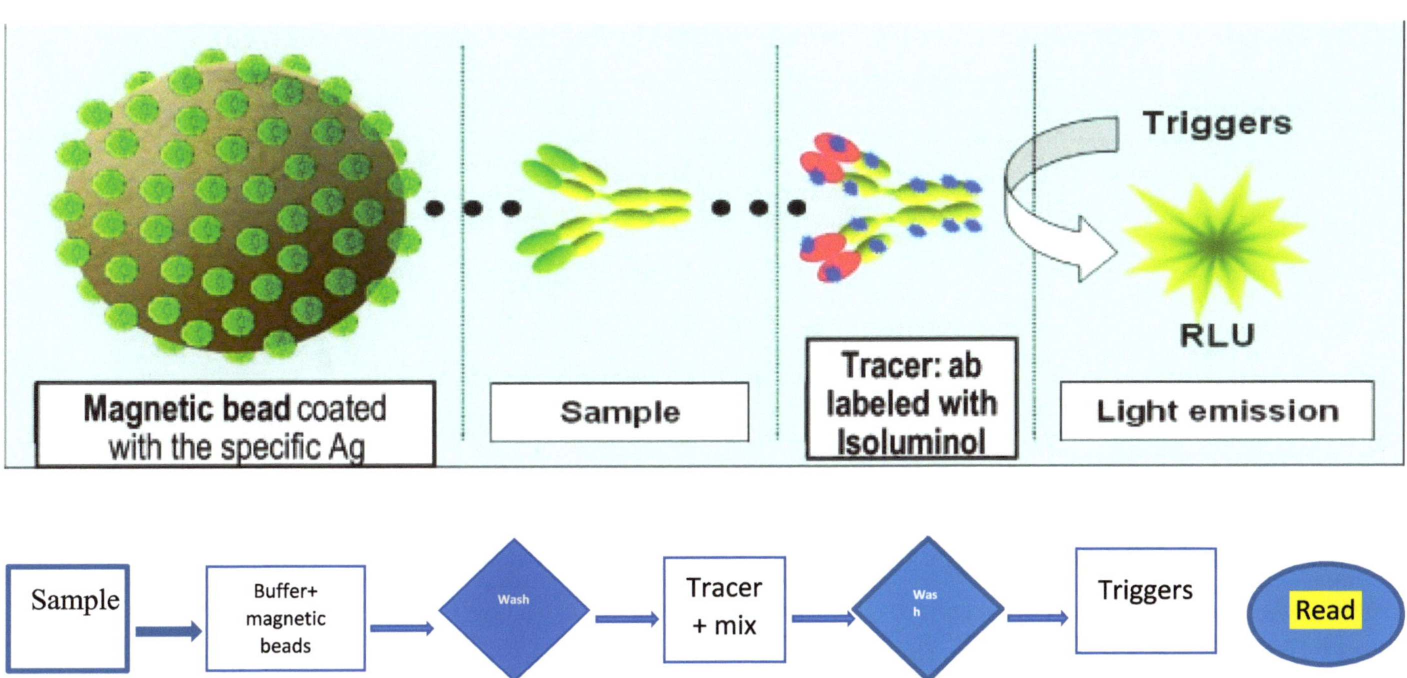

ELISA	Chemiluminescence	Radioimmunoassay
Stop solution required	No	No
Least sensitive	Most sensitive	Moderate
Requirement for a light source	Only filter	No

19.2 MANDATORY TTI INFECTION TESTING IN INDIA:

An infection in the recipient wherein there is evidence that it was acquired following transfusion with blood components, and there was no evidence of infection prior to transfusion and no evidence of an alternate source of infection and

At least one of the components received by the infected recipient was donated by a donor who had evidence of the same transmissible infection

Or

At least one component received by the infected recipient was shown to contain the infection

So TTI diagnosis requires all the following:

- Documentation of seronegativity of patients in the pretransfusion sample
- Investigations in both patients and implicated donors
- Exclusion of other modes of transmission
- Viral genotyping in the recipient and donor reveals the presence of the same genotype

Index donation: the product from the donation that the infected recipient received

Patient details	Clinical details
Full name	Consultant with speciality
Address	Likely timing of infection/transfusion
Date of birth	Reason for transfusion
Sex	Underlying diagnosis
Ethnic origin	Current condition
Travel history	Clinical evidence of post-transfusion infection
Laboratory details	**Transfusion details**
Laboratory reports for infectious markers	Components transfused, blood group,
Test results on samples prior to transfusion	Expiry date, the outcome of transfusion
Liver function test results (hepatitis cases)	Donor details of each component
	Test results of index and subsequent donations from each donor
	Additional testing
	If bacterial- colour change

Possible sources of infection: hospital admission, invasive medical procedures, infected sexual partner, IVDU, laboratory accident or vertical transmission

Investigating possible transmission by transfusion	
Viral infections	window period, error in testing
Parasitic infections	Travel history
Bacterial infections	Arm swab, donor illness in recent times, scarring or skin lesions at the venepuncture site

Investigation on Donor:

- Demographic information
- Travel history
- Outdoor activities
- History of exposure to the agent
- Clinical manifestations consistent with infection

Look Back: In 2 situations

1. When the donor is newly identified as infected
2. When a new screening test is applied to all blood donations

HIV

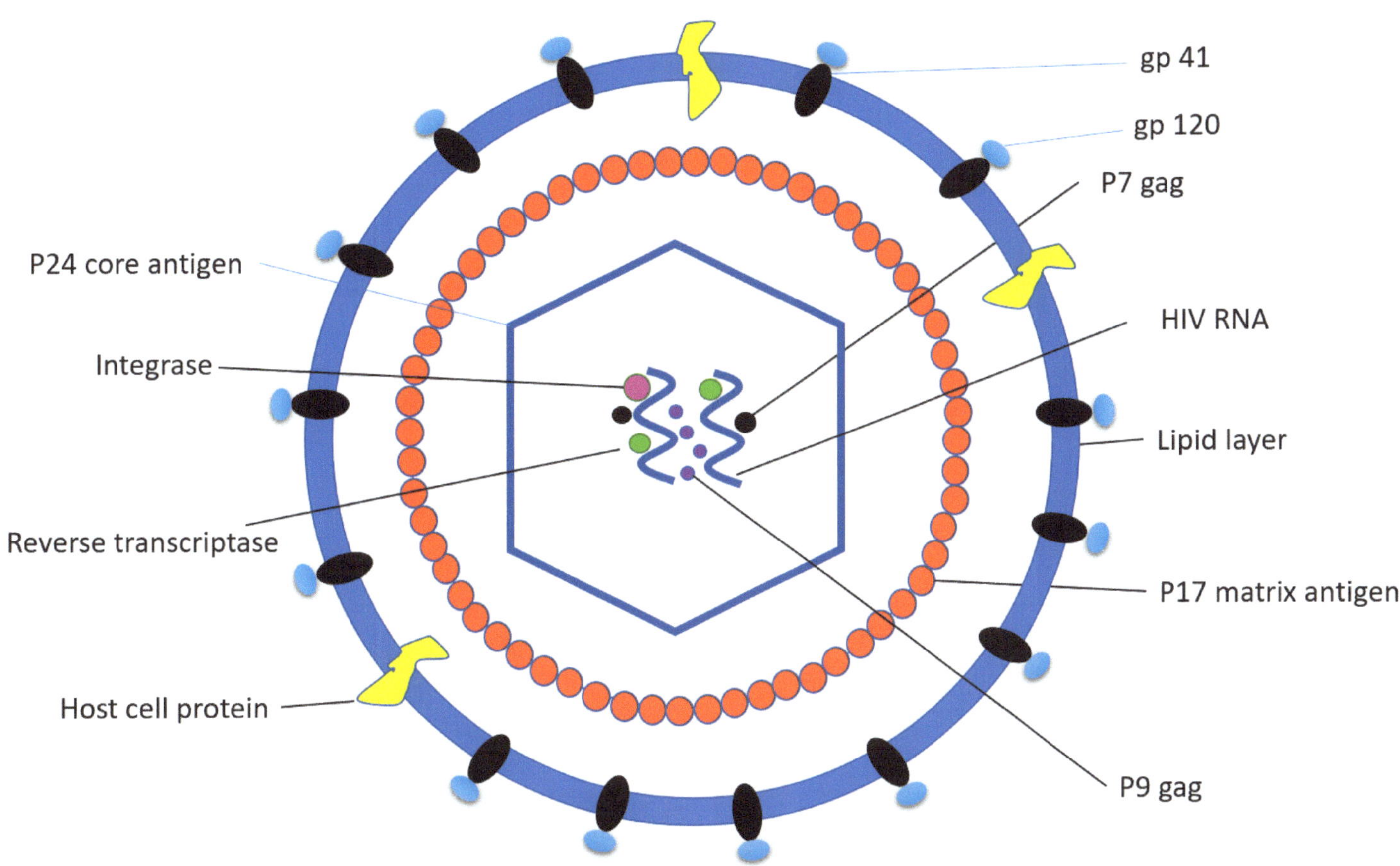

Retroviruses: Lentivirus(HIV 1 and 2), Oncovirus (HTLV 1 and 2)

HIV-1 and HIV-2

According to NACO guidelines, a Single test (enzyme-linked immunosorbent assay [ELISA] or rapid diagnostic tests) is mandatory for screening donated blood in blood banks.

Under the NACP, the most commonly employed rapid tests are based on the principle of

- Dipstick and comb assay based on Enzyme Immune Assay (EIA)
- Immunochromatographic assay (lateral flow),
- Immunoconcentration /dot-blot assays (vertical flow)
- Particle agglutination assay.

All these different rapid tests should have a sensitivity of ≥99.5% and a specificity of ≥98%.

Table 19.1 HIV

Test Generation	Antigen source	Window period (weeks)	Detects	Sensitivity (%)	Specificity
1st (1985)	Virus-infected cell lysate	8-10	IgG anti- HIV1	99	95-98%
2nd (1987)	Lysate and recombinant	4-6	IgG anti- HIV1& HIV2	>99.5	>99%
3rd (1992)	Recombinant and synthetic peptides (Antigen sandwich format)	2-3	IgG and IgM anti- HIV1, HIV2 and Group O	>99.5	>99.5
4th	Recombinant and synthetic peptides (Antigen/Antibody combo)	2	IgG and IgM anti- HIV1, HIV2 and Group O + HIV1p24 Ag	>99.8	>99.5
5th	Multiplex analysis with separate results for each analyte.	2	IgG and IgM anti- HIV1, HIV2 and Group O + HIV1p24 Ag	100	>99.5
P24	>10,000 RNA copies per ml	15 days			
NAT (2001)		9 days			
Id NAT	5 copies per ml				

Immunoconcentration / Dot Blot immunoassay (vertical flow)

This type of solid-phase immunoassay is where HIV antigens are immobilised on a porous membrane.

- Specimens with added reagents pass through a membrane and are absorbed into the underlying absorbent pad.
- As the specimen passes through the membrane, HIV antibodies, if present, bind to the immobilised antigens.
- The conjugate binds to the Fc portion of the HIV antibodies producing a distinct coloured dot against a white background.

Immunochromatography Tests

The strips/cards incorporate antigen and signal reagents into the nitrocellulose strip.

- The test device is incorporated with the following:
  - 1st band of purified gp120 and gp41 synthetic peptides, specific to HIV-1 at test region '1' and
  - 2nd band of purified gp36 synthetic peptide specific to HIV-2 at test region '2.'
  - 3rd band incorporated at region 'C' corresponds to the assay performance control.
- The specimen (with or without a buffer) is applied to the absorbent pad on the kit, which migrates through the strip.
- If present, antibodies to HIV-1 and/or 2 are captured by the respective antigens
- After washing with a buffer, the Protein A conjugated reagent is added to reveal the presence/absence of bound antibodies.

- A positive reaction results in a visual coloured line on the membrane at specific sites where the HIV antigen has been incorporated.
- The appearance of a control band validates the test
- The absence of bands at test regions '1' & '2' is a negative test result.

Particle Agglutination Tests

The antigen is coated onto a carrier particle, and the antigen-antibody reaction is observed in clumps.

- These assays incorporate various antigen-coated carriers, e.g., red cells, latex particles, gelatine particles and microbeads.
- During the agglutination reaction, an HIV antibody in the patient's sera combines with the HIV antigen on the carrier particles and appears in clumps.

Immunocomb Assay:

The comb test consists of a comb-like device with projections.

- Each tooth of the comb represents the solid phase and has three spots for the adsorption of a specific antigen/antibody.
    - HIV-1 and HIV-2 antigens are immobilised as circular spots at two sites.
    - The thi[rd] spot acts as an antibody control containing goat anti-human IgG.
- The test is carried out by sequentially immersing the comb in wells with ready-to-use reagents.
- When the comb is incubated with a serum containing HIV antibodies, these antibodies bind to the antigen on the comb.
- The complex is then visualised after the addition of antibody-enzyme conjugate and substrate.

Hepatitis B:

Belongs to Hepadna virus type 1(orthohepadna)

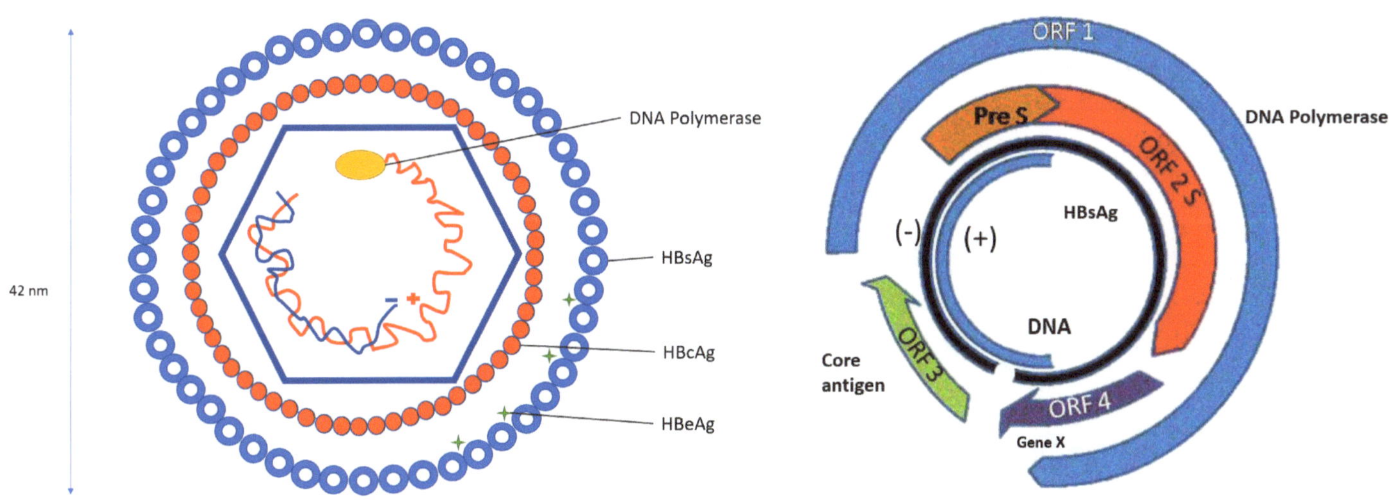

Gene		Protein	
S		HBsAg (Major Protein)	
S + Pre S2		Middle protein	
S + Pre S1+ Pre S2		Large protein	
P	Largest gene	DNA polymerase	directs replication and repair of HBV DNA
C	Initiation from pre-C	HBeAg (soluble, secreted protein)	Nucleocapsid proteins
	Initiation after pre-C	HBcAg (intracellular core protein)	
X		HBxAg	transactivate the transcription of cellular and viral genes

Three particulate forms:

1. Double-shelled virion (surface and core) spherical (42nm); antigens s,c,e
2. Nucleocapsid core (27nm); antigens c and e
3. Spherical and filamentous; represents excess virus coat material(22nm); s antigen only. Most numerous form

Genotypes: 10 (A to J)

Subtypes: 8, Common reactive antigen a with either *d* or *w,y* or *r*

Subtype A(adw) and D(ayw): the US and Europe

Subtype B (adw) and C (adr): Asia

Genotype B is associated with less rapidly progressive liver disease and cirrhosis, lower likelihood or delayed appearance, and hepatocellular carcinoma than genotype C or D.

Genotype A is more likely to clear circulating viremia and achieve hepatitis B e antigen (HBeAg) and HBsAg seroconversion, both spontaneously and in response to antiviral therapy

Host Factors	
Age	Propensity to Chronicity is inversely related to age Chronic hepatitis happens in 80-90% of perinatal, 30-50% of <6 yrs old and <5% of healthy adults Acute hepatitis happens in 1% of perinatal, 10% of 1-5 yrs old and 30% of >5yrs
High-risk groups	Surgeons, healthcare and laboratory personnel, blood transfusion recipients, commercial sex workers, LGBT, iv drug abusers, infants of HBV carrier mothers, immunocompromised patients, organ transplant recipients

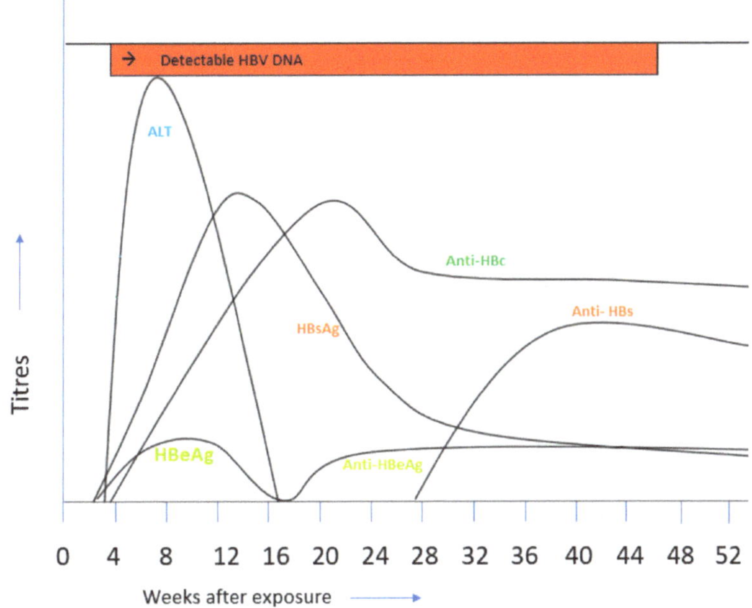

➢ HBcAg particles remain inside the hepatocyte: detectable by immunohistochemical staining. They are exported after encapsidation by an envelope of HbsAg; hence, naked core particles do not circulate in the serum.

➢ HBsAg-positive serum-containing HBeAg is more likely to be highly infectious. The persistence of HBeAg in serum beyond the first three months of acute infection may be predictive of the development of chronic infection

Surrogate markers	Aminotransferases	Up to 100 times normal
	Bilirubin levels	Mild to moderate elevation (5-10mg/dL)
Serological markers (By Enzyme Immuno Assays, Radioimmunoassay, OR Chemiluminescence)	HBSAg	Also, present in chronic HBV carriers but not consistently detectable
	Anti-HBs	Immunisation with HBSAg (after vaccination), Hepatitis B in the remote past or False-positive
	HBcAg	They are exported after encapsidation by an envelope of HbsAg, and hence, naked core particles do not circulate in the serum
	Anti-HBc	Typically persists for the lifetime. Identifies "escape mutants."
	HBeAg	Marker of active disease and high infectivity
	Anti-HBe	It appears with the disappearance of HBeAg
Molecular Assays	HBV DNA	By RT PCR, the limit of detection is 10 to 20 international units/mL

Problems with using Antibody to HBcAg as a screening method:

- Poor specificity, high false positivity
- Usage is limited to low-prevalence countries only, as donor loss rates would be unacceptably high in endemic areas

Common serological patterns and their interpretation

HBsAg	Anti-HBs	Anti-HBc	HBeAg	Anti-HBe	Remarks/Interpretation
+	-	IgM	+	-	Acute hepatitis B, high infectivity
+	-	IgG	+		Chronic hepatitis B, high infectivity
+	-	IgG	-	+	Late acute or chronic hepatitis B, low infectivity HBeAg-negative ("pre-core-mutant") hepatitis B (chronic or, rarely, acute)
+	+	+	±	±	HBsAg of one subtype and heterotypic anti-HBs Process of seroconversion from HBsAg to anti-HBs
-	-	IgM	±	±	Acute hepatitis Anti-HBc "window"
-	-	IgG	-	±	Low-level hepatitis B carrier Hepatitis B in remote past
-	+	IgG	-	±	Recovery from hepatitis B
-	+	-	-	-	Immunisation with HBsAg Hepatitis B in the remote past False-positive

Occult Hepatitis B Infection(OBI): (Silent infection)

International workshop (2008) Italy definition: "detection of HBV DNA in the liver or tissues (with or without HBV DNA in serum) without HBsAg."

OBI

Seropositive(80%): detection of anti-HBc antibody with or without anti-HBs antibody

The detection of anti-HBc is a good test for this

Seronegative(20%): both anti-HBc and anti-HBs antibodies undetectable

screening of HBV by the NAT is effective for this subgroup

Mechanisms of OBI:

- A mutation in the "a" determinant of the surface antigen brings a structural arrangement of the protein, leading to undetectable HBsAg by commercially HBsAg test kits
- Mutations in the S region lead to reduced expression of HBV surface proteins
- Substitution of nt (no turning) G-to-A at position 458 of the surface gene interferes with the splicing of S gene mRNA and is associated with a lack of HBsAg expression

The prevalence of OBI among blood donors in India is about anti-HBc, 10.22%; HBV DNA, 0.15%.

Test Generation	Test Description	Window period	Infective Dose
1st Generation	Gel diffusion		
2nd Generation	Counterimmuno electrophoresis		
3rd Generation	RIA, ELISA, RPHA		
4th Generation	HBsAg and Anti-HBcAg	38-44	

HCV

	In India	Global
Prevalence	1-2% in blood donors	High prevalence: Eastern Mediterranean (Egypt, Greece, Turkey etc.)- >2% Moderate prevalence (1-2%) Asia,Africa Low prevalence: Americas, Australias- <1%
Transmission	Blood Transfusion (MC) Therapeutic injections iv drug use Dialysis and renal Transplant iv drug abuse Blood transfusion Body piercing, scarification Perinatal transmission, Immunoglobulins	
High-risk groups	Healthcare workers Household contacts Prisoners Sexual contacts iv drug users Homosexuals	

Test Generation	Antigen source	Window period	Remarks	Sensitivity (%)	specificity
1st (1989)	c100-3 (recombinant NS4)	12-26 weeks	Only 12% of the genome	~ 80	99.6
2nd (1992)	NS4(C200,HC-31)+ core(c22-3) and NS3(c33c)	10-24 weeks (Avg 82 days)		> 99	99.7
3rd (1996)	+NS5	7-8 weeks (66 Days)		~100	97.4
4th (2003)	Ag+Ab	26 days		~100	~99

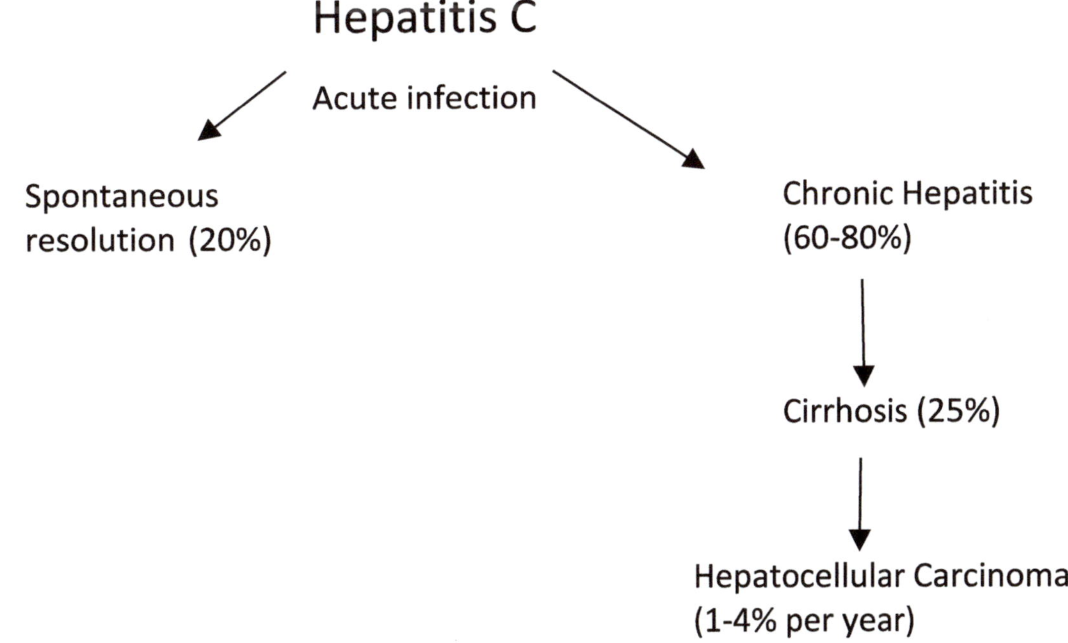

Figure 19. Natural history of Hepatitis C

ELISA	Chemiluminescence
"Splashing" of wells	Fewer false positives (more specific)
	Fewer low-positives (Better positive predictive values)
	Shorter turnaround time
	Higher throughput
	Fully automated
	Technically simpler, reliable and precise

False positives: Cross-reactive antigens/antibodies in Pregnancy, HIV, HBV, Herpes simplex

In blood centres, Viral nucleic acids are detected by one of the two technologies

1. PCR; and
2. Transfusion-mediated amplification (TMA).

PCR: This is an ideal method for DNA amplification. However, as RNA amplification is required for HCV, a reverse-transcription step is needed to generate cDNA. It is possible to incorporate reverse transcriptase and DNA polymerase in the same reaction into a single step.

TMA technology: uses two enzymes-RNA polymerases and reverse transcriptase (RT). The RT enzyme creates cDNA.This serves as a template to generate RNA by the activity of the enzyme RNA polymerase. About a billion RNA amplicons can be produced in less than an hour.

ID-NAT: detects as low as 2.0 to 9.4 IU/mL.

NAT testing reduced the infectious pre-seroconversion period dramatically to 4 to 6 days

It also helped to detect immunosilent carriers

Occult hepatitis C infection (OCI): The presence of HCV RNA in hepatocytes or peripheral blood mononuclear cells (PBMCs) and the absence of HCV RNA in serum.

The gold standard for OCI diagnosis: The detection of HCV RNA by nucleic acid amplification testing (NAT) from hepatocytes of biopsied liver

At-risk populations:

- patients with treated hepatitis C liver disease
- hemodialysis patients

Serologic window period:

Phase I: nucleic acid and antigen are not detectable

Phase II: nucleic acid and antigen are potentially detectable, but antibodies are not

The window period for HCV NAT itself has recently been reported to be 2.5 and 4.9 days, respectively, for NAT individual and mini-pool testing

Malaria

Indian Scenario: It is described as unstable transmission as it is seasonal with an increased intensity related to rains. Hence the immunity is also uncertain. Transmission is intense in forest areas, and the burden is concentrated in children. Semi-immune individuals may harbour parasites without having any symptoms.

High transmission areas	>1 case/1000 population	Northeastern states, Jharkhand, Chhattisgarh, Madhya Pradesh, Orissa, Andhra Pradesh, Gujarat, West Bengal, Rajasthan, Karnataka
Low transmission areas	<1 case/1000 population	Rest of the states

Parasite	Prevalence	Distribution	Incubation period	Communicability	Relapse
Plasmodium vivax (Pv)	40%, 8%(mixed Pf+Pv)	Throughout India	8-17 days	4-5 days	3 yrs
Plasmodium falciparum (Pf)	50%	Throughout India	9-14 days	10-12 days	1-2 yrs
Plasmodium malariae	<1%	Karnataka (Tumkur,Hassan)	18-40 days		40 yrs
Plasmodium ovale	-	-	16-18 days		3 yrs

Vectors in India	
Species	**Areas**
Anopheles culicifacies, Species A for P. Vivax and P. Falciparum Species B for P. Falciparum	Rural and peri-urban
Anopheles stephensi	Urban and industrial
Anopheles fluviatilis	Hilly, forest
Anopheles minimus	Foothills(Northeast)
Anopheles dirus	Forest (Northeast)
Anopheles epiroticus	Andaman and Nicobar

Laboratory diagnosis of Malaria		
Direct Methods	Light microscopy	*Sensitivity: 4 to 20 parasites/mcL of blood*
	Fluorescent microscopy	*Dyes like acridine orange detect RNA and DNA contents of parasites. Cheap and sensitivities up to 90%*
	Quantitative Buffy coat (QBC) Becton-Dickinson	*Useful for screening a large number of samples quick. The capillary tube is filled with 50-100 µl of blood and centrifuged. Parasites are concentrated below the granulocyte layer in the tube.* ***Disadv:*** *cost, cannot be stored for reference later*
Serologic	Antigen based	1. Histidine-rich protein 2 (HRP2, for detection of P. falciparum) 2. Plasmodium lactate dehydrogenase (pLDH, for detection of all species or specific detection of P. falciparum or P. vivax) 3. Aldolase (for detection of all species)
	Antibody-based	*It becomes positive two weeks after infection, and mostly the donor is no more infectious*
Molecular	PCR LAMP assays (Loop-mediated isothermal amplification)	*generally limited to reference laboratories and is primarily for research and epidemiologic purposes*

Host Factors	
Age	Affects all ages. Newborn infants are resistant to Pf(due to HbF)
Sex	Males (outdoor life, lesser clothing)
Race	Sickle cell trait has a milder illness, Duffy negative are resistant to Pv
Pregnancy	Higher infectivity causes IUD, preterm labour and miscarriage
Socioeconomic status	Predominantly agriculture, ill-ventilated and lit houses, sleeping outdoors, lower socioeconomic status

Peripheral smear: Smears should be prepared as soon as possible after collecting venous blood to avoid changes in parasite morphology

	Thick film	Thin film
Threshold of detection	5-20 parasites/L	100 parasites/L
RBCs	Lysed	Fixed
Volume required	Comparatively larger 0.25µl/100 fields	Smaller 0.005µl/100 fields
Blood elements	Concentrated	Single layer spread out
Utility	Screening test	Species differentiation
Time required to examine	Shorter	Longer

Malaria Serology		
Features	**PfHRP-2**	**pLDH**
Principle	Uses Monoclonal Antibody	Both monoclonal and polyclonal
Detection threshold	10 parasites/ µl	≥100 parasites/µl
Cross-reaction with other species	No	Yes, with all Pv, Po, Pm
Sensitivity	94-100%	Pf 88-98%, Pv 89-94%
Specificity	88-100%	Pf 93-99%, Pv 99-100%

Acceptance criteria for RDTs

P. falciparum panel detection score > 75% at 200 parasites/µl

P. vivax panel detection score > 75% at 200 parasites/µl

False positive rate < 10%

Invalid rate < 5%

Band intensity: Usually given a score of 0 to 4, with 4 being a perfectly visible band to 0 being no band at all.

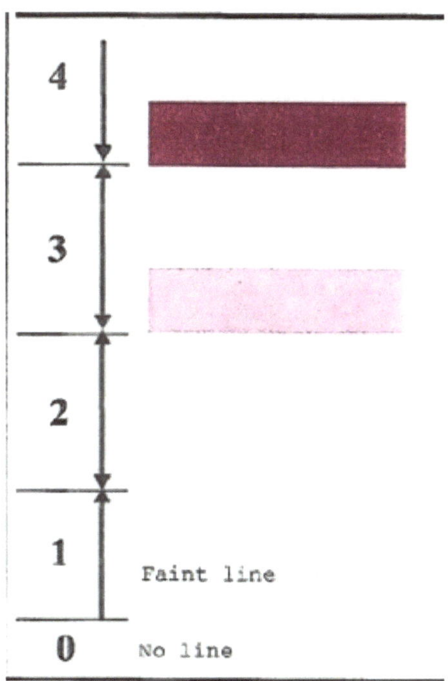

Worked Example: 3 samples of blood, namely A, B, and C, known to have a P.falciparum parasitic density of 200/µl, were used to evaluate a new Rapid Card test introduced into the market. Two cards, each from 2 different lot numbers, were tested. The results obtained are tabulated below.

	LOT NO 20180101		LOT NO 20180103	
	KIT 1	KIT 2	KIT 1	KIT 2
A	C [Pan Pv Pf] A☐ ⊙B	C [Pan Pv Pf] A☐ ⊙B	C [Pan Pv Pf] A☐ ⊙B	C [Pan Pv Pf] A☐ ⊙B
B	C [Pan Pv Pf] A☐ ⊙B	C [Pan Pv Pf] A☐ ⊙B	C [Pan Pv Pf] A☐ ⊙B	C [Pan Pv Pf] A☐ ⊙B
C	C [Pan Pv Pf] A☐ ⊙B	C [Pan Pv Pf] A☐ ⊙B	C [Pan Pv Pf] A☐ ⊙B	C [Pan Pv Pf] A☐ ⊙B

Calculate the   a) Positivity rate

                 b) Panel Detection Score

The positivity rate: calculated as the percentage of all tests of a particular product that returned a positive test result at the manufacturers' recommended minimum reading time when tested against a P. falciparum or P. vivax sample.

i.e 9/12 = 75%

(9 is the number of tests that yielded positive results total, and 12 is the number of total tests done)

Panel detection score: The percentage number of samples that were positive all the time it was tested.

i.e 1/3 = 33%

(Only 1 of the sample, C, turned out to be positive in all 4 tests amongst the three samples tested A, B and C)

> ➤ The positivity rate is always greater than the PDS, except when the PDS and the positivity rate are both 100%

Syphilis

Laboratory diagnosis of Syphilis		
Serologic	Non-Treponemal tests	Rapid plasma reagin (RPR)
		Venereal Disease Research Laboratory (VDRL) assays
		Toluidine Red Unheated Serum Test (TRUST)
	Treponemal tests	Fluorescent treponemal antibody absorption (FTA-ABS)
		Treponema pallidum particle agglutination (TP-PA)
		Microhemagglutination test for antibodies to T. pallidum (MHA-TP)
		Enzyme immunoassay (EIA)
		Multiplex flow immunoassay (MFI)
		Chemiluminescence immunoassay (CIA)
Direct Methods		Darkfield microscopy
		Direct fluorescent antibody (DFA) testing
		Polymerase chain reaction (PCR) tests

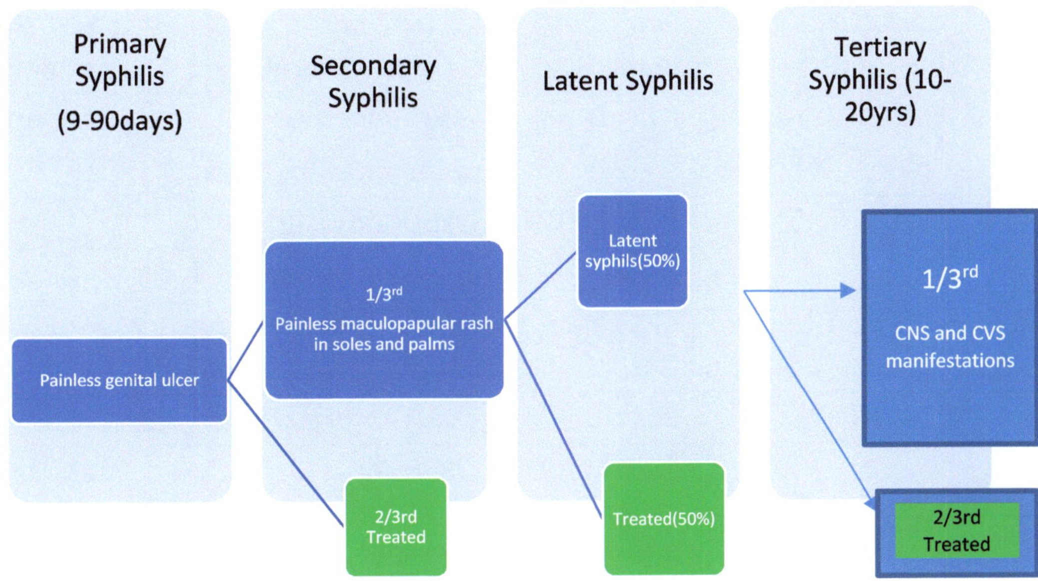

Figure 20. The natural history of Syphilis

Traditional Algorithm	Reverse Algorithm
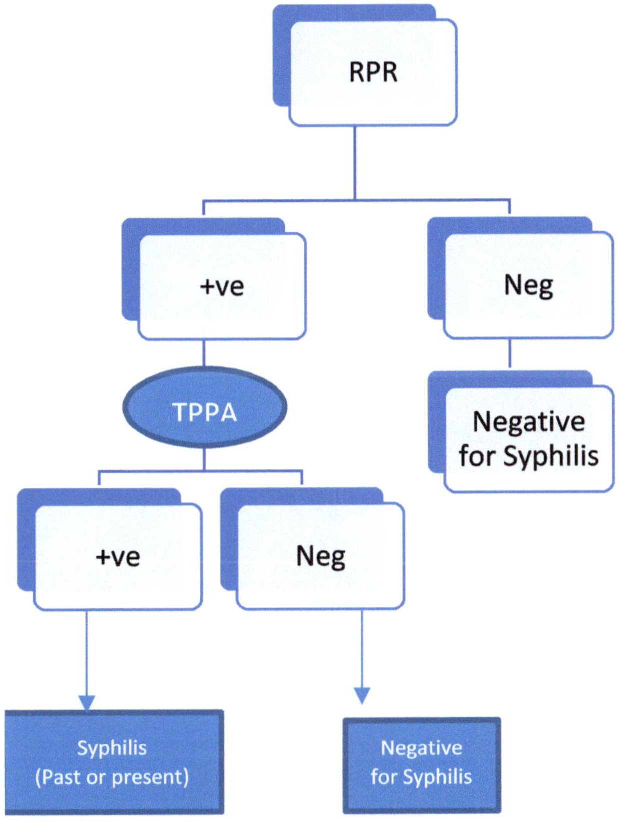 RPR → +ve → TPPA → +ve → Syphilis (Past or present); TPPA → Neg → Negative for Syphilis. RPR → Neg → Negative for Syphilis	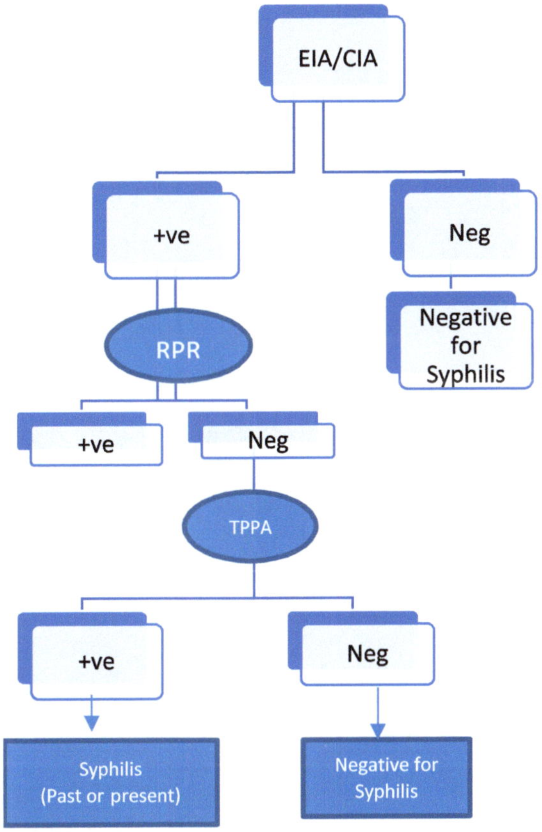 EIA/CIA → +ve → RPR → +ve → Syphilis (Past or present); RPR → Neg → TPPA → +ve → Syphilis (Past or present), TPPA → Neg → Negative for Syphilis. EIA/CIA → Neg → Negative for Syphilis
Reliable, especially in high-prevalence settings	More specific – better for low prevalence areas
Rapid, easy, and economical	Higher cost
Low throughput	Amenable to automation
Subjective interpretation	Objective interpretation
Non-specific, High false positives	Enhanced sensitivity to late and latent infection

Agent	Markers detected	Screening tests	Confirmatory/ supplemental tests	Additional information
HTLV I/II	Anti-HTLV-I/II (IgG) antibodies	EIA or ChLIA	Western Blot Line immunoblots	Diagnostic window = 51 days
West Nile virus	RNA	PCR or TMA	Antibody (IgM or IgG)	
Zika	RNA	PCR or TMA	Antibody (IgM or IgG)	
Trypanosoma	(IgG) antibodies	EIA or ChLIA	Enzyme strip assay	
Babesia	DNA/RNA	PCR or TMA	Research antibody	
CMV		EIA, Latex agglutination test	PCR	IgM antibodies indicate recent infection
Parvovirus		NAT	Antibody (IgM 6-10 days) (IgG 12th day onwards)	Low virus concentration detectable for up to 12 months

19.3 L J CHART:

– Dr. Remi R

- **Label the charts.** Include

  Name of the test, Name of the control material

  The measurement unit (in the label or the label for the y-axis)

  Name of the analytical system, the lot number of the control,

  Current mean and standard deviation, Time period covered by the chart.

- x-axis: label as days, date of run- typically 1 to 30
- y-axis: label as control value(E-ratios) -from -4 SD to +4SD

The rule of thumb is to collect 20 values over preferably 4 weeks or 20 working days

Calculations

Calculate the Mean $(\bar{x})$

Calculate the variance, and square the variance $(x - \bar{x})^2$

Calculate the sum of the square of the variance $\sum (x - \bar{x})^2$

Calculate Standard deviation (SD) = $\sqrt{\dfrac{\sum (x - \bar{x})^2}{n-1}}$

Now calculate mean+1SD, mean+2SD, mean-1SD, mean-2SD and so on

Draw a green horizontal line at the mean, yellow at 2 SD and red at 3SD

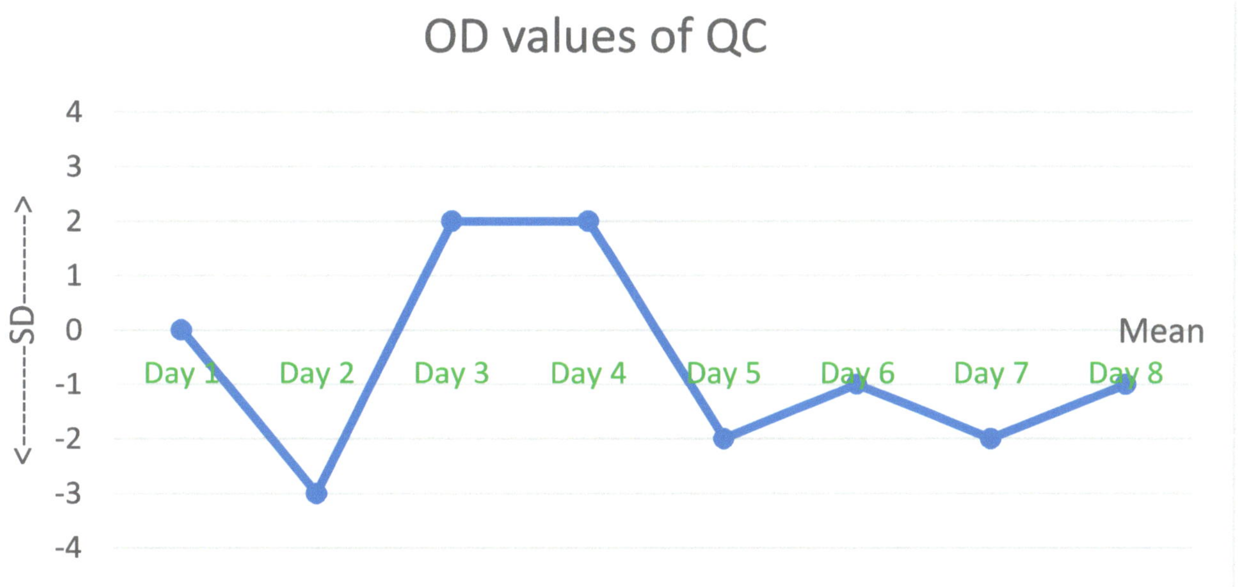

Westgard Rules (Ref Fig 1)				
Rule	**Description**	**Action**	**Remarks**	**Fig**
13S	One value of ± 3 SD	Reject		Day 2
12S	One value of ± 2 SD	Warning	Careful inspection	Day 3
22S	Two consecutive values of ± 2 SD	Reject		Day 3 & 4
R4S	control measurement in a group exceeds the mean plus 2s, and another exceeds the mean minus 2s	Reject	Only within the run and not in different runs	Day 4 to 5
41S		Reject		Day 5 to 8
10X	10 consecutive control measurements fall on one side of the mean.	Reject	Only when two different control materials are measured 1 or 2 times per material.	
8X	8 consecutive control measurements fall on one side of the mean.	Reject		
Other Multi rules (Ref Fig.2)				
2 of 32S	Two out of three control measurements	Reject		Day 1 to 3
7T	7 control measurements in the same direction (increasing or decreasing)	Reject		Day 4 to 10

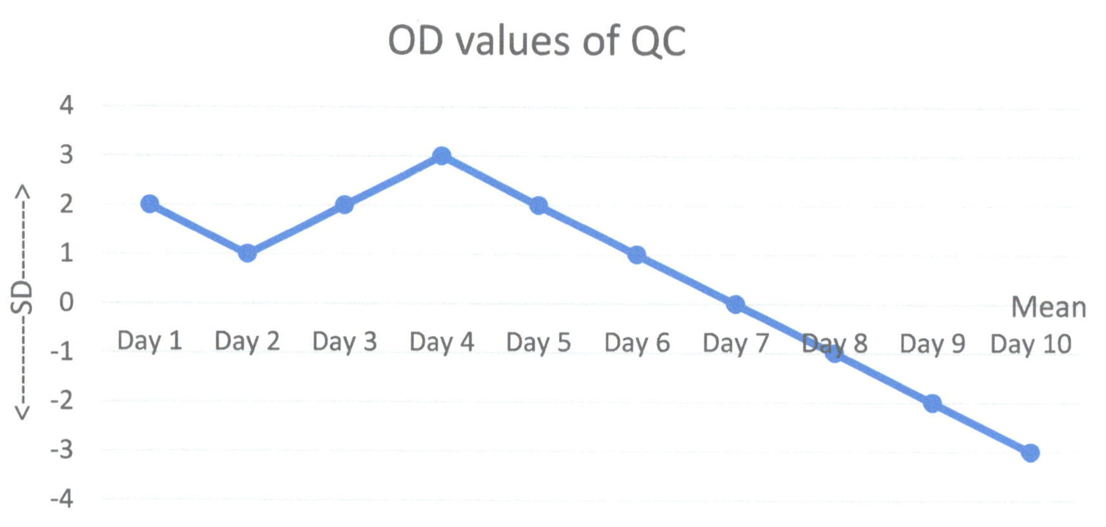

	Shift	**Trend**
Definition	Abrupt changes in the control mean (sudden and dramatic) positive or negative change	A gradual loss of reliability in the test system
	Causes:	Causes:
Light source	Failure/change	Deterioration
Tubings	Sudden blockage	Debris accumulation
Electrode surface		Corrosion
Reagents	Change in lot	Ageing
Calibration	Inaccurate	Gradual deterioration
Machine	Major maintenance issues	Minor
	Failure of sampling or dispensing system	
Incubation	Change in room temperature/humidity	Enzyme deterioration

19.4. NUCLEIC ACID AMPLIFICATION TESTING

– Dr. Veena

Background

Screening blood products by sensitive serological tests and nucleic acid amplification tests (NAT) brings us closer to providing the safest blood. NAT performs sequence-specific viral genome detection. Many blood transfusion services across the globe started using NAT assay in blood donor screening to minimize the residual risk of transfusion-transmitted infections.

NAT in developed countries:

Germany started using NAT screening in1997 when many transfusion-transmitted HIV and HCV infections were reported. HIV-1 NAT was made mandatory in Germany in 2004;anti-

Hepatitis-B core antibody testing in 2006. However, HBV NAT is not a mandatory test in Germany. Today, 100% blood supply in the US is screened with NAT for HCV, HIV-1, HBV and West Nile Virus.

In a survey by ISBT working party on Transfusion transmitted infectious diseases, the data from 33 countries which performed NAT screening of 300 million donations revealed a total of 2808 virus-contaminated donations worldwide from 1999 to 2009.

Indian Scenario:

Seroprevalence of transfusion-transmitted infections (TTI) in India is 0.26% for HIV,2-4% for HBV and 0.46% for HCV. Indian blood banks started establishing NAT testing facilities in 2008. Even now, approximately 2% of blood banks are performing NAT tests covering 7% of the blood collected in India per annum. It is not mandatory to screen donors using NAT according to Indian regulatory requirements. With its high seroprevalence of TTI and a high proportion of first-time and replacement donors, India will benefit from performing additional assays like NAT.

What is Nucleic acid amplification testing

It is a qualitative nucleic acid amplification test for detecting Transfusion transmitted viruses like HIV 1 & 2, HCV or HBV in blood, organ and tissue donors. It is based on amplifying a targeted viral RNA or DNA region. As the viral particles are detected by NAT earlier than the detection of antigens or antibodies by other screening methods, it can considerably reduce the window period.

It involves the following steps:

1. Sample preparation, viral concentration & nucleic acid extraction
2. Amplification of target DNA or RNA
3. Detection of the amplified product.

Molecular methods like a polymerase chain reaction and transcription-mediated amplification are commonly used for viral nucleic acid amplification in blood screening.

1. **Polymerase chain reaction**

   Kary Mullis developed the polymerase chain reaction in the 1980s. It is a molecular technique which involves thermal cycles to amplify the target DNA template. High temperatures (94-96 degrees) separate the DNA double strands in the first step. In the cooling phase, the primer oligonucleotides anneal to the complementary DNA target. In the third step, temperature-dependent DNA polymerases like Taq polymerase adds nucleotides to the end of the annealed primers. This generates a DNA strand complementary to the target DNA strand. Again this three-step cycle repeats. After each cycle, the copy number is doubled. For amplification of RNA targets, reverse transcription PCR is employed in which the reverse transcriptase enzyme makes a cDNA from the RNA template.

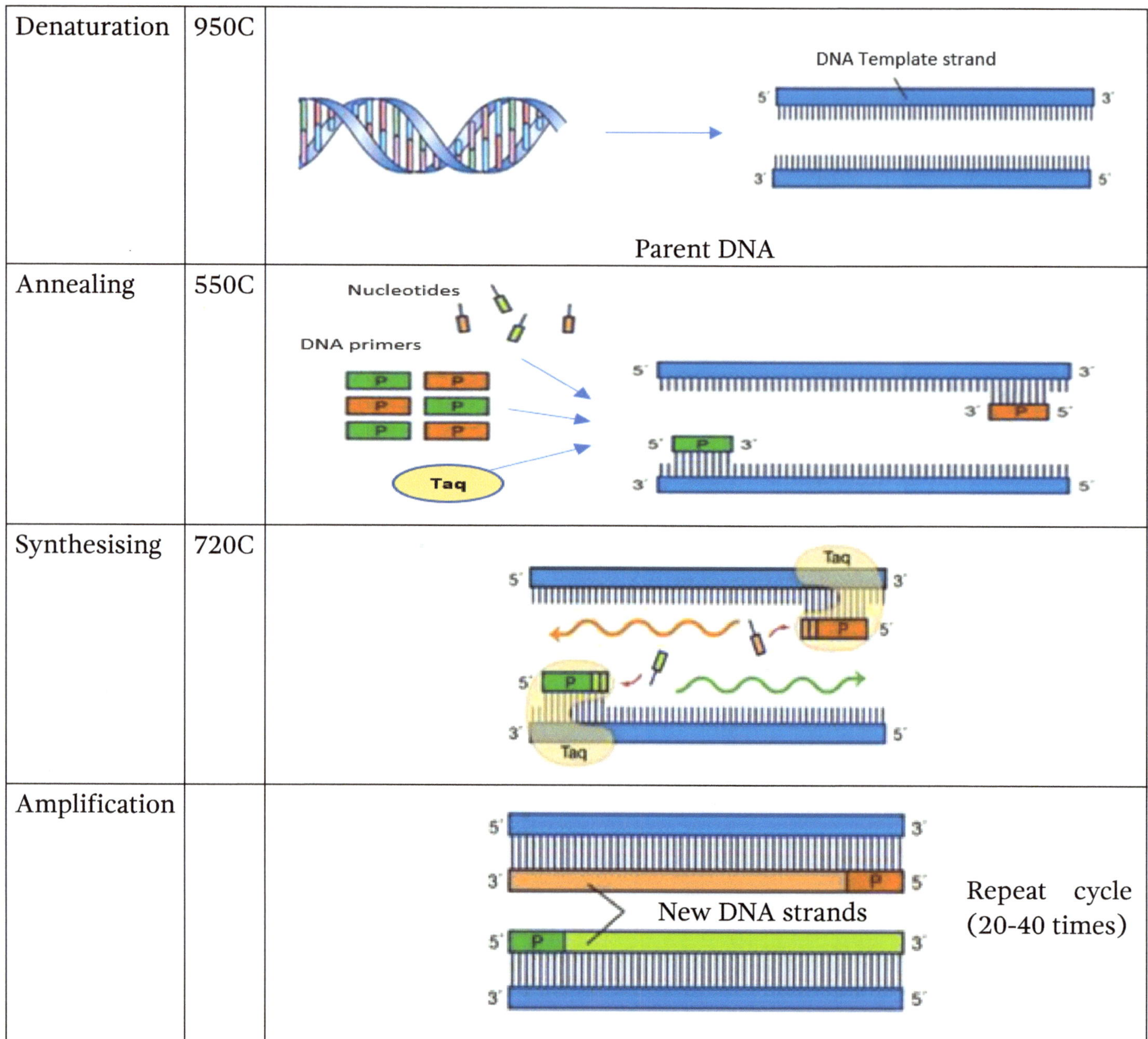

Fig 1:Principle of PCR

Real-time PCR

Real-time PCR is different from traditional PCR as the amount of nucleic acid present in the sample is being quantified as the reaction proceeds and hence does not require post-**PCR** methods.

The detection of fluorescent labelled sequence-specific DNA oligonucleotide probes is enabled when the probe hybridizes with its complementary sequence.

Specimen preparation: The Lysis reagent releases RNA or DNA from viral particles. The released nucleic acids bind to the positively charged **magnetic glass particles. Wash reagent** removes the unbound substances. Purified nucleic acids are eluted from the magnetic glass particles at high temperature with **Elution Buffer.**

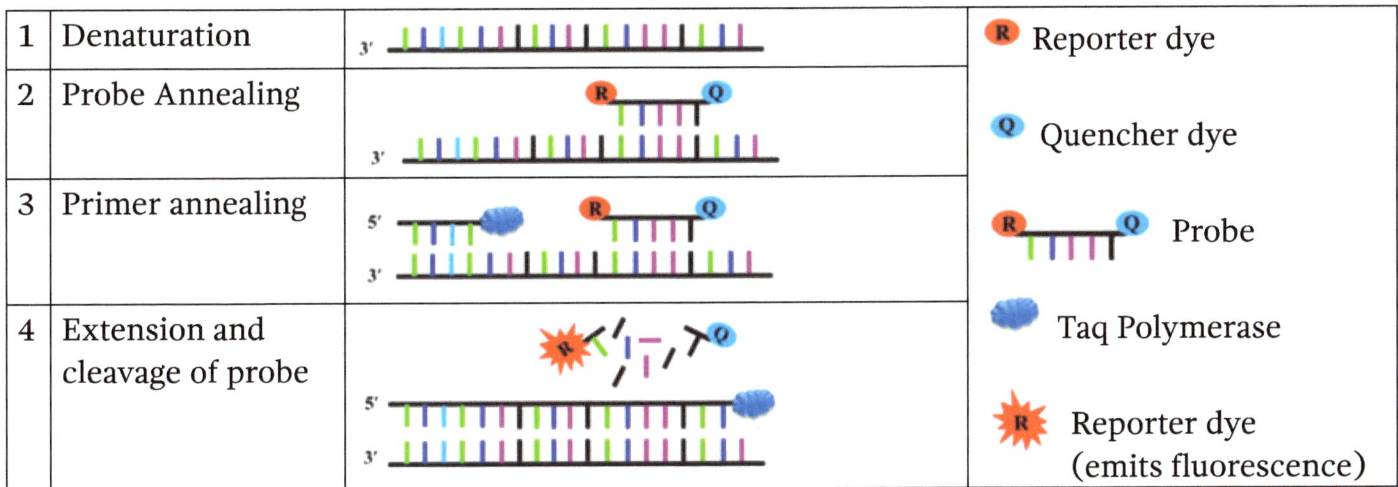

1	Denaturation		R Reporter dye
2	Probe Annealing		Q Quencher dye
3	Primer annealing		Probe
4	Extension and cleavage of probe		Taq Polymerase
			Reporter dye (emits fluorescence)

Figure 2: Principle of Real-time PCR

Amplification:

Master mix is the mixture of enzymes and cofactors required for the amplification.

Selective amplification is achieved by the use of **Amp Erase enzyme and deoxyuridine triphosphate** nucleotides. Deoxy uridine triphosphate nucleotides are one of the dNTPs in the master mix. Amp Erase enzyme causes selective destruction of DNA strands containing deoxyuridine. Hence unwanted amplicons are removed before the amplification of the target. Z05D DNA Polymerase having both reverse transcriptase and DNA polymerase activity, in the presence of manganese (Mn2+), performs both reverse Transcription and PCR amplification in the same reaction mixture. High temperature during the thermal cycling denatures the target amplicon and forms single-stranded DNA. The **oligonucleotide detection probes** hybridize with the single-stranded, amplified DNA.

Detection: Specific Probes labelled with unique fluorescent dyes are used for internal control, and each target, such as HIV-1 (Groups M and O), HIV-2, HCV, and HBV. Before the amplification process, the reporter dye on the probes is suppressed by the quencher dye. During amplification, probes hybridize into single-stranded DNA amplicons. The 5'-3'nuclease activity of the DNA polymerase separates the Reporter and quencher dye. This unmasks the reporter dye, and fluorescent signals are generated. Discrimination of viral markers is possible with the initial run itself. All three HIV targets are detected using the same fluorescent dye and hence cannot be discriminated against each other.

2. **Transcription-mediated amplification** (TMA)

TMA involves the reverse Transcription of RNA by isothermal amplification to generate multiple RNA copies by RNA polymerase.

The sample is treated with **Target capture Reagent** (TCR):

a. *Detergent* solubilizes viral envelope and releases RNA or DNA
b. *Oligonucleotides* in the reagent hybridize to the target RNA/DNA of HIV/HBV/HCV if the target is present in the specimen. These oligo-nucleotides are homologous to highly conserved regions of the viruses.

c. *Magnetic microparticles* present in the TCR capture the hybridized target. They are then separated from the unhybridized oligonucleotides in a magnetic field.

3. **Target enhancer reagent** enhances the denaturation of viral particles due to its alkaline nature. It is a concentrated solution of lithium hydroxide.

4. **Transcription mediated Amplification**: Enzyme reagent contains two enzymes. Reverse transcriptase makes a DNA copy to the target viral material (MMLV Reverse transcriptase). Multiple copies of RNA amplicons are made from the DNA copy using T7 RNA polymerase. It is an Isothermal amplification. Amplification reagent contains Primers and nucleotides.

Detection is by Hybridization protection assay: **Probe reagent** having single-stranded nucleic acid strands with chemiluminescent labels, which are complementary to RNA amplified products, is added. Hence labelled probes will get bound to the amplicon.

The selection reagent inactivates all the probes which are not hybridized to RNA amplicons. It is a borate-buffered solution with detergent.

Hybridized probe releases a chemiluminescent signal, and a luminometer measures it. Measurement is given in terms of Relative light unit (RLU). The signal from the internal control and the target can be differentiated using the dual kinetic assay (DKA). Internal control emits a signal with rapid light kinetics called a flasher signal. Target emits a signal with slower light emission kinetics and is referred to as a glower signal.

Step	Description	Illustration
Step 1	A sequence-specific downstream primer hybridizes to the 3' end of the target rRNA, and RT synthesizes a cDNA copy	Hybridisation of primer 1 / rRNA target / Reverse transcriptase(RT)
Step 2	Primer 1(promoter primer) contains a sequence at its 3' end that hybridizes to the target RNA and a specific sequence at its 5' end that serves as a promoter for the T7 polymerase. *	RNAse H / cDNA / RNA
Step 3	A second primer (primer 2) then binds to the newly synthesized cDNA	Hybridisation of primer 2 / DNA / DNA polymerase
Step 4	Utilizing DNA polymerase, a dsDNA is synthesised	
Step 5	The T7 promoter at one end (from primer 1) drives the transcription of new RNA	T7 polymerase / Multiple copies of RNA antisense to original mRNA

*** The RNA template is degraded either by RT itself (TMA assay) or by RNAseH (NASBA assay)**

Figure 21. Principle of Transcription mediated amplification.

A discriminatory test (for HIV-1, HCV & HBV) is performed to detect the reactive marker in every *Initial reactive* sample. All the steps are the same as multiplex assay, except the HIV-specific/HBV-specific and HCV-specific probes are utilized in discriminatory assay.

- An algorithm is developed with the consensus of the users in India, which is given in Figure 1

1. NAT ASSAY ALGORITHM & TESTING PROTOCOL

- **Invalid Tube:** Repeat the Test in the next run. If Positive on the repeat run, then Discriminatoryassay to be done.
- **Invalid Run:** Repeat the full batch of samples
- **NAT Negative and Sero Negative:** No further test is required. This sample is termed **Concordant Negative**

NAT Reactive and Seroreactive

a. After confirming the serology result by duplicate or triplicate testing as per blood centre protocol, perform a discriminatory assay once(1X) for each virus.
b. If the Discriminatory assay is reactive, the sample is termed **Concordant Positive HXV.** (X is the virus).
c. If the Discriminatory assay is non-reactive, then the sample will be termed **Concordant Positive discriminatory non-reactive (DNR).**
d. Repeat the serology test if discrimination becomes reactive for more viruses than in the serology. If the serology test has the same result, repeat the discriminatory assay in duplicate (2X). If any duplicate discriminatory assay is reactive, the sample is a NAT yield. This sample will be termed NAT Co-Infection and NAT Yield for the virus, which is sero non-reactive.

NAT Reactive and Sero Negative

a. Repeat the NAT test in triplicate (3X) from the sample tube.
b. If all three are non Reactive, then the sample is called repeat non-reactive and Discriminatory Not Done **(RNR DND).** No further testing is required.
c. If one of the three repeats is reactive, perform a NAT test on a sample from the plasma bag in triplicate.
d. If one of the six repeats is reactive, proceed with a discriminatory assay for each virus in triplicate (3X).
e. If one of six repeats and one of the discriminatory tests comes reactive, the sample is termed **NAT Yield for the discriminatory reactive virus.**
f. If one of the six repeats is reactive, and none of the discriminatory tests is reactive from them, the sample is denoted as repeat reactive discriminatory non-reactive **(RR DNR).**

Serology positive and NAT negative:

a. Repeat the serology test
b. If Serology Repeat Reactive, perform NAT in triplicate (3X) from the sample Tube.
c. If repeat serology is reactive and NAT is non-reactive, then the sample will be denoted as **Sero Yield.**
d. If repeat serology is negative, then the sample will be a **Serology false positive.**
   Quantitative viral load estimation may be performed for the NAT yield samples if feasible.

3. Nucleic acid sequence-based amplification

It involves isothermal amplification to produce multiple copies of RNA/DNA. The critical point is that amplification starts from a single-stranded RNA and the amplicons are also RNA. In order to amplify DNA, it should be translated into RNA. Enzymes used are Avian Myeloblastosis Reverse Transcriptase (AMV-RT), RNase H, and RNA polymerase.

- The primer is annealed to the RNA template.
- After this primer annealing, AMV-RT generates a complementary DNA strand (cDNA) from the RNA template.
- RNase H removes the RNA from the RNA-DNA hybrid.
- The second primer binds to the cDNA to form double-stranded DNA using the DNA polymerase activity of reverse transcriptase.
- The T7 promoter is identified by the T7 RNA polymerase and produces a large number of single-strand RNA.

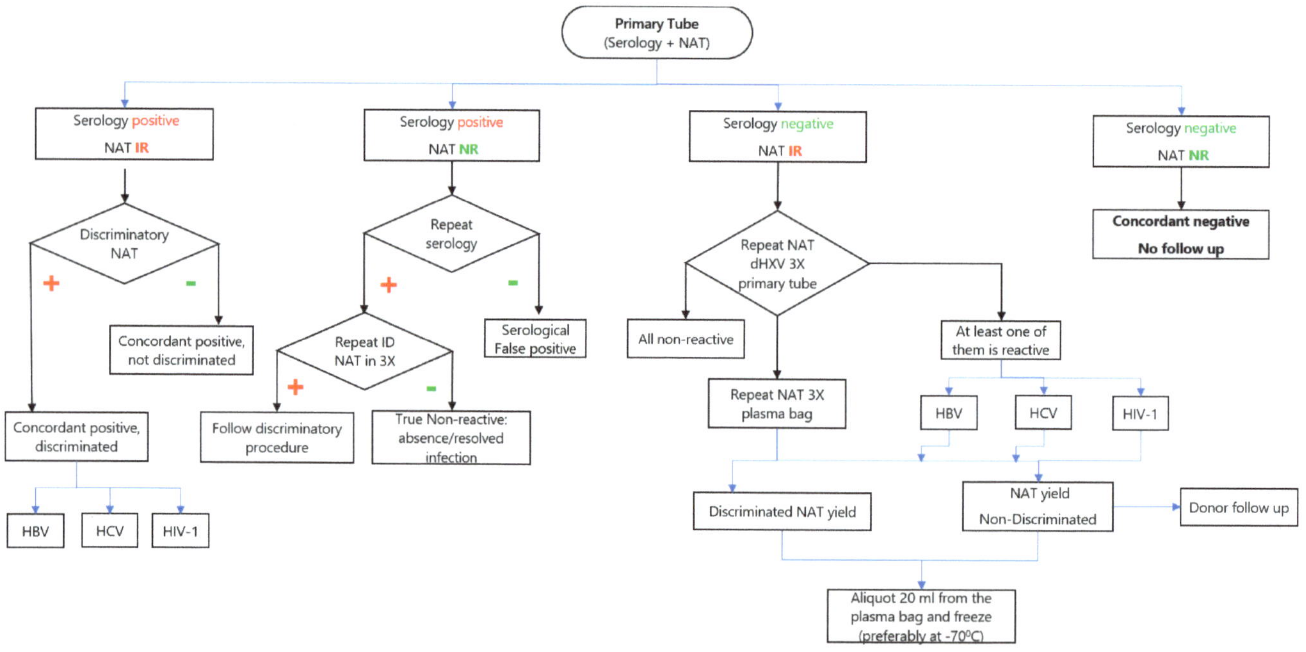

NAT IR: NAT initial reactive, NAT NR: NAT non-reactive, d HBV R: discriminatory HBV reactive

Fig 4: Nat Assay Algorithm & Testing Protocol

4. Branched DNA assay (b-DNA)

Synthetic branched DNA is added to the sample to be tested. Target DNA needs no amplification for detection. Capture oligonucleotides bind to the target and immobilize it to a solid support. The branched DNA, coupled with the enzymes, bind to the target, which is fixed to the support. The enzyme acts on the chemiluminescent substrate and generates light that is detected by a luminometer.

All these blood donor screening assays are qualitative.

- The light emitted by the hybridized ruthenium-labelled probe is detected and proportional to the number of amplicons.

Table 19.2 Comparison of NAT assay platforms available in India

NAT systems available in India	PANTHER system	Tigris system	eSAS-system	NATSpert ID TripleH detection assay	Cobas s201 system
Kit used	Procleix ultrio elite kit Grifols Diagnostic Solutions, Inc.	Procleix Ultrio Plus assay Grifols Diagnostic Solutions, Inc.	Procleix Ultrio Plus assay Grifols Diagnostic Solutions, Inc.	NATSpert ID TripleH detection assay Mylab Discovery Solutions, India)	TaqScreen MPX 2.0 Test Roche diagnostics
Automation	Automated System with a single chamber	Automated System with a single chamber	Semi-automated modular system	Semi-automated system	Automated system with multiple processing units
Sample testing	Individual donor testing	Individual donor testing	Individual donor testing	Individual donor testing	Mini pool testing (Pool of 6)
Method	Transcription-mediated amplification (TMA) assay	Transcription-mediated amplification (TMA) assay	Transcription-mediated amplification (TMA) assay	Real-time PCR	Real-time PCR
Number of tests per run	With the continuous testing platform, no need for a batch run. Can perform 275 tests in 8 hours	500 Tests/ Run	91 samples per run	8 samples per run	108 samples in pools of 6 per run
Turn around time	For 100 tests,5 hrs required	For 100 tests,5 hrs required	For 91 samples, 5 hrs required	2.5 hrs	4 hrs
Number of tests in discriminatory assays	200 tests in the discriminatory assay	200 tests in the discriminatory assay	200 tests in the discriminatory assay	The discriminatory assay is not required. Detection and discrimination are performed in the initial multiplex assay.	The discriminatory assay is not required. Detection and discrimination performed during positive pool resolution

Viruses detected	HIV1M/N, HIV1 O, HIV2, HCV, HBV Two region detection of HIV-1. Enhanced detection of HBV.	Does not detect HIV- 2	Does not detect HIV- 2	HIV1M/N, HIV1 O, HIV2, HCV, HBV	HIV-1 Group M, HIV-1 Group O, HIV-2, HCV, HBV
Limitations	Cannot differentiate HIV1 &2 in	Does not detect HIV 2. Batch System.	Does not detect HIV 2. Batch System. Manual pipetting of reagent	Multiple systems need to be networked for large blood centres. Batch system. Multiple hands-on operations	It does not discriminate between HIV-1 Group M, HIV-1 Group O and HIV-2. Batch System Heparin inhibits PCR. Do not use the heparin sample
Remarks	A walk-away automated system with a continuous testing facility and 24 hours calibration stability	It is a walk-away automated system	Suitable for small blood centres	Suitable for small blood centres	No reagent needs freezer storage

Common terms in NAT:

- ✓ **Individual donor test:** Tests run on every individual sample.
- ✓ **Mini pool test:** Test run on a pool of 6-8 samples
- ✓ **Multiplex assay:** Simultaneous detection of multiple markers in a single tube-like HIV, HBV, HCV.
- ✓ **NAT Reactive:** The sample is reactive in NAT (It may or may not be reactive in serology).
- ✓ **NAT yield:** The sample is reactive in NAT and non-reactive in the serology test.
- ✓ **Sero yield:** The sample is reactive in serology and non-reactive in the NAT test.
- ✓ **Yield rate:** Number of samples tested/Number of NAT yield. E.g., 3 NAT yield out of a total of 45000 samples tested. Yield rate:45000/3=15000, i.e. 1 in 15000
- ✓ **Concordant reactive:** Serology and NAT test is reactive for a marker.

Note :

Yield rates vary depending on the

- The assay used for baseline serology testing
- The sensitivity of the baseline serology assay
- Prevalence of the infection in the population: High prevalence regions will yield more window period donations.
- Stringent donor screening, provision of donor self-deferral and donor notification.

Advantages of NAT

NAT reduces the window period of infection by detecting

- Pre-seroconversion window period infections
- Immunologically variant Mutants
- Chronic occult infections
- Immunosilent donors with a long serological window period
- Blood centres can utilize the NAT test to resolve the false reactive serology results before notifying the donor.

Window period reduction

The window period is the period during which the immunological assays are not able to detect the presence of antigen/antibody. NAT reduces this window period by detecting the viral genome.

Table 19.2 Window period with serology and NAT assays

	3RD Gen ELISA	4TH Gen ELISA	Individual donor NAT	Mini pool NAT
HIV	22 d	15 d	2.93 days	8
HBV	43.6 d	38.3 d	10.34 days	16.7
HCV	50.9 d	27 d	1.34 days	3.9

The marker which obtained a maximum reduction in window period with NAT: HCV

- ✓ Studies with seroconversion panels were used to assess the infectious window period for these viral markers.
- ✓ Detection of infection during the window period depends on the analytical sensitivity of the NAT assay.
- ✓ The residual risk of virus transmission during the window period depends on
    - Probability of NAT detection
    - Probability of infectivity

Occult Infections:

Donors with occult hepatitis B infection (OBI) are negative for the HBsAg serology test and reactive for HBV-DNA in NAT (levels below 200 IU/ml.) They often have concomitant anti-HBc and anti-HBs antibodies and hence have a low risk for HBV transmission.

Quality control and validity of assay:

- **Internal control** is to be added to each specimen to validate the test. It has an RNA transcript.
- Negative and positive calibrators determine the cut-off and validity of the run.
- Calibrators are lot-specific.
- A sample result is valid if the internal control signal is greater than the internal control cut-off and timeless than the limit defined for the assay.
- The sample is non-reactive when the analyte signal is less than the analyte cut-off (Analyte S/CO < 1.00).

- The sample is Reactive when the analyte signal is more than the analyte cut-off. (Analyte S/CO >1.00)
- **External quality control** may be performed for quality assurance.

Performance characteristics of assays

Performance characteristics of the available assays may be compared in terms of specificity, clinical and analytical sensitivity. The **specificity** of the assay is the ability of the test to detect a sample which is a true negative, or it is the ability of the assay to detect the analyte with accuracy. **Clinical sensitivity** is the ability of the assay to detect the reactive samples correctly.

Analytical sensitivity is the ability of the assay to detect a target analyte which is expressed as the minimum detectable concentration of the analyte (IU/ml). **Analytical sensitivity** is determined by testing the panels containing serially diluted WHO Standards of HIV1/HCV/HBV with the NAT assays. The predicted 95% detection probability in IU/ml for each target is given in table 3.

Table 19.3 Performance characteristics of the NAT assays

Assay	Specificity	Clinical sensitivity	Analytical sensitivity
Ultrio elite assay	99.9%	100% for HIV1,HCV,HBV 54% FOR HIV 2	HIV 1: 18 IU/ml HIV 2: 10.4 IU/ml HBV: 4.3IU/ml HCV: 3 IU/ml
Ultrio elite discriminatory assay	100%	100% for HIV1,HCV,HBV	HIV 1: 17.3IU/ml HIV2: 9.6 IU/ml HCV: 2.4 IU/ml HBV: 4.5 IU/ml
Ultrio Plus Assay	99.87%	100% for HIV1,HCV,HBV	HIV1:21.2 IU/ml HCV:5.4 IU/ml HBV:3.4 IU/ml
Ultrio Plus discriminatory Assay	100%	100% for HIV1,HCV,HBV	HIV1:18.9 IU/ml HCV:4.4 IU/ml HBV:4.1 IU/ml
Cobas Taqscreen MPX test	99.99%	100% for HIV1,HCV,HBV	HIV 1: 50.3 IU/ml HIV2:7.9 IU/ml HCV: 6.8 IU/ml HBV: 2.3 IU/ml (when the test is done individually)
NATspert assay	100%	100% for HIV1,HCV,HBV	HIV-1 M: 17.5 IU/ml HIV-1 O: 18.5 copies/ml HIV-2: 8.17 IU/ml HCV: 7 IU/ml HBV: 2 IU/ml.

Dual target NAT in HIV 1 is mandated to prevent false-negative results owing to the mutations in the genomic region.

Selection of NAT assay

Some aspects that may be considered while selecting a NAT assay are:

- Analytical sensitivity
- Availability of automation
- Turn around time
- Approval from regulatory authorities

Automation in NAT Available automated systems: Procleix panther system (Grifols), Tigris (Grifols), Cobas s201 (Rosche),

Advantages

- Continuous testing
- Stat sample entry
- Calibration is valid for 24 hours
- The system automatically prompts at each step
- The chances of manual errors are low

Lab requirements

Space requirements :

- Around 200-250 Sq feet area required for the NAT lab
- Semi-automated procedures require segregating the three steps in three different rooms and restricted movement of personnel and materials to avoid contamination. The lab is to be compartmentalized into Ante Room, Pre amplification Room, and Post amplification room. However, automated systems allow all procedures in one single room.
- Temperature 15° to 30°C and humidity requirements have to be met.
- Air quality: Clean air supply is required.
- Unidirectional workflow to be followed: Movement should be from reagent preparation to sample preparation to amplification and then to detection areas.
-

Surface cleaning :

- To prevent the cross-contamination of lab surfaces and equipment with the Amplicons.
    - The semi-automated system requires cleaning surfaces and equipment with 0.5% Sodium Hypochlorite solution. After using hypochlorite, thoroughly rinse the equipment with water to avoid corrosion of metal surfaces.
    - In automated systems, only lab surfaces are to be cleaned. The decontamination process is in-built for the parts within the machine.

As RNA is an unstable molecule, it will degrade soon; hence, RNA amplification methods are less prone to amplicon contamination.

Sample requirement

- Plasma sample
- Storage :2-8 ^{0}C
- Avoid frothing or bubbling during sample preparation.

Practical issues:

➢ Test-related issues:

- Initial reactive samples may not be reactive in the discriminatory assay. This could be false positives.
- Sero reactive and NAT non-reactive (sero yield): Repeat serology in the same platform and /or another platform. Repeat NAT in triplicate. The serology test could be false positivity if the same result is obtained.
- Other causes of Sero yield :
    - ✓ Undetectable viral load
    - ✓ Presence of Dane Particles (without HBV DNA)
    - ✓ Resolved Infection: Donor no longer infected (No RNA/DNA) but with antibodies

➢ Donor related issues

- Notifying donors who are NAT yield or indeterminate results, their counselling and follow-up testing.
- Counsel about the reactive result and advise not to donate blood in future.
- Helps the donor to seek medical advice and treatment at the right time.
- Prevent secondary transmission of infection to the partner.
- Reduces the chance of vertical transmission.
- Those who do not respond to notification may continue to donate blood at other blood centres and hence pose a danger to the safety of the blood supply.

➢ Recipient related issues

- Notification of recipients of NAT reactive blood components.
- Post-exposure prophylaxis for recipients of NAT reactive components.
- Counselling & follow-up of NAT reactive components.

Limitations of the NAT assay

- Very low viral loads may result in false-negative reports. Hence additional tests and donor follow-up is essential.
- Mutations in the primer binding regions cause false-negative NAT Results. Mutations continue to occur, and antibody assays may give reactive results in such cases.
- False-positive test results are often attributed to cross-contamination.

Some frequently asked questions related to NAT:

- **NAT & HbCore antibody testing**

HBV NAT will be useful in countries where HBcore antibody testing is not routinely done. NAT will be beneficial in high and intermediate endemic areas. HBcore antibody prevalence is high in such areas, ranging between 10-15%, leading to high discard rates. In India, most blood centres which perform NAT have given up HBcore antibody testing to reduce the discarding of blood units.

- **NAT and antigen testing:**

NAT tests replace HIV P24 antigen tests and HCV antigen tests. Replacement of HBsAg assay by HBV NAT along with anti-HBc is debated. In countries with a high anti-HBc prevalence, the positive units have to be tested by a quantitative anti-HBs assay to recover units positive for anti-HBc but negative for HBV-DNA and containing protective titres of anti-HBs. The Japanese red cross society follows this.

Challenges in establishing NAT testing facilities

- Expensive: 5 to 10 times the cost of an ELISA test
- The requirement for qualified technical staff
- Dedicated Infrastructure
- Prevention of cross-contamination
- Turnaround time for blood release into inventory increases

Impact of NAT on Inventory Management:

- Distribution & issue of components is done after the results of the NAT test are available. Hence processing time is increased. In cases where a component has to be issued within a few hours of the collection, like granulocytes, consider collection from already tested donors. If a component has to be issued before NAT testing due to the urgency of the situation, the testing status of the component should be informed to the treating physician.
- Turnaround time in the lab should be kept to a minimum to allow maximum shelf life for the components with short expiry, like platelets.
- Pool testing involves withholding the issue of the units till the resolution of reactive pools
- Breakdown and inventory management
- Service of engineers and standby equipment should be available in a short time
- Backup testing facilities should be identified to get the samples tested in the shortest possible time during the breakdown of the system.

NAT testing available for other viruses :

Westnile virus, dengue virus, Chikungunya virus, Cytomegalo virus, Zika Virus, Hepatitis A, Parvo virus B-19.

Regulatory requirement

In India, it is not a mandatory screening test for detecting Transfusion transmitted infection in blood donors as per the Drug and Cosmetics Act of 1940

Other countries: Germany has mandated HIV and HCV NAT for blood screening.

Cost-effectiveness: In countries with a high prevalence of viral infections in donors, the NAT assay will be cost-effective, considering the cost saved by preventing the Transfusion of NAT yield donations.

Centralized testing centre for NAT:

- Helps to maintain the quality standards of testing
- Helps to lower the cost to make it affordable for smaller blood centres
- Helps to bring uniformity in testing, reporting and quality control
- Limitations: Transportation of samples in good condition. It is challenging to obtain samples for additional testing, if any.

In India, centralized testing is performed by states like Karnataka, Orissa, Uttar Pradesh, and Rajasthan.

NAT testing for plasma fractionation units: Plasma fractionation units in Europe were the first to start utilizing the NAT assay to screen Transfusion transmitted pathogens. The European Union mandated NAT for HCV and HIV for all plasma for fractionation in 1997 and 1999, respectively. According to the current guidelines, NAT is not mandatory for fractionation units in India.

FUTURE

Small benchtop versions with automation and multi-parameter assays will allow small and medium blood banks to adopt NAT. Implementation of pathogen inactivation and NAT will take us to the goal of zero-risk transfusion.

19.5 BACTERIAL CONTAMINATION OF BLOOD COMPONENTS

– Dr. Ketan

Susceptibility of Blood components to Microbial Contaminations

Compared to other blood components, platelet concentrate (PC) are highly susceptible to bacterial contamination due to the following:

- The recommended storage temperatures of 20–24°C facilitate the proliferation of many bacterial species from human microflora and environmental sources.
- Bacterial growth is promoted by the comparably high oxygen supply supported by the continuous mixing of the gas-permeable PC bags.
- Frequently employed additives in the storage solution might serve as an additional energy source for some microorganisms resulting in a growth advantage

Source of blood products contamination

The Source of blood products contamination with microorganisms is as follows:

1. At the time of donation:
    a. Bacteraemic donor
    b. Improper skin disinfection of donor

2. Post-collection during storage

Bacterial vs viral contamination:

The virus does not proliferate in the blood bags, so their load and detection are constant. However, bacteria proliferate on storage. Thus, the initial bacterial counts can increase tremendously over time & hence the risk of adverse reaction increases with prolonged storage—also, the chances of bacterial detection increase with late sampling in contrast to early sampling.

Early vs late sampling;

There are two major approaches for bacterial testing based on the sampling time, e.g.,

1. **"Early sampling"** - is defined as sampling within 36 h after blood donation. The rationale is to obtain microbiological results as early as possible. However, due to the low initial concentration of microbial contaminants, the detection of pathogens within the first 24 h bears the risk of sampling errors and false-negative results.
2. **"Late sampling"** - is defined as sampling when cultivation is initiated later than 36 h. It improves the possibility of the detection of replicating bacterial contaminants. If performed on day 4 or 5 of storage, this serves as an additional safety measure that allows extension of the PC shelf life.

Indications of performing microbiological testing

Indications, where microbiological testing can be performed, are as follows.

1. **Sterility testing:** testing of unused new blood bags routinely for bacteriological sterility
2. **Testing of donor's blood:**

   a. Virological screening of donor's blood
   b. An early sampling of donor's blood (<36hours of collection) for bacteriological contamination
   c. A late sampling of blood products (<36hours of collection) for bacteriological contamination
   d. Near-use screening of blood products using rapid diagnostic tests

3. **ATR:** Testing is indicated in the event of an adverse transfusion reaction (ATR).

   a. Testing of the residual amount of blood products in the transfused bag
   b. Testing for blood culture of the recipient's blood

Bacterial Screening Strategies

The ideal test should have an extremely high diagnostic sensitivity and specificity and be inexpensive, reliable, and fast.

In general, diagnostic methods for the detection of bacteria in blood products can be divided into:

- Culture-Based Methods in combination with an early sampling strategy.
- Culture-Based Methods in combination with a late sampling strategy.
- Methods using rapid direct detection in combination with an early sampling strategy.
- Methods using rapid direct detection in combination with the late sampling strategy

Culture-Based Methods

The culture of blood products can be carried out in conventional or automated blood culture systems, depending on the availability in the microbiology laboratory.

Collection of culture samples from the blood bag:

The blood from the blood bag is collected in the following manner.

- Stored blood and blood product bags are thoroughly mixed, and the end of the tied tubing is swabbed, disinfected, and cut with sterile scissors.
- Some of the mixed blood from the main bag is allowed to seep into the line.
- The end of each line is clipped with sterile forceps to prevent blood from flowing back into the main bag.
- These cut ends are directly transported to the Microbiology for sample processing and laboratory analysis
- Two knots are made on the line, and the last knot is swabbed with 70% ethanol and punctured with a sterile needle with a syringe to draw 5 - 10 mL of blood product.
- Alternatively, a residual blood bag or unused blood bag is sent directly to the laboratory, where the sample is drawn out using a sterile syringe

An alternative method to collect the sample from residual blood bag:

The following steps need to be followed while sending the residual blood bag to the microbiology laboratory:

- A blood component bag suspected of being bacterially contaminated should be handled in an aseptic manner.
- The priority is to create a closed system by sealing the transfusion tubing. Options for sealing include heat sealing, clamping, or, if these are not available, placement of a tight slip knot in the tubing (i.e., tighten until the tubing in the knot is a white colour).
- The culprit bag is sent to the microbiology laboratory as soon as possible. If a delay in transport is expected, the bag should be refrigerated as soon as possible until bacteriologic testing can be performed.
- With the help of a syringe and needle, a sample can be obtained aseptically through the outlet ports of the blood bag directly or through a sampling site coupler.
- If no adequate sample is left in the used blood bag, sterile normal saline can be used for irrigation of the blood bag aseptically using a syringe and needle through the outlet ports, and then the saline is aspirated back after proper mixing in the bag
- The blood product sample should be inoculated directly into automated blood culture bottles or in-house prepared conventional blood culture bottles for qualitative culture
- If possible, samples are to be serially inoculated into dilution blanks (e.g., undiluted, 1:10, 1:1000, 1:100,000) of sterile 0.9% saline so that spread plate (e.g., chocolate agar) quantitative cultures can be performed.
- Dilution methods are preferred for quantitative culture, but semi-quantitative methods may be used if unavailable.

Conventional blood culture system:

The conventional blood culture media are of two types:

- **Monophasic medium:** It contains a sterile screw-capped glass bottle (e.g. McCartney bottle) [Fig. 1A, 1B, 1C] containing 50mL of Brain Heart Infusion (BHI) broth
- **Biphasic medium:** It has a liquid phase containing BHI broth and a solid agar slope made up of BHI agar.[Fig. 1D]

Processing Workflow of conventional blood culture

The Processing workflow of conventional blood culture is as follows.

- The blood product is inoculated into BHI broth in the approximate ratio of 1:5 to 1:10.
- At the same time, the samples are inoculated using standard methods onto culture media plates viz blood agar (BA), chocolate agar (CA), and MacConkey agar (MAC).
- Gram staining is performed from a direct sample & looked for any microorganism
- Culture plates & BHI broth are incubated at 37°C aerobically for 2 days & 7 days, respectively.
- BHI broth is daily looked for visible turbidity and sub-cultured on BA, CA & MAC when visible turbidity is seen or at the end of seven days
- Plates are inspected for bacterial growth at 24 h and 48 h.

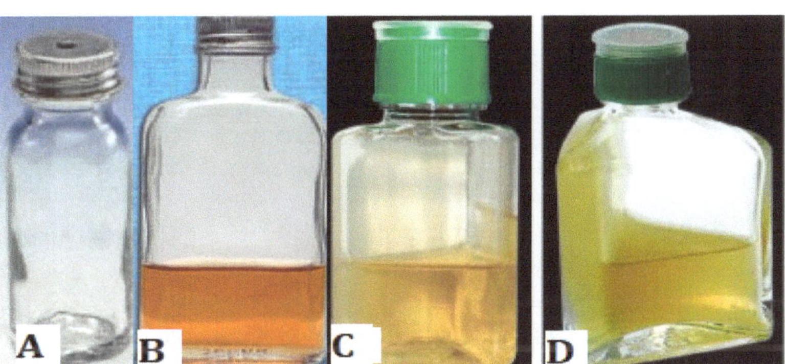

Fig1: Conventional blood culture system

The automated blood culture system

Alternatively, the blood products can be inoculated & cultured into automated blood culture bottles.

- The culture bottles are loaded inside the automated culture system machine following inoculation.
- There is a provision for continuous automated monitoring of microbial growth.
- Once detected positive for microbial growth, the instrument gives a positive signal/alarm
- The culture bottles are then brought out from the instrument.
- Gram staining was performed from bottle broth & looked for any microorganisms
- At the same time, the broth was inoculated using standard methods onto culture media plates viz blood agar (BA), chocolate agar (CA), and MacConkey agar (MAC).
- Culture plates were incubated at 37°C aerobically for 48 - 72hours & inspected for bacterial growth periodically.

Automated blood culture systems

Three automated blood culture systems have been in routine use or have been validated for blood products quality control:

BacT/ ALERT system

BacT/ ALERT system (BioMérieux, France) is one of the most commonly used automated blood culture systems (Fig2B).

- It is based on the colourimetric detection principle.
- A sensor (liquid emulsion sensor) which is pH sensitive is bonded to the bottom of each bottle and separated from the broth medium by a differentially permeable membrane
- When bacteria multiply, they produce CO_2 that diffuses through the permeable membrane & leads to lower pH, which changes the colour of a gas-permeable sensor at the bottom of the culture bottle from greenish-grey to yellow, detected by colourimetry.

Virtuo

Virtuo is an advanced version of the BacT/ALERT System (Fig3). It is different from other systems in the following aspects:

- Real-time notifications on the blood volume.
- Robotics is used for loading and unloading bottles.
- Provides notifications for under-filler and overfilled bottles.
- It has a scanning station that automatically scans the label (patient details)
- Quicker time to detection.
- Contamination tracking
- Safer waste disposal

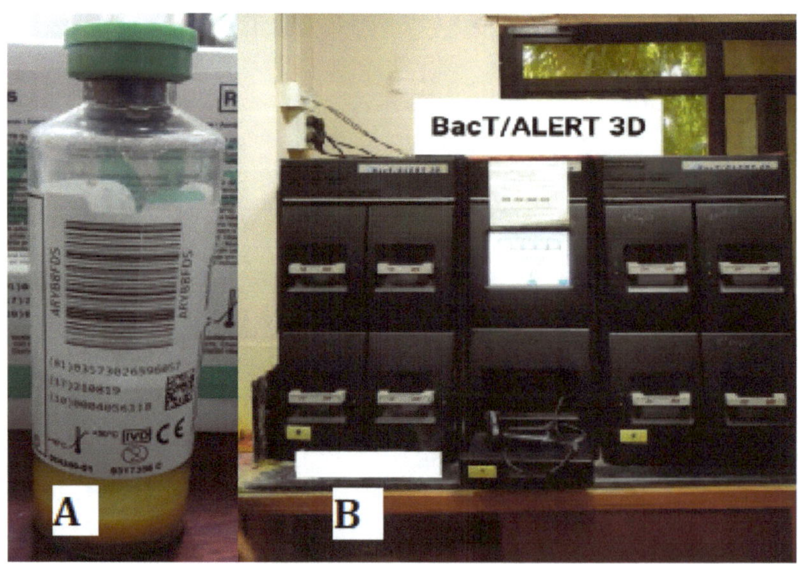

Fig2A: BacT/ALERT blood culture bottle Fig2B: BacT/ALERT 3D System

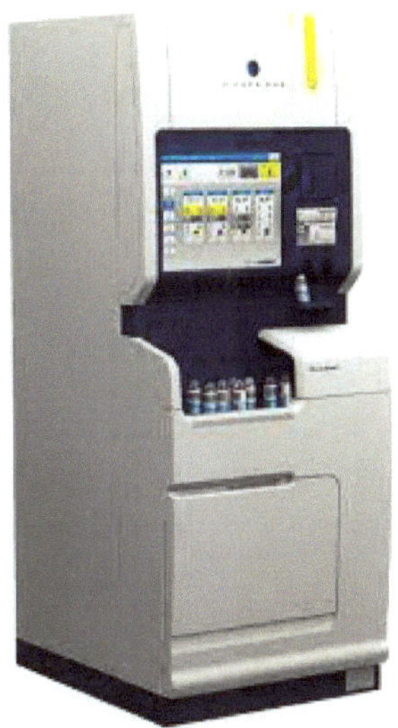

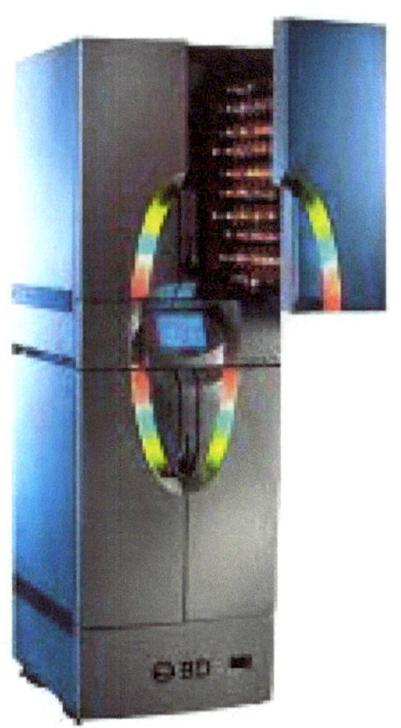

Fig3: Virtuo BacT/ALERT System   **Fig4: BACTEC system**

BACTEC system

BACTEC system (BD Diagnostics, USA) is another commonly used automated blood culture system (Fig4).

- It is based on the fluorometric detection principle.

There is a fluorescent dye presence in the bottle and an O2-sensitive quencher.

- Quencher blocks the fluorescence of the dye in the presence of abundant dissolved O2 in the broth
- On microbial growth, there is depletion of O2 leading to inactivation of the quencher and the dye fluoresce. This is detected & a positive flagged signal is given when fluorescence crosses a threshold value.

VersaTrek system

VersaTrek system (Trek Diagnostics, USA) is based on the barometric detection principle & monitors bacterial growth by detecting pressure changes in the headspace of the blood culture bottle secondary to gas consumption/production.

Composition of the automated blood culture bottle

The composition of the automated blood culture bottle (Fig 2A) includes the following:

- Tryptic soy broth
- Adsorbent beads- to neutralise the effect of antimicrobials present in the blood
- Sodium polyanethol sulfonate- as an anticoagulant

Identification of microbial pathogens using automated identification systems

Microbial pathogen identification needs to be performed on getting visible colonies on the culture agar plates or sometimes directly from the flagged blood culture bottle broth.

Two methods can do this:

1. **Conventional biochemical methods:** This is time-consuming, sometimes inaccurate, and often unable to identify the correct pathogen.
2. **Automated identification systems:** These are rapid, accurate and reliable microbial identification methods. Two methodologies that are most commonly employed are:

   - Matrix-Assisted Laser Desorption Ionization Time of Flight Mass Spectrometry (MALDI-TOF MS): based on the principle of proteomics
   - Automated Systems based on a panel of phenotypic biochemical identification: e.g. VITEK-2, Microscan Walkaway etc.

MALDI-TOF MS

MALDI-TOF (Matrix-Assisted Laser Desorption Ionization Time of Flight Mass Spectrometry) technology has revolutionised the identification of organisms in clinical microbiology laboratories, with a turnaround time of a few minutes and with absolute accuracy (Fig5).

3. Two systems are commercially available: VITEK MS (bioMérieux) and Biotyper system (Bruker)
4. MALDI-TOF examines the patterns of ribosomal proteins present in the organism.
5. A single colony of an organism is smeared at the designated spot on the slide, followed by the addition of a matrix solution (composed of cyanohydroxy-cinnamic acid). The slide is then loaded into the system.

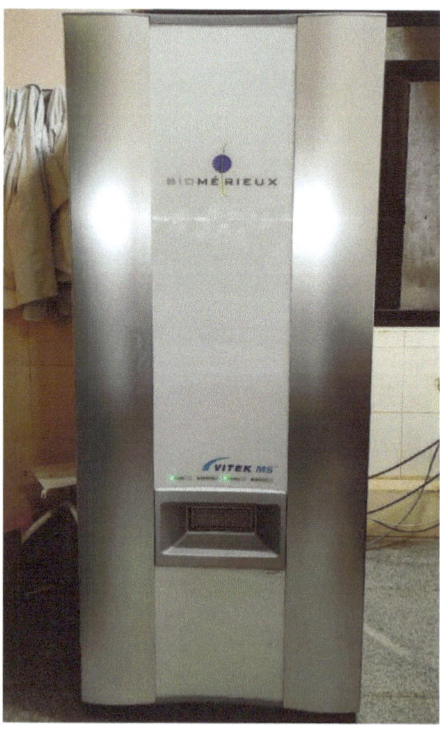

Fig5: MALDI-TOF MS (Vitek MS)

VITEK 2 Automated System

The VITEK 2 is an automated system to identify and perform antimicrobial susceptibility testing (AST) bacteria and yeast (Fig6).

- It uses a colourimetric reagent card containing 64 wells; each well contains an individual test substrate. Separate cards are available for gram-negative, gram-positive, fastidious, and yeasts.
- **Identification:** Substrates in the well measure various metabolic activities such as acidification, alkalinisation, enzyme hydrolysis etc., which helps identify the organism. The reaction pattern obtained from the test organism is compared with the database, and the identification is reported with a confidence level of matching (excellent matching to the unidentified organism).
- **AST:** It works on the principle of micro broth dilution. The wells in the card contain a doubling dilution of antimicrobial agents. The organism suspension (of the turbidity as recommended by the manufacturer) is added to the wells. The MIC is determined as the highest dilution of the antimicrobial agent, which inhibits organism growth.
- The reading is taken once every 15 minutes by the optical system of the equipment, which measures any coloured products of substrate metabolism (for identification) or turbidity (for AST).
- The result of identification is usually available within 4-6 hours, and AST within 16-18 hours

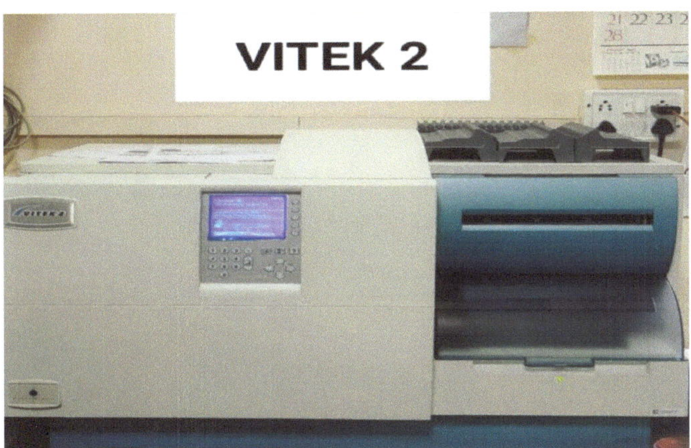

Fig6: VITEK 2 system

Antimicrobial susceptibility testing

It is not routinely performed for the pathogens isolated from blood products unless needed to treat bacteremia in the donor or the recipient post-transfusion.

"Negative-to-Date" concept

The blood products with negative virological screening reports and ongoing culture by early sampling are released as "Negative-to-Date" as needed, but culture is continued.

- The policy for a minimum hold time of blood products before use & maximum storage duration varies from country to country.

- If the culture result status changes from negative to reactive, physicians must be informed immediately, and products must be recalled.
- If already transfused, a look-back procedure has to be initiated

Disadvantages of culture screening methods with early sampling:

The disadvantages of culture screening methods with early sampling are as follows.

- High risk of sampling error and false negativity or delayed positivity due to the low number of contaminating bacteria at the beginning of PC shelf life, particularly when slow-growing bacteria are involved in the contamination, as a relevant percentage of platelets, had already been transfused by the time a positive signal occurred.
- Detection of bacterial contamination with non-transfusion relevant bacterial species, e.g. non-pathogenic skin commensal like *Propionibacterium acnes*, diphtheroids, Aerobic spore bearers etc., which either do not multiple in blood bags or usually die due to auto-sterilisation on storage, resulting in a higher rate of positive PCs accompanied by high diagnostic efforts and irrelevant discard of products.

RAPID automated diagnostic modalities

Direct detection of bacteria in blood products using rapid detection methods in combination with early sampling

The following are the various recent automated diagnostic modalities used, along with early sampling.

Haemonetics eBDS (Formerly Pall eBDS)

This monitors the concentration of oxygen in the headspace of a satellite bag that is incubated at 37 °C

- The eBDS system comprises:

  - A disposable sample set with a pouch containing a readily dissolvable tablet of sodium polyanethol sulfonate to avoid platelet aggregation
  - Trypticase soy broth as a source of nutrition for microorganisms
  - Others: Flatbed agitator, an incubator and an oxygen analyser.

- This system is based on the principle that the growing aerobic and facultative anaerobic bacteria consume oxygen in the plasma and that the oxygen in the air of the sample pouch will equilibrate with the plasma.
- After the collection of a 3-ml sample, the automated culture system should be run for a minimum of 24 h
- before the pouch is heat-sealed and incubated at 35 °C with constant agitation and subsequent oxygen concentration measurement.
- Bacterial contamination is assumed if the O2 reading is less than 12.5%, which is the cut-off value between a positive and negative reading

- Using this technology, only bacteria that can grow under aerobic conditions will be detected, which confers a risk of false-negative screening results
- The sensitivity of the Pall eBDS system is similar to the BacT/ALERT system in the order of 1 CFU/ml

Microcalorimetry

A microcalorimetry thermostat is used to measure the heat due to replicating microorganisms in culture to detect bacteria in PCs. Any heat generated or absorbed by the sample is measured continuously over time.

Direct Detection of Bacteria in blood products using Rapid Detection Methods in Combination with Late Sampling

The following are the direct detection methods of bacteria in PCs using rapid detection methods combined with late sampling.

Real-Time PCR

Conserved nucleic acid sequences in the two target regions, 16S rDNA and 23S rDNA, have been used to develop real-time PCR assays to detect bacterial contamination in PCs. However, NAT testing is more laborious and expensive (equipment, reagents) compared to other methods.

PGD (Pan Genera Detection)

The test principle of the FDA-licensed, qualitative PGD (Verax Biomedical Inc., Worcester, MA, USA) assay is based on a lateral-flow immunoprecipitation of bacterial cell wall antigens (lipopolysaccharide or lipoteichoic acid), which are present at high copy numbers (>200,000 copies/cell).

The short hands-on time and the minimum requirement for laboratory instrumentation provide the opportunity for a point-of-issue bacterial detection test immediately before the transfusion of PCs. The analytical sensitivity of this assay is specified as $10^3 - 10^4$ CFU/ml for Gram-positive bacteria and $10^3 - 10^6$ CFU/ml for Gram-negative bacteria. Further disadvantages of the PGD assay are the costs, high false-positive results, and subjective result interpretation.

BacTx Peptidoglycan Assay

The BacTx assay is a rapid, qualitative, colourimetric assay for detecting the presence of peptidoglycan in bacteria cell walls.

The PC sample (0.5 ml) is added to a microfuge tube containing a lysis reagent and is centrifuged to pellet insoluble platelet debris and bacterial cell wall fragments.

The pellet is then homogenised by adding an extraction reagent to release peptidoglycan from the bacterial cell walls for optimal detection.

After neutralisation, the mixture is added to a tube containing the lyophilised detection reagents placed in the BacTx photometer reader, which monitors the detection reaction and interprets the result using software installed on the laptop provided.

The test has a sensitivity of approximately 10^4 CFU/ml, provides results within one hour and is suitable for use near the time of issue of PCs. The BacTx received FDA clearance for bacterial contamination of PCs in 2012.

Flow Cytometry

Labelling bacterial components with fluorescent dyes presents another approach for detecting and quantifying bacteria in PCs by flow cytometry.

(1) The BactiFlow assay

It detects and enumerates bacteria by fluorescent labelling viable cells. A non-fluorescent fluorochrome passes the cell membrane of cells with intact membrane integrity and enzymatic activity and is cleaved by intracellular esterases. To reduce the background noise, the esterase activity of platelets is selectively eliminated by enzymatic digestion. The analytical sensitivity of this assay is validated to be 300–500 CFU/ml. This technology is used for routine bacterial screening of PCs.

(2) Scansystem

The FDA-cleared solid-phase flow cytometric method, Scansystem, was based on the filtration of PC samples followed by picogreen staining of bacteria and detection using a laser-based, solid-phase scanning cytometry. It is no longer being marketed.

A method based on reagents from BD Biosciences has been evaluated for investigating PCs. The membrane-permeable fluorescent dye thiazole orange binds specifically to bacterial nucleic acids and emits a bright green-orange fluorescence. In a two-step procedure, platelets are lysed, and bacteria are labelled. The result is available in less than 15 min. The low sensitivity of 104 CFU/ml could be increased by an additional short pre-incubation of the platelet sample at 37 °C. Unfortunately, reagents are no longer commercially available.

LEXSAS system:

It uses a spore-based biosensor for detecting bacteria in real-time, which exploits the ability of spores to produce fluorescence when sensing neighbouring bacterial cells. The LEXSAS contains microbial spores suspended in an enzymatic substrate that produces a germinant upon enzymatic catalysis combined with diacetate fluorescein, a component that fluoresces when hydrolysed by esterases.

PCR with lateral-flow dipstick (LFD) technology:

This detects specific nucleic acid fragments by combining universal PCR with lateral-flow dipstick (LFD) technology. This assay utilises the amplification of genes followed by hybridisation by a set of probes specific to the conserved region of the target. Colloidal gold-labelled avidin and specific anti-FITC (fluorescein isothiocyanate) antibodies immobilised on the LFD nitrocellulose membrane then capture a probe-amplicon complex, producing a visible red line on the membrane.

According to the results, the total analysis time of LFD technology is only about two hrs, but the sensitivity varies depending on the bacterial species, from 5 to 10^4 CFU/ml.

Conclusion

No single test can detect bacteria in platelet units, and regardless of the method, bacterial screening of platelets is unlikely to detect all pathogens. In practice, the tests employed should be as per the national & local guidelines and available resources.

It is essential to investigate reports of potential infectious disease transmission and reports of adverse reactions and errors or incidents associated with blood transfusions to prevent transmission of infectious diseases through blood transfusions and other transfusion-related adverse events.

Bacterial species identified in platelet concentrates

Gram-positive	Gram-negative
Bacillus species	Klebsiella species Serratia species
Staphylococcus species	Escherichia coli Acinetobacter species
Streptococcus species	Enterobacter species Providencia rettgeri
Propionibacterium acne	Yersinia enterocolitica

Bacterial species identified in Packed Red Blood Cells

Gram-positive	Gram-negative	
Bacillus cereus	Klebsiella species	Serratia species
Staphylococcus Aureus	Escherichia coli	Acinetobacter species
Streptococcus species	Enterobacter species	Providencia rettgeri
Propionibacterium acne	Yersinia enterocolitica	Proteus mirabilis
Coagulase-negative Staphylococci	Pseudomonas species	Pantoea agglomerans
Enterococcus Faecalis		

Bacterial species identified in Fresh Frozen Plasma/Cryoprecipitate
Pseudomonas cepacia Pseudomonas aeruginosa
Stenotrophomonas multophilia Enterococcus gallinarum E.cloacae.

APHERESIS

– Dr. Shahida

VEINS OF LOWER LIMB

Groups of Veins of the lower limb

- The lower limb veins are grouped anatomically as follows:

Superficial veins

- They lie in the superficial fascia. They include small and great saphenous veins. These are thick-walled veins with numerous valves. The valves are more in the lower part than in the upper part of the veins.

Deep veins

- They lie along the anterior and mostly under cover of muscles. They include medial plantar, lateral plantar, dorsalis, femoral veins, their tributaries, and venae comitantes of arteries.

Perforating veins

- They connect the superficial veins to the deep veins. The valves of the perforating veins permit the blood to flow unidirectionally from superficial to deep veins

The common femoral vein is the ideal to puncture when performing central venous access at the femoral site. The common femoral vein lies within the "femoral triangle" in the inguinal-femoral region. This region is bordered by the inguinal ligament superiorly, the adductor longus medially, and the sartorius muscle laterally. the relationship of structures within the inguinal-femoral region can be remembered using the mnemonic "NAVEL." Moving laterally to medially, (N) femoral nerve, (A) femoral artery, (V) femoral vein, (E) space, (L) lymphatics.

The key anatomical landmarks in the inguinal-femoral region are the inguinal ligament and the femoral artery pulsation.

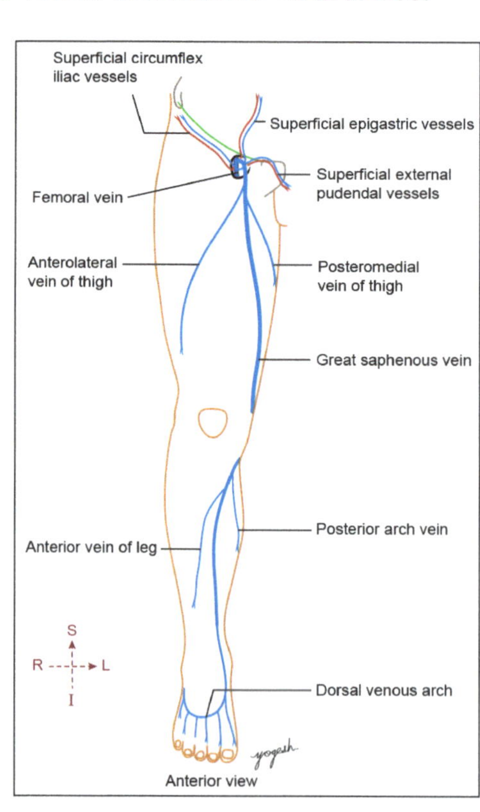

Technique: Use your index finger to locate the arterial pulsation along the inguinal ligament at the midpoint between the anterior superior iliac spine and the pubic symphysis. Then move 1 cm to 2 cm inferior to this position as the needle puncture must be performed below the inguinal ligament. Next, move 1 cm to 2 cm medially.

Use your index and middle fingers to locate the distal and proximal pulsations of the femoral artery. Just medial to your fingertips should be the general course of the femoral vein. Hence, you should puncture just medial to your index finger in a medial direction to your middle finger.

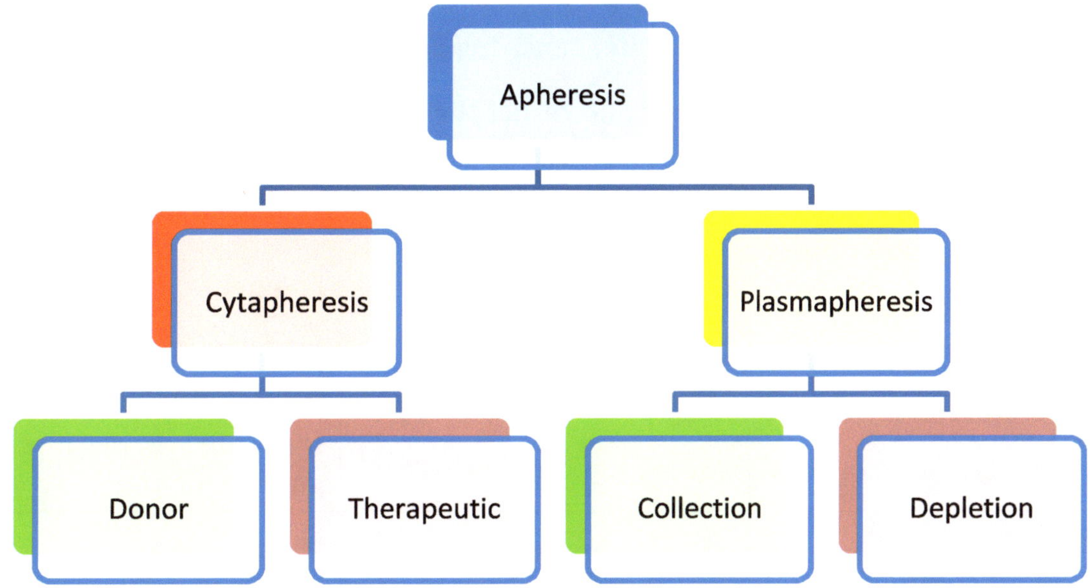

Figure 22. Classification of apheresis procedures

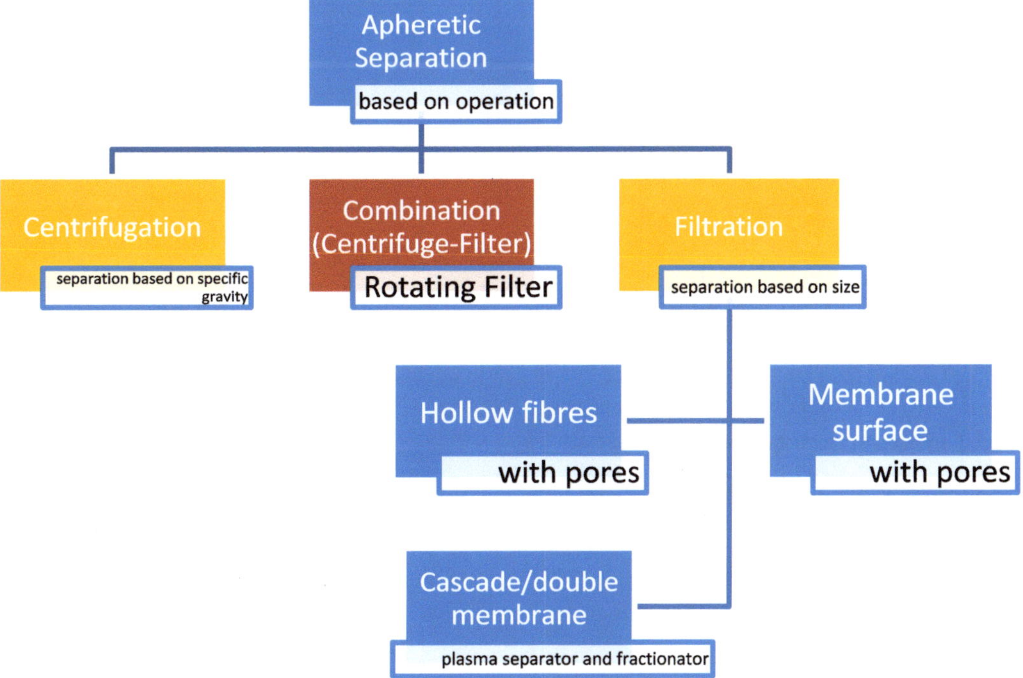

Figure 23. Principles of Apheresis separation

Leading segments of apheresis equipment:

Pumps:
a. Roller pumps – Trima accel, Haemonetics

b. Pneumatic pumps – Therakos UVAR XTS, Fenwal Alyx

c. Syringe pumps – Kaneka MA-03 for Heparin

Valves: Pinch clamps, offset rollers, pistons

Sensors: Air sensors, Pressure sensors, Optical sensors, Fluid sensors

Separation devices: Hollow fibres, flat plate, centrifuge chambers

Microprocessors: monitor safety sensors and direct the procedure, troubleshooting advice through interactive screens or buttons

Anticoagulation:

	Citrate	Heparin
Risks	Hypocalcemia Metabolic alkalosis	Heparin Induced thrombocytopenia Bleeding risk because of systemic anticoagulation
An additional risk with citrated blood components	Yes	No
Half-life	Variable (18-52 minutes)	90 minutes
Flow rates	Slow	Fast
Reversal	Calcium	Protamine

Donor Apheresis

Blood components collected by apheresis:

1. Granulocytes
2. Hematopoietic progenitor cells
3. Plasma: single or multiple doses
4. Platelet: single, double, or triple
5. Double platelet and single plasma
6. Platelet and single or double plasma
7. Red blood cells: single or double
8. Red blood cells and plasma
9. Red blood cell and platelet
10. Red blood cells, platelet, and plasma
11. Convalescent plasma

Advantages of Apheresis derived blood components:

- Total transfusion dose: reduced donor exposure
- Pedigreed donor: frequent repeat donor
- Better quality of components/products: because of automation
- Consistent yield and standardized products
- Matched donor-recipient program
- Reduced donor reactions
- Multiple yield/dose blood components
- Enhanced safety for the patients

History taking in a donor:

General Health

Lifestyle

Social history

Travel History

Medical History

Medication

Apheresis-specific donor criteria:

	NBTC/DnC Criteria	WHO Criteria	AABB Criteria
Age	18-60 yrs.		
Donation Interval	At least 48 hrs. interval (*not more than two times a week, limited to 24 times in one year*) From whole blood to plateletpheresis or vice versa – 28 days If the reinfusion of red cells could not be completed during apheresis- 90 days *For any donation* From marrow donation, one year From PBSC donation six months	Sixteen weeks for double red cell donation. The minimum interval between donations of platelets should be four weeks The minimum interval between donations of plasma should be two weeks	Defer for 16 weeks after 2-unit red cell collection. Defer for four weeks after infrequent plasmapheresis. Defer two days after plasmapheresis, plateletpheresis, or leukapheresis.

Factors associated with Hypercalcaemic Symptoms in Adult Allogeneic PBSC Donors	
Female gender	Smaller Body Surface Area
Older age	Smaller blood volume
Lower body weight	Large volume of blood processed
Lower Initial Mg²⁺ levels	

Acute adverse effects specific to apheresis:

Acute:

   i. **Venepuncture-related complications:**

  ii. **Citrate toxicity (0.4%)**

      Signs and symptoms: perioral and acral paresthesias, Shivering, Lightheadedness, Twitching, Tremors, Nausea and vomiting, Hypotension, Carpopedal spasm, Tetany, Seizure

  iii. **Vasovagal reactions**

Table 20.1 Comparison of reaction rates in apheresis collection to whole blood collection

Reaction	Apheresis donation (%)	Whole blood donation (%)
Hematoma	1.15	9-16
Vasovagal reactions	0.05	2-5
Vasovagal reactions with LOC	0.08	0.1-0.3

Granulocyte collections:

A tendency for the bilateral occurrence of cataracts exclusively among glucocorticoid-stimulated granulocyte donors

Long-term issues for platelet donors /multicomponent collections:

- Risk for iron depletion
- Higher risk for fracture: citrate anticoagulant might chelate serum calcium and alter the bone mineral density
- Lymphopenia: increased risk for bacterial infection in a dose-dependent manner
- Progressive decreases in platelet counts
- Serum protein, albumin, and IgG concentration are statistically lower in frequent plasmapheresis donors compared to nondonors

Managing Hypocalcemia due to citrate:

- Reduce the reinfusion
- Increase blood-to-citrate ratio
- Administer oral calcium
- Administer iv calcium gluconate or calcium chloride

Table 20.2 Donor eligibility based on total RBC lost during apheresis procedures

Blood lost in the First procedure (ml)	Blood loss total (First + subsequent donation)	Deferral period
<200	<200	No deferral
<200	200- 300 ml	Eight weeks from the second procedure
200-300		Eight weeks from the first procedure
<200	>300	Sixteen weeks from the second procedure
≥ 300		Sixteen weeks from the first procedure

Therapeutic Apheresis

Possible mechanisms of action of plasma exchange

- Removal of pathogenic antibodies.
- Sensitisation of antibodies-producing cells to immunosuppressant and chemotherapeutic agents.
- Removal of pathogenic immune complexes that could prevent splenic blockade and improve monocyte/macrophage functions.
- Removal of cytokines and adhesion molecules.
- Replacement of missing plasma component (e.g. TTP).
- Alteration of the cellular immune system, which may include:

  - changes in lymphocyte numbers and distribution (decline in B-cells and increase in T-cells)
  - changes in NK cell numbers and activity
  - increased in T-suppressor or T-regulatory cell function
  - shift from Th2 to Th1 predominant pattern.

Fraction of the target removed per volume exchanged

Plasma volume removed	Fraction of the target removed (%)
0.5	40
1.0	62
1.5	78
2.0	85
2.5	91
3.0	94

McLeod's Criteria for evaluation of Apheresis Efficacy:

Mechanism	The current understanding of the disease pathophysiology supports the use of apheresis as a treatment
correction	The abnormality involved in pathogenesis can be corrected with apheresis
Clinical effect	Evidence exists that apheresis confers a clinical benefit and not just a significant change in a laboratory parameter

Diseases that require emergent apheresis treatment

Disease characteristic: rapidly worsening or progressive, e.g., TTP
Imminently life or limb-threatening: Myasthenic crisis, Respiratory paralysis in GBS
Acute conditions: Diffuse alveolar haemorrhage
Treatment can immediately reverse disease progression. e.g., poisoning

ASFA Categories

Category	Description	Examples
I	First-line therapy, either as a stand-alone or in conjunction with another mode of treatment	GBS, CIDP, Erythrodermic Sezary, Homozygous hypercholesterolemia
II	Second-line therapy, either as a stand-alone or in conjunction with another mode of treatment	Acute disseminated Encephalomyelitis, severe Cold Agglutinin disease, Major ABO-incompatible transplant
III	The optimum role is not established; individualised decision	Henoch Schonlein Purpura, Aplastic anaemia, HIT, Crohn's disease
IV	Ineffective or harmful, Institutional Review and approval required	SLE Nephritis, Schizophrenia, Rheumatoid Arthritis, POEMS

The intensity of treatment: categories for TPE

Category	Schedule	No of cycles	Indications
Aggressive	Daily	3- indefinite	Myasthenia Gravis, TTP, HUS, PTP, Acute hepatic failure, poisoning, ABO-incompatible transplant
Routine	Alternate day	5-7	GBS, Lambert-Eaton, Multiple sclerosis, ITP, Transplant rejection of the heart, RFGN, AIHA
Prolonged	Once or twice a week	3-8 weeks	CIDP, Peripheral neuropathy with monoclonal gammopathy
Chronic	Every 1-4 weeks	Indefinite	Hyperviscosity syndromes, cryoglobulinemia, Neuromyotonia and limbic encephalitis

Comparison of Apheresis to Dialysis:

	Apheresis	Hemodialysis
Mechanism	Separates whole blood into fractions and removes the entire fraction	Plasma is passed through a semipermeable membrane with the use of counter-current flow with the exchange of molecules and electrolytes
Applicability, when a pathologic agent is	High molecular mass (>15000D) A slow rate of formation Low volume of distribution	Small and medium-sized diffusible molecules

Separation mechanism	Centrifugation generally	Membrane separation
Volume depletion	Always needs replacement	Can perform ultrafiltration restoring euvolemia
Hypotension	Common	Rare
Flow rate (ml/min)	Low (15-165)	High (100-500)
Vascular access	Subcutaneous ports and peripheral lines	Tunnelled dialysis catheters AV fistulas or grafts
Duration	Short interval	Usually for long term (years)
Type of Disease	Usually, for acute illness	Chronic illnesses
Anticoagulant	Citrate, sometimes heparin	Heparin
Effects	Immunological as well as rheological	Usually, metabolic

Factors to be considered while starting Apheresis treatment

- Blood volume and status of volume (hyper/hypovolemia)
- Cardiovascular stability
- Availability of vascular access: central vs peripheral
- Impact on other treatments: removal of drugs, fall in therapeutic concentration, Interactions with medications
- Change in haemostasis: thrombocytopenia, fall in coagulation factors if planning surgery
- Effect on accuracy and interpretation of laboratory tests

Special considerations while using citrate:

- Sedated patients and children: cannot remark on hypocalcemia-associated effects
- Liver and kidney disease: cannot metabolise and excrete citrate

Advantages of peripheral vascular access over central:

- Routinely done by trained staff
- Minimal maintenance
- Immediate availability
- Low cost
- Lesser complications
- Preservation of patient lifestyle and comfort
- Ideal for short-term and infrequent procedures

Replacement fluids used in therapeutic apheresis

Products	Advantages	Disadvantages
Normal saline (0.9%)	It can be used in combination with other replacement fluids	Risk of third spacing Hemolysis if osmolality is not accurate
Albumin (5%)		Risk of hypotension with ACE inhibitors

Hetastarch	Effective red cell sedimenting agent It can be used in Jehovah's witness Low cost	Causes coagulopathy Caution for use in critically ill patients and those with kidney injury
Pentastarch	No coagulopathy It can be used by those who refuse human-derived blood products	Results in hypoalbuminemia
Plasma	It can be used in patients with ACE inhibitors	Transfusion reactions
Blood	Increases oxygen-carrying capacity	It May exacerbate hyperviscosity if used too early in apheresis

	Allergic reactions	Coagulation factors	Source	Osmolality	Compatibility	Sterility	Cost	Hypocalcemia risk
Normal saline (0.9%)	----	--		Isosmotic	Not required	Yes	Low	
Albumin	++	--		Isosmotic Hyperoncotic	Not required	Yes	High	++
Hetastarch	-----	--	Natural		Not required	Yes	Low	
Pentastarch		--	Prepared from HES		Not required	Yes	Low	
Plasma	++	++			Required	No		++
Blood	++	+			Required	No		---

Complications of therapeutic apheresis and their management		
Procedure-related		
Complication	**Signs and symptoms**	**Management**
Anxiety/ Hyperventilation	Tachycardia, hyper/ hypotension, diaphoresis Tingling of fingers/toes	Reassurance Breathing into a paper bag For Hypotension: trendelenberg position and saline bolus Consider anxiolytics for subsequent procedures
VVR	Bradycardia, hypotension, diaphoresis, pallor, nausea	Put the patient in the Trendelenburg position and saline bolus Cool, moist towels on the forehead Stimulation: Physical/ammonia spirits

Hypocalcemia	Paresthesias: circumoral and progress to other parts Jaw vibration, tetany Nausea, vomiting, diarrhoea Chest tightness, hypotension ECG: Prolonged QT interval	Pause procedure Slow citrate infusion Administer calcium: oral or iv. Add calcium to colloid/crystalloid replacement fluid (continuous replacement)
Hypovolemia	Hypotension, diaphoresis, tachycardia	Put the patient in the Trendelenburg position and saline bolus Increase colloid and decrease crystalloid Withhold routine antihypertensive medications prior to the procedure
	If using ACE- inhibitor: flushing, hypotension	Withhold apheresis for 24-48 hours after the last dosage for non-urgent procedures
Reaction to ethylene oxide	Burning eyes, periorbital oedema, allergic symptoms	Stop procedure. Perform double prime for subsequent procedures
Replacement fluid-related		
Allergic	Itching, urticaria, facial oedema, change in voice, difficulty swallowing, wheezing, shortness of breath, hypotension	Administer iv diphenhydramine, methylprednisolone Subcutaneous epinephrine
Transfusion reactions	Varied depending on the reaction type	Stop transfusion and follow transfusion reaction protocol
Vascular access-related		
Sepsis	Hypotension, positive blood cultures	Antimicrobial therapy, Place new catheter, Use peripheral access if feasible
Thrombosis	High-pressure alarms	Radiograph to assess the placement of the catheter
	Unable to flush the catheter	Instil thrombolytic agent

Clues suggestive of inadequate oxygenation

Resting tachypnea

Dyspnea, either at rest or on modest exertion

Any state of confusion, lethargy, or obtundation

Persistent dizziness or light-headed feeling

Any unexplained state of anxiety, irritability, or restlessness

Any unexplained headache, especially if chronic or recurring

Cardiomegaly or heart failure of unknown cause

Polycythemia of unknown cause

Causes of hypoxia: a general classification

1. **Hypoxemia (reduced arterial oxygen content)**

   a. Reduced PaO2*
   b. Reduced SaO2**
   c. Reduced haemoglobin content (anaemia)

2. **Reduced oxygen delivery**

   a. Reduced cardiac output
   b. Left to right systemic shunt (e.g., septic shock)

3. **Decreased tissue oxygen uptake**

   a. Mitochondrial poisoning (e.g., cyanide)
   b. Left shifted haemoglobin dissociation curve (e.g., abnormal haemoglobin structure)

Patients at risk of citrate toxicity:

Liver/kidney diseases

Older age

Female sex

Lower body weight

Blood volume<4 litres

In case of citrate toxicity:

- Decrease the rate of exchange
- Reduce citrate infusion rate
- Monitor ionised calcium level
- Calcium supplementation- oral or iv
- Use non-citrated replacement fluid- albumin
- Add alternative anticoagulant- heparin

Hypocalcemia:

Abnormalities of parathyroid hormone

Vitamin D deficiency/resistance

Chronic renal disease

Pancreatitis

Hyperphosphatemia – tumour lysis syndrome, rhabdomyolysis

Selective removal systems in comparison to Therapeutic Plasma Exchange	
Advantages	Disadvantages
Removes selectively, leaving behind the normal and beneficial plasma constituents	Not helpful when the pathophysiology or agent is not clear
Minimal requirement of replacement fluids, if any, and hence avoid associated reactions, expenses	Blood is exposed to biologically active columns and materials, Clogging, clotting, hemolysis
More efficient removal of the target	Systems are complex and expensive to operate
Some systems do not require RBC and plasma separation	Limited availability of the systems
	Need a higher flow rate

Table 20.3 Specialised therapeutic apheresis procedures

Technique	Equipment	Description	Indication
Extracorporeal Photopheresis	UVAR XTS (Therakos), Therakos Cellex	Buffy coat is separated from the patient blood, treated with a photoactive compound (Psoralen) and exposed to UV light A and reinfused to the patient	Cutaneous T-Cell Lymphoma, GVHD, Transplant Rejection-Heart, Lung
Rheopheresis		Apheresis separates high molecular weight components such as fibrinogen, α2-microglobulin, LDL-cholesterol, and IgM to reduce plasma viscosity and red cell aggregation and improve flow and tissue oxygenation	Age-related macular degeneration, peripheral artery occlusive disease, angina, stroke
Double Filtration plasmapheresis		Removing pathogenic substances based on their size (molecular weight and 3-D configuration) like lipoproteins, immune complexes	SLE, RA, Myasthenia Gravis, GBS, TTP, MS, ITP, Goodpasture Syn, Pemphigus
Specific Immunoadsorption (IA)			
LDL-Apheresis	Liposorber LA-15 system	Ligand: Dextran sulphate carrier: Cellulose	Familial hypercholesterolemia, Steroid-resistant Nephrotic Syndrome by FSGS, Sudden sensorineural hearing loss
	MONET	Fresenius polysulphone membrane	
	Therasorb	Sepharose coupled with sheep antihuman apoB-100 antibodies	
	DALI	Porous polyacrylamide beads coated with anionic polyacrylate ligands	

ABO-specific IA Glycosorb	Glycorex Transplantation AB	A synthetic blood group A or B trisaccharide bound to Sepharose removes anti-A or anti-B antibodies	ABO-incompatible Liver or Kidney Transplantation
IgE IA	IgEnio	Recombinant protein-ligand BM10 binds to IgE with a high affinity	Atopic dermatitis, severe allergic asthma
β2 microglobulin column	Lixelle	Cellulose porous microspheres coated by hexadecyl hydrophobic group	Dialysis related amyloidosis
Nonspecific Immunoadsorption			
Staphylococcal protein A columns	Prosorba (silica) Immunosorba (Agarose)	Binds and removes IgG	ITP, RA, TTP, Paraneoplastic CNS syndromes Factor VIII or IX inhibitors, Wegeners, Dilated cardiomyopathy
Anti-human polyclonal Immunoglobulin (AHPI) Column	Ig-Therasorb	Sheep AHPI bound to a matrix	APLS, SLE, Dilated cardiomyopathy, coagulation factor inhibitors
Dextran sulphate column	Selesorb	Removes DNA antibodies, cardiolipin antibodies, and immune complexes	SLE with RPGN or CNS disease
Polyvinyl alcohol gel column	Tryptophan (Immunosorba-TR) Phenylalanine (Immunosorba-PH)	Immunoglobulins are removed by hydrophobic and ionic interactions	RA, Myasthenia Gravis, GBS, CIDP, MS, Pemphigus, acquired haemophilia

Steps in undertaking Therapeutic Apheresis

1. Assessment: Clinical History, Physical Examination, laboratory testing, imaging Complicating factors: Severity of illness, pregnancy, obesity, young age
2. Plan

Diagnosis	Working, Final
Type of procedure	Red cell exchange, plasma exchange, Leukacytapheresis
Goals	
Number of procedures planned	
Scheduling of procedures/ Intensity	Plasma volumes (single or double), therapeutic targets
Vascular access	
Laboratory tests required	Before/through/after

Other Communications/ consulatations	Requirement of a paediatrician or anaesthesiologist
PRN (pro re nata)	(Pre-medications/SOS orders)

PRN= prescription as needed

3. Consent: Discuss risks vs benefits of the procedure,

Clearly state the rationale for performing the procedure, expectations, and plan

Treatment alternatives, if any

Consent for transfusion

Consent for the emergency procedure, if any required

4. Procedure

Procedure Documentation for Therapeutic Apheresis		
Type of Procedure		Procedure number
Procedural targets(Vol)		Processing required
Replacement fluids		Anticoagulation
Medications	Pre/Intra/post	Vascular access
Patient condition	Pre/Intra/post	Events if any
Target achieved or not		If not, why?
Subsequent plan		

Patient evaluation for Therapeutic Apheresis:

Considerations: **1.** Safety

    2. Efficacy

General physical: Age

    Vital signs

    Height and weight

    Current vascular access

Hematologic: Hemoglobin and hematocrit (concern for anemia)

    Platelet count (exclude thrombocytopenia)

Coagulation status and anticoagulation therapy (exclude coagulopathy, assess the risk of bleeding)

History of thrombosis or hypercoagulable state

Cardiopulmonary: Adequate oxygenation

    Adequate cardiac function (blood pressure, ejection fraction, if known)

    History of or current cardiac disease, arrhythmias, or coronary artery disease

Hemodynamic stability

Sepsis/systemic inflammatory response syndrome

Renal/metabolic: Volume status and fluid balance

Electrolyte abnormalities (Ca, K, Mg)

History of renal or hepatic dysfunction

Neurologic: Mental status, including the ability to participate in the informed consent process and ability to report symptoms during procedure

History of seizures or cerebrovascular accidents

Autonomic dysfunction or neuropathy that may impact peripheral access

Medication: Allergies, Protein-bound drugs

Angiotensin-converting enzyme inhibitors, Other blood pressure medications

Anti-seizure drugs

Immunoglobulin preparations

Anticoagulants (heparin, coumadin, clopidogrel, ASA), Vasopressors

Consideration of timing of drug dosing

Disease-specific testing:

ADAMTS13, LDH, and reticulocytes for TTP

Anti-GBM for Goodpasture syndrome

Acetylcholine receptor antibodies for myasthenia gravis

ABO and/or HLA antibody titers for incompatible kidney transplant recipients

Percent haemoglobin S for patients with complications of sickle cell disease

Replacement volume, type and frequency of exchange

Utility:

i. **In Hematological disorders**

TPE: AIHA, Hyperviscosity syndromes

Leukacytapheresis: Hyperleukocytosis

Erythrocytapheresis/Red cell exchange: Malaria, Babesiosis, Hereditary hemochromatosis, Sickle Cell disease with iron overload, Polycythemia Vera

Thrombocytapheresis: Thrombocytosis, thrombotic microangiopathies

Condition	Threshold count for hyperleukocytosis (per μL)
Monoblastic or monocytic subtypes	50,000
AML	1,00,000
ALL	4,00,000

Condition	Threshold concentration at which hyperviscosity syndrome appears
IgM	4 (grams per dL)
IgA	6-7
IgG3	4

ii. **In Neurological disorders**

AIDP: GBS, CIDP, Myasthenia Gravis

iii. **In Renal disorders**

TPE: Goodpasture syndrome, Berger's disease (IgA nephropathy)

Immunoadsorption or lipoprotein apheresis: FSGS

iv. **In Rheumatological disorders:**

TPE: Antiphospholipid syndrome, ANCA-associated vasculitis

Immunoadsorption or lipoprotein apheresis: Behcet's disease

v. **In Endocrinological disorders:**

Thyroid storm, characterised by severe clinical manifestations of thyrotoxicosis. TPE helps by reducing cytokines, antibodies(Graves disease), catecholamines and protein-bound thyroid hormones.

Typical schedule: every 1-3 days for 3-6 procedures

vi. **In Transplantation**
vii. **In cardiac and vascular disorders:**

Lipoprotein apheresis: Familial hypercholesterolemia

TPE: Autoantibody-associated cardiomyopathy

Immunoadsorption: Thromboangitis obliterans

Double filtration plasmapheresis: Calciphylaxis

Format for Allogenic Donor Screening

Directed donation: Yes/No

> **If yes: Patient details in Brief: Diagnosis of the patient:** CR Status of Patient
>
> **If No: Collection intended for:**

Name: **Age/Gender:**

Hospital No:

Relationship with Patient: **Level of HLA Compatibility:**

The blood group of Donor: **Blood group of Patient:**

Current clinical status of Donor: Any current illnesses – DM, HTN, CAD, Asthma

Past history: Significant medical or surgical illnesses

Personal history: Diet/Addictions: Menstrual History/Marital status/Obstetric History:

Transfusion/Transplant History:

General Examination:

   PR: BP: RR:

   Pallor   icterus   cyanosis   clubbing   oedema   lymphadenopathy

Systemic Examination:

   CVS: RESP: GIT: CNS:

General parameters:

   Weight: Height: TBV:

Vascular/vein status:

Fitness from other departments:

   Psychiatry   Cardiology

Basic investigations:

   DAT/IAT: CBC: RFT: LFT:

   Calcium level: Serum electrolytes: Coagulation profile:

Procedure explanation:

Transplant Concerns:

   Degree of HLA Compatibility:

   ABO Mismatch: Anti-A/B Titer:

   Procedure Modifications: Priming: Flow rate: Target volume:

Ability to give consent: **Advice to the Donor:**

Format for Autologous Donor Screening

Name: **Age/Gender:**

Hospital No: **Unit/Ward:**

Diagnosis of the patient:

Brief H/o Patient condition:

Treatment Details:

Past history:

DM, HTN, TB, Asthma, CAD, CVD, Congenital diseases

Personal history:

Diet/Addictions:

Menstrual History/Marital status/Obstetric History:

Transfusion/Transplant History:

General Examination:

PR: BP: RR:

Pallor: Icterus: Cyanosis: Clubbing: Edema: Lymphadenopathy:

Systemic Examination:

CVS: RESP: GIT: CNS:

General parameters:

Weight: Height: TBV:

Vascular status: Peripheral/Central

Fitness from other departments:

Cardiology   Pulmonary Medicine   ENT   Psychiatry   Dental

Investigations:

Blood group: DAT/IAT: CBC: BM Status:

RFT: LFT: Calcium level: Serum electrolytes: Coagulation profile:

PETCT: GFR: ECHO:

Ability to give consent: (Procedural explanation)

Advice to the Patient:

Transplant Concerns: CR Status:

Procedure Modifications: Priming: Flow rate: Target volume:

Format for Plasma Exchange History Taking

Name: Age/Gender:

Hospital No: Unit/Ward:

Presenting complaints:

H/o presenting illness:

Treatment Details:

Past history:

Personal history:

Diet/Addictions: Menstrual History/Marital status/Obstetric History:

Transfusion/Transplant History:

Probable Diagnosis:

General Examination:

PR: BP: RR:

Pallor: Icterus: Cyanosis: Clubbing: Edema: Lymphadenopathy:

Systemic Examination:

CVS: RESP: GIT: CNS: Skin:

General parameters:

Weight: Height: TBV:

Vascular status:

Investigations:

Blood group: DAT/IAT:

CBC: Peripheral smear (For TTP):

RFT: LFT:

Calcium level: Serum electrolyte level:

Coagulation profile: CSF Analysis:

Radiological evaluation: Autoimmune Ab Panel: LDH:

Ability to give consent:

Vascular Assessment: **Replacement Fluid:**   **Anticoagulant:**

Modifications of any medications:

Priming: Flow rate:

Format for Leukapheresis History Taking

Name: **Age/Gender:**

Hospital No: **Unit/Ward:**

Presenting complaints:

H/o presenting illness:

Treatment Details:

Past history:

Personal history: Diet/Addictions: Menstrual History/Marital status/Obstetric History:

Transfusion/Transplant History:

Probable Diagnosis:

General Examination:

PR: BP: RR:

Pallor: Icterus: Cyanosis: Clubbing: Edema: Lymphadenopathy:

Systemic Examination:

CVS: RESP: GIT: CNS: Skin:

General parameters:

Weight: Height: TBV:

Vascular status:

Investigations:

Blood group: DAT/IAT:

CBC: Peripheral smear:

RFT: LFT:

Calcium level: Serum electrolyte level:

Coagulation profile: Uric acid: LDH:

Radiological Investigations:

CT/MRI Brain: HRCT Thorax: USG Abdomen:

Ability to give consent:

Vascular Assessment: **Replacement Fluid:**   **Anticoagulant:**

Modifications of any medications:

Priming: Flow rate: Target Volume:

Chapter
21

QUALITY MANAGEMENT

"Quality" is a Latin word that means "of what kind" or "character."

It is a measure of excellence.

Quality: Quality may be defined as the degree to which an object/entity, like a process, product, or service, fulfils a specified set of attributes or requirements.

The fundamental components of Quality management are Quality system, Quality assurance and Quality control.

1. **Quality System:** Organizational structure, procedures, processes, and resources needed to implement quality management
2. **Quality Assurance:** Planned, systematic activities implemented within the quality system to provide confidence that requirements for quality will be fulfilled
3. **Quality Control:** Operational techniques and activities used to fulfil the requirements for quality

Quality management systems (QMS):

A collection of processes that are put in place to achieve quality while also meeting end-user requirements concerning the products or services.

Comprises of

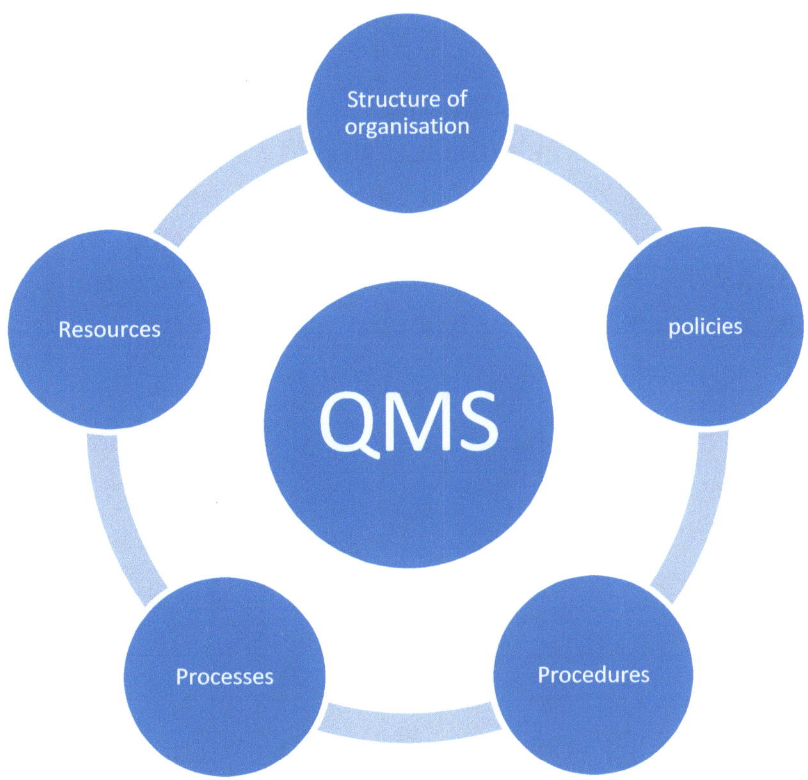

Customer requirements are defined, processes are designed to meet those requirements, and processes are in place to manage and improve the service level.

Why QMS?

* They assure that the products and services produced and provided are safe and effective for their intended use.
* To meet the expectations of regulators
* To operate most cost-effectively- A good QMS will reduce rework, wastage and inefficiencies
* Provides confidence to the organisation and other interested parties

How does QMS work?

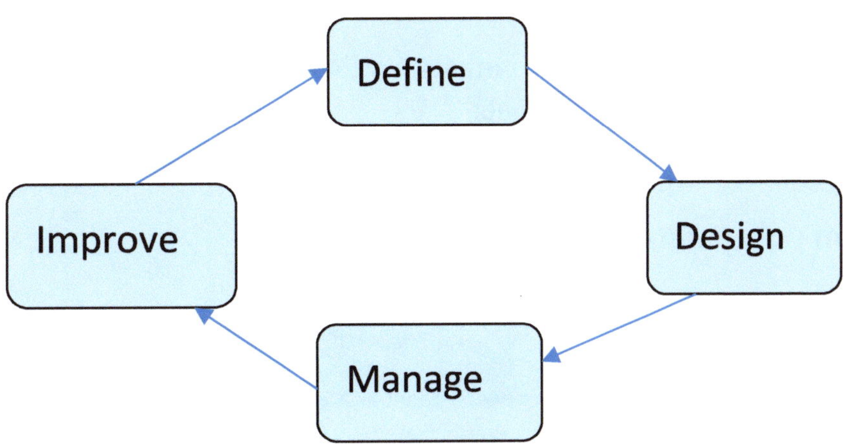

Essential elements of QMS are:

1. **Organisation and leadership:** the organisation must be structured so the QMS can be well implemented and facilitate communication. Leadership must create an environment where individuals are fully engaged in the QMS and monitor it to ensure that the system operates effectively. The key here is that no individual should review his or her work.
2. **Customer focus:** Customer requirements need to be established and documented. There should be a mechanism to receive feedback from the customer at regular intervals from an analysis of critical metrics developed in conjunction with the customer (e.g., fill rates, on-time delivery, customer complaint rates) or from customer surveys
3. **Human resources:**

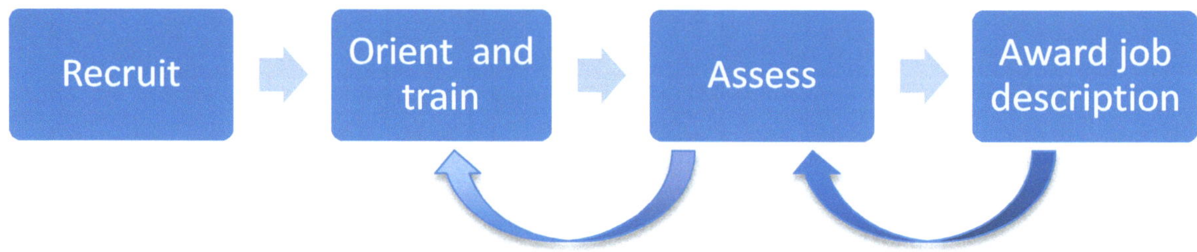

4. **Equipment management:** Selection, Identification, Maintenance, calibration, QC
5. **Suppliers and materials management:** supplier qualification, contracts and agreements, receipt and inspection of incoming supplies
6. **Process control and management:** process control is the sum of activities involved in ensuring a process is predictable, stable, and consistently operating at the target level of performance with only normal variation.
   The components are

   - SOPs
   - Process validation
   - Computer system validation
   - Test method validation
   - QC
   - Training
   - Tracking and trending

7. **Documents and records:** Quality manuals, Policies and process documents, SOPs, Work instructions, Job aids, Forms, and Labels.
8. **Information management:** confidentiality, the integrity of data, data protection, backup and retention
9. **Management of nonconforming events:**

10. **Monitoring and evaluation:** Quality indicators, Blood utilisation, External assessments, Proficiency testing
11. **Process improvement:** should have processes in place that allow for continuous improvement in operations and patient safety
12. **Facilities, work environment, and safety:** fire safety, biological and chemical safety, radiation safety, disaster preparedness, response, and recovery.

Quality Assurance: maintenance of a desired level of quality in a service or product, especially through attentiveness to every stage of the process of delivery or production. The program designed and implemented to ensure that it is achieved is called the Quality Assurance Program

Goals:

- ❖ To decrease errors
- ❖ Ensure Credibility
- ❖ Implement safe and effective processes and controls
- ❖ Ensure continued product safety and quality

Quality Assurance Program: includes Retrospective reviews and analysis of operational performance data

Error Prevention:

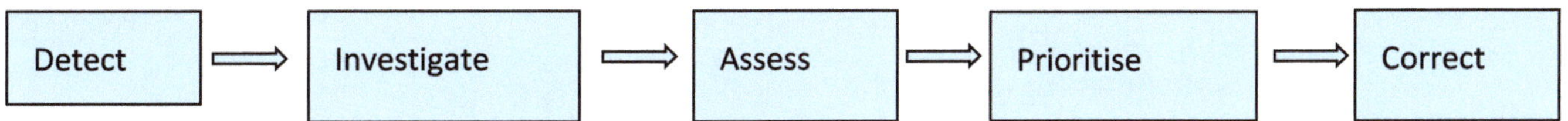

Tool: A chart, device, software, strategy, or technique that supports quality management efforts

Calibration: Comparing a measurement device to a known standard and then adjusting it, if necessary, to measure the same as the standard.

Validation: Demonstration through objective evidence that the requirements for a particular application or intended use have been met.

Quality Control

Operational techniques and activities that are used to monitor and eliminate causes of unsatisfactory performance at any stage of a process.

It usually involves sampling and testing.

E.g., reagent QC, product QC, clerical checks, visual inspections, and regular measurements like temperature monitoring

- ❖ Trends in QC indicate the potential for a problem in the future

Reagents

Reagent Red Cells

Parameter	DGHS	Frequency
Appearance	No hemolysis or turbidity in the supernatant by visual inspections	Daily
Reactivity and specificity	Clear cut reactions	Daily

ABO antisera

Parameter		DGHS	Frequency
Appearance	No turbidity, No precipitate No particles No gel formation		Daily
Specificity	Clear-cut reactions with Positive and Negative Controls		Daily and for each new lot
Reactivity	No immune hemolysis, No rouleaux formation No Prozone.		Each new lot
Avidity	Macroscopic agglutination with 50% red cells suspension on the slide at Room Temperature(R.T.)	10 sec with A1 or B cells 20 sec with A2 or A2B cells	Daily and for each new lot
Potency	Undiluted serum should give +++ or above reaction in the saline tube test using a 3% red cell suspension at R.T.	Titre 128 with A1 or B cells 64 sec with A2 or A2B cells	Each new lot

			A1 Cells	A2 Cells	A1B Cells	A2B Cells	B cells	O Cells
Monoclonal	anti-A	Titer	1:256	1:128		1:64	-	-
		Avidity(Sec)	3-4	5-6		5-6	-	-
		Intensity	3+	2+/3+		3+/4+	-	-
	anti-B	Titer	-	-	1:128	-	1:256	-
		Avidity(Sec)	-	-	5-6	-	3-4	-
		Intensity	-	-	3+ to 4+	-	4+	-
	anti-AB	Titer	1:256	1:128			1:256	-
		Avidity(Sec)	3-4	5-6			3-4	-
		Intensity	4+	3+			4+	-

Polyclonal	anti-A	Titer	1:256	1:128		1:64	-	-
		Avidity(Sec)	10-12	15-18		15-18	-	-
		Intensity	3+	2+/3+		2+	-	-
	anti-B	Titer	-	-	1:128	-	1:256	-
		Avidity(Sec)	-	-	12-15	-	10-12	-
		Intensity	-	-	1+	-	3+	-
	anti-AB	Titer	1:256	1:64			1:256	-
		Avidity(Sec)	10-12	15-18			10-12	-
		Intensity	3+	2+			3+	-

Anti- Rh antisera(anti-D,C,E)

Parameter		DGHS		Frequency
		O(R1r or R1R2)	O	
Appearance	No turbidity, No precipitate No particles No gel formation			Daily
Specificity	Clear cut reactions	+++	-	Daily and for each new lot
Reactivity	No immune hemolysis, No rouleaux formation No Prozone.	3+		Each new lot
Avidity	Macroscopic agglutination with 40% red cells suspension on the slide at Room Temperature(R.T.)	5-10 sec for IgM (Monoclonal Blend) 10-20 sec for IgG+IgM (Monoclonal Blend)		Daily and for each new lot
Potency	Undiluted serum should give +++ or above reaction in saline tube test using a 3% red cells suspension	Titre IS: 64 -128(IgM) 128-256(IgG+IgM) 37^0C(30 min): 128-256		Each new lot

Type of reagent		Type of red cells Immediate spin	Titres		Avidity (sec)	Intensity
			30-45 min Incubation			
Monoclonal	IgM	O (R1r or R1R2)	1:64 to 1:128	1:128 to 1:256	5-10	3+
	IgM + IgG		1:32 to 1:64	1:128 to 1:256	10-20	3+
Polyclonal	IgG		-	1:32 to 1:64	60	3+
	Blend		1:32 to 1:64	1:128 to 1:256	10-20	3+

Antiglobulin antisera(anti-IgG,C3D)

Parameter		DGHS	Frequency
Appearance	No turbidity, No precipitate No particles No gel formation		Daily
Specificity	Agglutination of red cells sensitized with anti-D serum containing not more than 0.2 mg/ml antibody activity Agglutination of red cells sensitized with a complement-binding antibody (e.g.anti-Lea) Agglutination of red cells coated with C3b and C3d. No/ weak agglutination with C4-coated red cells.		Daily and for each new lot
Reactivity	No immune hemolysis, No rouleaux formation No Prozone.		Each new lot
Potency	Anti-IgG Anti-C3d	1:64 1:4	

Albumin

Parameter	QC Requirement	Frequency
Appearance	No precipitate, particles or gel formation by visual inspection	Every day
Purity	> 98% albumin, as determined by electrophoresis	Every batch
Reactivity	No agglutination of unsensitized red cells; no hemolytic activity; no prozone phenomenon.	Every batch
Potency	IgG anti-D should give a titer of 32-64 with red cells R1r	Every month

Enzymes

Parameter	QC Requirement	Frequency
Appearance	No precipitate, particles or gel formation by visual inspection	Every day
Reactivity	No agglutination or hemolysis using inert A.B. serum Agglutination (+++) of cells sensitized with a weak IgG (Anti-D)	Every batch
Potency	An IgG antibody, preferably anti-D standardized to give a titer of about 32-64 by the protease technique, should show the same titer on repeated testing with different batches. The 2-stage enzyme titer should at least be equal to the titer obtained with IgG (anti-D) by the AHG test.	Every batch

Parameter	Normal Saline	LISS	Distilled Water	Frequency
Appearance	Clear, no particles on visual inspections			Every day
pH	6.0-8.0	6.65-6.85	6.0-7.0	Every batch
Nacl content	0-154 mol/l(=9g/I)			Every batch
Serological assessment	No hemolysis should be seen when a mixture of 0.1 ml saline and 0.1 ml of 5% red cells suspension centrifuged after 10 min	A weak IgG anti-D (0.25 IU/ml) should give a +/++ reaction with R1r red cells by the routine LISS-AHG test		Each new batch
Osmolarity		270-285 (mmol)		
Conductivity		3.6-3.7mohm/cm at 23°C		

A Nonconformance event is when things do not go as planned or failed to meet a requirement. They are also called accidents, adverse events, errors, events, incidents or occurrences.

Processes and procedures for managing events	
Processes	**Procedures**
Document: classify, severity	
Effect: on the product, services	
Effect on interrelated activities/ organization's operations	
Investigation and Root Cause analysis	Staff interview, review records/data, direct observation, review SOPs
Selection of appropriate corrective action	
Implementation of corrective action (CA)	
Quarantine, Notification and recall	
Implementation of preventive action (PA)	
Evaluation of the effectiveness of CAPA taken	
Reporting to external agencies if required	

Root cause analysis: Root causes are those which are:

- specific underlying causes
- Reasonably identifiable
- Fixable
- Effective Recommendations can be generated for preventing recurrences

Tools for Root cause analysis	
Brainstorming	Generates potential causes
Fishbone diagram (Ishikawa charts)	For determining causes and contributing factors
Failure mode effects analysis (FMEA)	Step-by-step approach for identifying all possible failures
Five Whys	Drilling down to the true cause

Brainstorming: can be structured or unstructured.

Unstructured – everyone is free to give ideas

Structured – each one gives one idea by turn or in his section of expertise

FMEA sample Proforma:

Analysis				Actions				
Process name/ causes	Potential failure/ probability	Potential effect of failure/ criticality score	Severity	Action type- control, accept, eliminate	Action	Outcome	Person responsible	Management concurrence

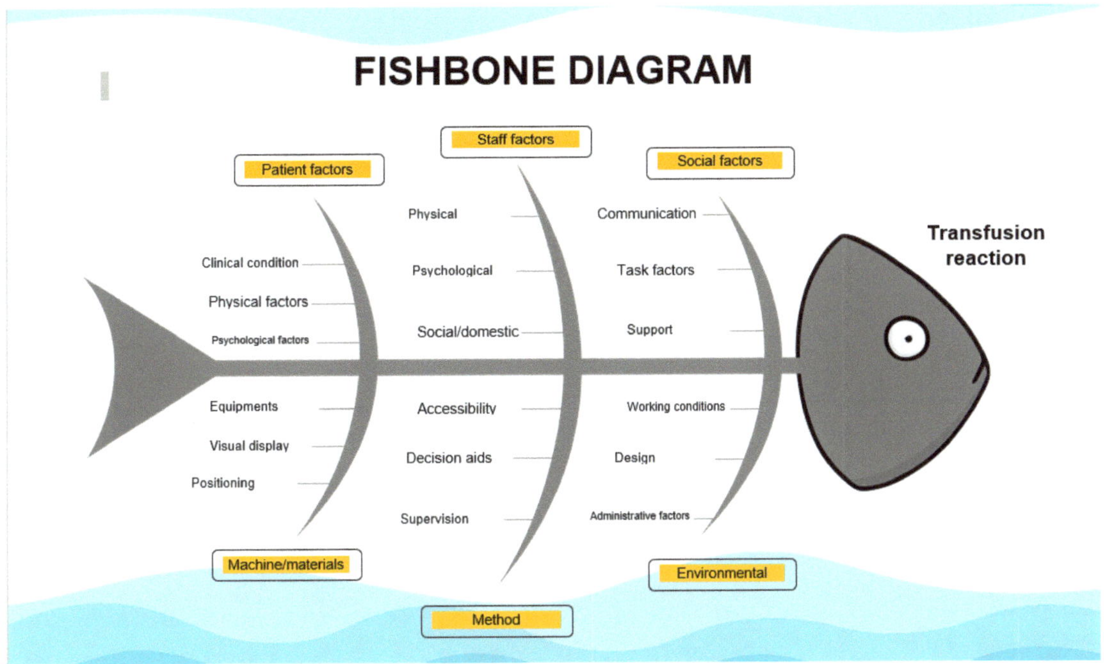

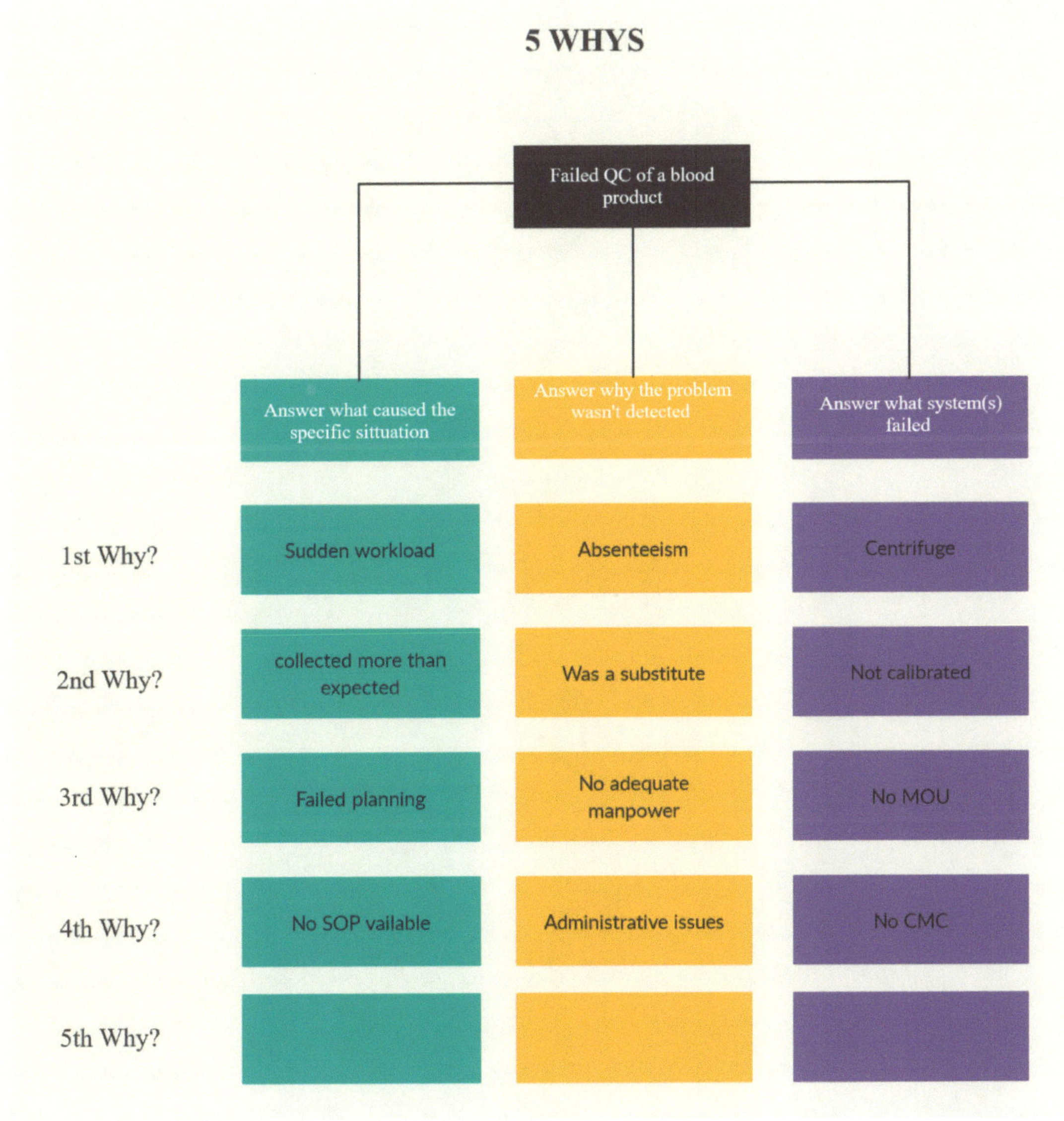

5 WHYS

	Failed QC of a blood product		
	Answer what caused the specific sittuation	Answer why the problem wasn't detected	Answer what system(s) failed
1st Why?	Sudden workload	Absenteeism	Centrifuge
2nd Why?	collected more than expected	Was a substitute	Not calibrated
3rd Why?	Failed planning	No adequate manpower	No MOU
4th Why?	No SOP vailable	Administrative issues	No CMC
5th Why?			

System: An organised, purposeful structure that comprises interrelated and interdependent elements

Process: a set of activities that use resources to transform inputs into outputs

Inputs	Process	Output
Trained phlebotomist Approved collection set Approved arm scrub Phlebotomy SOP	Blood collection	A unit of Whole blood

CLINICAL TRANSFUSION

Pretransfusion Considerations:

	Components	Details
1	Obtaining an informed consent	A description of the risks, benefits, possible side effects, and alternatives (including nontreatment)
		Opportunity to ask questions
		The right to accept or refuse transfusion
2	Transfusion history	Previous transfusions, the timing and the types of blood Products that were transfused, previous transfusion reactions, if any
		Documentation of alloantibodies to red blood cell antigens identified in the patient
3	Compatibility testing	ABO and RhD blood type of the transfusion recipient and identifying any unexpected antibodies in the plasma
4	Other preparations	Modifications to the product
		Premedication if required
		Venous access

At the bedside: transfusion administration

- Verify all pertinent pieces of information before the transfusion is initiated:

  - Positively identify the recipient in their presence using two unique identifiers and confirm the recipient's ABO group and Rh type
  - donation identification number, ABO group and Rh type of the blood unit crossmatch interpretation, documentation of special transfusion requirements and processing (e.g., irradiation), and the unit expiration
  - check for any visual abnormalities in the unit

- Record vitals, including temperature, pulse, blood pressure, and oxygen saturation, before starting the transfusion as a baseline
- Check for a valid order for transfusion and confirm the presence of an appropriately signed consent form

- Blood administration sets and filters
- Coadministration of fluids and blood components
- Coadministration of medications
- Patient monitoring
- Infusion flow rates

Blood warming:

Indications:

1. Rapid transfusion (trauma, surgery settings)
2. Neonatal transfusions
3. Patients with cold agglutinins
4. Transfusion through the central vein

Prerequisites for warmers:

- Equipped with a temperature-sensing device
- Warning system to detect malfunctions and prevent hemolysis or other damage to blood and blood components
- Validated as per manufacturer's suggestions
- Education and competency assessment for the user must be documented

➢ Never to be used for platelets transfusion.
➢ Never should be warmed to more than 42^0 C

DO NOT USE THESE FOR WARMING BLOOD AND BLOOD PRODUCTS

Bedside blood pumps

Post-transfusion:

- check for any signs of an adverse reaction to the blood component
- a final set of vital signs should be taken
- monitored for at least 4–6 hours after the infusion is completed
- proper disposal of empty bags and administration set
- completion report to the blood centre

Techniques for rapid transfusion:

a. The cannula used: smaller length and larger internal bore, faster the infusion
b. Decrease the viscosity of the product (for a fall in Hct by 3%, flow rate increases by 5%)
c. Warming the blood: to the body temperature almost doubles the rate of flow
d. Warming the patient: cold causes vasospasm
e. Positive pressure infusion devices (pressure cuff at 300 mm Hg doubles the rate)
f. Have Multiple infusion sites

Internal bore (SWG)	Rate of infusion (ml/min)- for distilled water, run under a pressure of 76 mm Hg, 220C via 110 cm tubing.
14	286± 35
16	162± 35
18	91± 17
20	54 ± 14

Transfusion in Burns:

Body part	Percentage of area	
Head and neck	9	
Front of chest	9	
Back of chest	9	
Front of abdomen	9	
Back of abdomen	9	
Upper limb	9 each	
Lower limb (Thigh)	9 each	
Lower limb (leg)	9 each	
Genitalia	1	

Parkland's formula: 4 ml/kg × % of burns

Half of this is given in the first 8 hrs and the rest within the next 16 hrs

Red cells are destroyed in burned tissue. A Hb of more than 7 gm% is to be maintained.

Physiologic adaptions in Anemia	
Increased cardiac output	Increased heart rate Increased stroke volume
Increased coronary artery blood flow	
Redistribution of blood flow	Shunting blood flow from high-flow, low-extraction areas to tissues with high oxygen requirements
Increased oxygen extraction	From 0.2 to 0.75
Increased red cell 2,3-DPG	A rightward shift in oxyhemoglobin dissociation curve (better offloading to tissues)

Critical oxygen delivery levels 4 to 10 mL/kg/min

Critical Hb Concentration 3.5- 5.0 g/dL

Patient category	Thresholds	Outcomes	Evidence
Critically Ill	Restrictive group (7g/dL) vs Liberal group(10g/dL)	No difference in 60-day mortality. Restrictive better rate for 30-day mortality. Lesser RBC transfusions	TRICC 1999
Mechanically ventilated	Restrictive group (7g/dL) vs Liberal group(9g/dL)	Higher mortality in the liberal group	CRIT 2004
Cardiac patients	8 gm/dL or 24% Hct		CRUSADE 2005
Cardiovascular surgery	7.5 g/dL	Important risk factors for transfusion: 1. Advanced age (>70 yrs.) 2. Small body size, preoperative anaemia 3. Prolonged Bypass	STS Guidelines
Orthopaedic surgery	8g/dL vs 10g/dL	Wound infection, DVT, Length of stay	FOCUS 2011
Trauma		Restrictive in stable trauma except those with MI or unstable cardiac ischemia. Interventions: tourniquet, avoidance of crystalloid Hemodilution	Transfusion in adult trauma 2009
Elective general surgery	C:T ratio ideally <2.0	OSBOS: Optimal Surgical Blood Order Schedule	
Traumatic brain Injury	>10 g/dL in the acute phase	No difference in neurological outcomes 7g/dL vs 10g/dL	CRASH 2008
Congenital anaemias	To maintain a pretransfusion threshold of 9-10.5 g/dL		

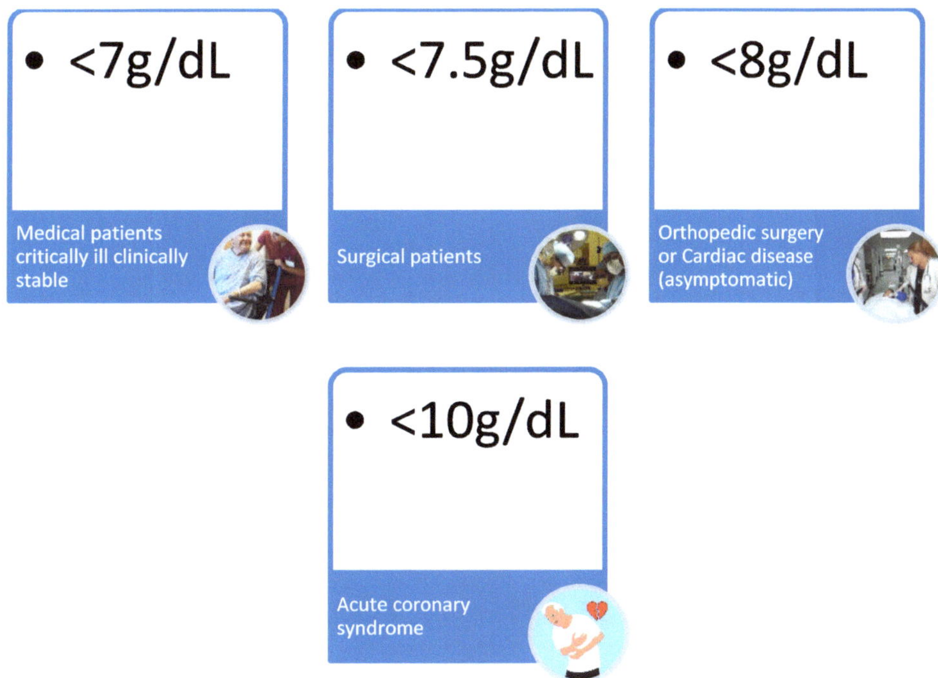

Figure 25. Transfusion Thresholds for PRBC transfusion

RBC Transfusion

Whom to transfuse in Thalassaemic?

Haemoglobin level (Hb)<7g/dL on 2 occasions more than 2 weeks apart (excluding all other contributory causes such as infections)

OR

Haemoglobin > 7 g/dl with any of the following:

Facial changes, Poor growth, Fractures, Clinically significant extramedullary haematopoiesis

Plasma Transfusion

Aspects of the INR and aPTT make these tests poor predictors of haemorrhage:

➢ The relationship between coagulation factors and the prothrombin time (PT) and aPTT is EXPONENTIAL and not non-linear
➢ Mild abnormality in test results occurs among patients with biologically normal coagulation
➢ INR and aPTT tests overestimate deficiencies in the upper limb of the cascade(dominated by factor VII) and underestimate deficiencies in the lower limb
➢ The tests overestimate the extent of coagulation factor depletion if more than one factor is reduced
➢ INR and aPTT are tested to analyze the defect in patients with disorders of fibrin formation; neither test was designed to predict bleeding
➢ These tests are insufficient to assess global hemostasis

Problems with PT and aPTT as predictors of bleeding	
Observation	**Comments**
Non-linear relationship between the tests and coagulation factor levels	Correlation is good between INR 5 TO 1.8. Once the INR is fallen below 1.8, it is not easy to correlate with the response to plasma therapy
Abnormal results are expected in patients with normal biological coagulation	40-50% activity is usually enough for normal haemostasis in people
Overestimates the deficiencies of the factors in the upper limb of the cascade and underestimates those in the lower limb	Especially factor VII
If more than one factor is deficient, then the deficiency is overestimated	If two factors are deficient by 25%, the INR is more prolonged compared to when a single factor is 50% deficient
Designed to evaluate the formation of fibrin only and not bleeding	Bleeding is dependent on the interrelation between the vessel wall, cellular elements of blood, platelet number and function, fibrinolysis

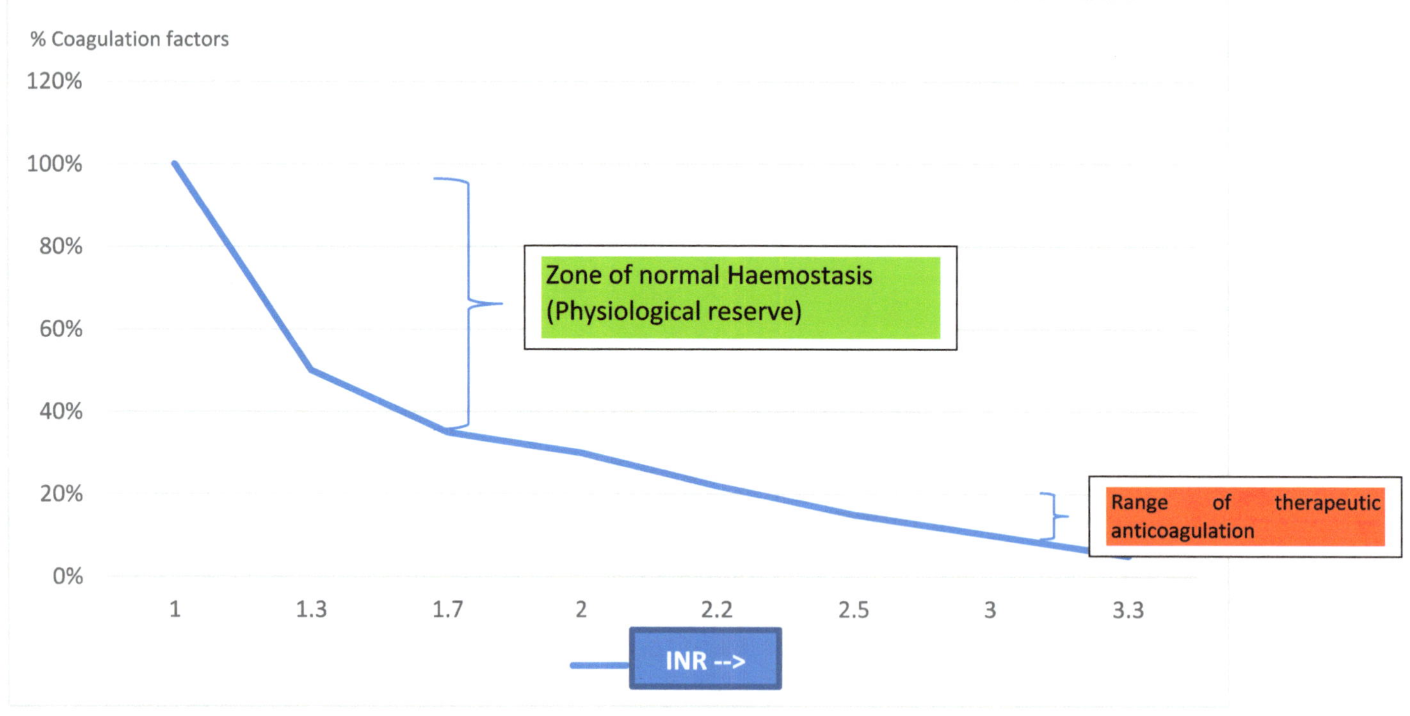

Figure 26 Relationship between coagulation factors concentration and PT/INR results

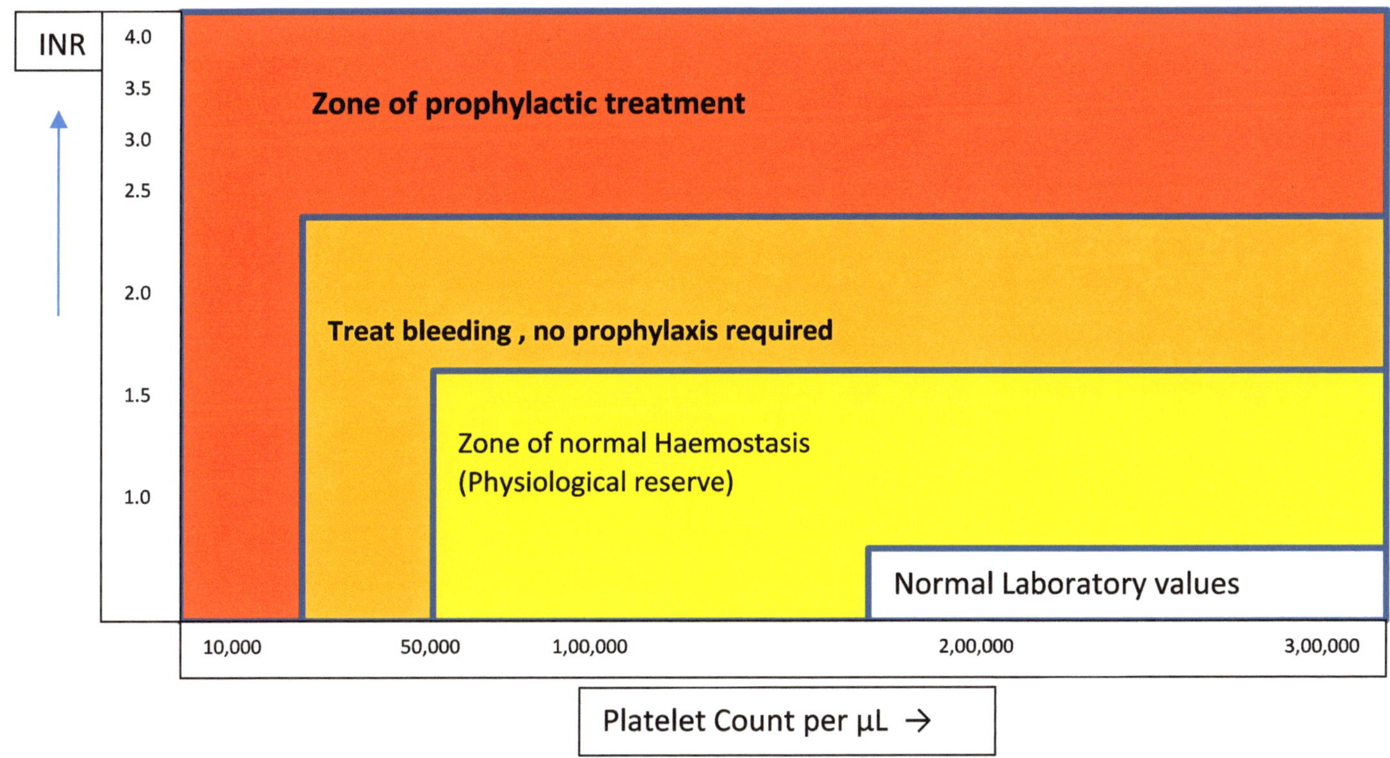

Figure 2 . Zones of response to bleeding risk at the time of invasive procedures

Transfusion in neonatology and paediatrics

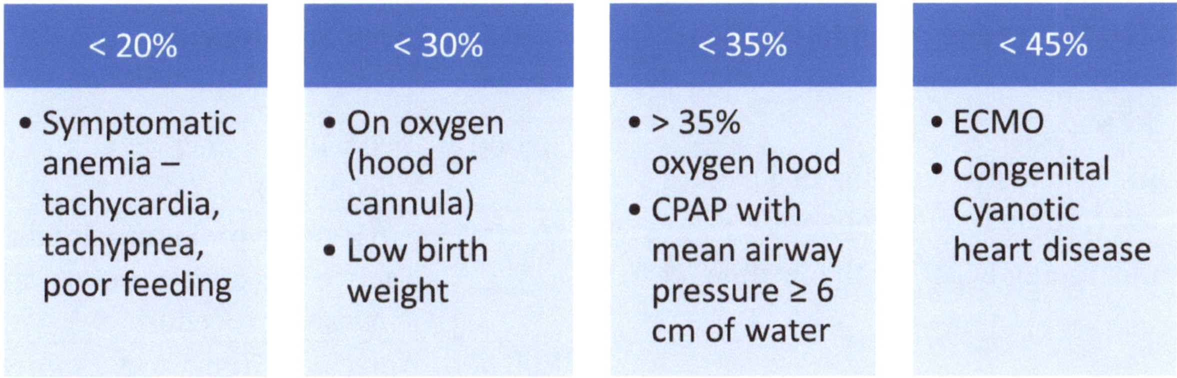

< 20%	< 30%	< 35%	< 45%
• Symptomatic anemia – tachycardia, tachypnea, poor feeding	• On oxygen (hood or cannula) • Low birth weight	• > 35% oxygen hood • CPAP with mean airway pressure ≥ 6 cm of water	• ECMO • Congenital Cyanotic heart disease

Figure 1. Transfusion threshold guidelines for infants younger than four months

Indications for transfusion in paediatric population aged more than 4 months:

- Preoperative anaemia, when another corrective therapy is not available.
- Intraoperative blood loss >15% of total blood volume
- Emergency surgical procedure in a patient with significant postoperative anaemia.
- Acute blood loss with hypovolemia not responsive to other therapy
- Chronic transfusion programs for disorders of red cell production (e.g., β-thalassemia major or Diamond-Blackfan syndrome)
- Sickle cell disease with any of these: Cerebrovascular accident, acute chest syndrome, splenic sequestration, aplastic crisis, recurrent priapism

<table>
<tr><td>Hct < 24</td><td>Hct < 30</td><td>Hct < 40</td></tr>
<tr>
<td>

- In perioperative period, with signs and symptoms of anemia.
- While on chemotherapy/radiotherapy
- Chronic congenital or acquiredsymptomatic anemia

</td>
<td>

- Preoperatively when general anaesthesia is planned

</td>
<td>

- With severe pulmonary disease
- On ECMO

</td>
</tr>
</table>

Table 22.1 Dosing of blood components and expected increment in the paediatric population

Component	Dose	Expected increment
Red blood cells (60% Hct)	5 ml/kg	1 g/dl of Hb
Fresh Frozen plasma	1 ml/kg	Raises factor level by 1% (assuming 100% recovery)
Platelets	5-10 ml/kg or 1 unit per 10 Kg	50,000/μL
Cryoprecipitate	1 unit /10 kg	Raises fibrinogen level by 60-100 mg/dL (assuming 100% recovery)

Transfusion Guidelines for Platelets in Children

Even in the absence of thrombocytopenia in	In Thrombocytopenia (per μL)	
Active bleeding in association with qualitative platelet defect. Unexplained excessive bleeding in a patient undergoing cardiopulmonary bypass. Patient undergoing ECMO with bleeding	< 10,000	Platelet production failure
	< 30,000	Platelet production failure (in neonates)
	< 50,000	in a stable premature infant with active bleeding or before an invasive procedure
	< 1,00,000	in a sick premature infant with active bleeding or before an invasive procedure (with DIC) or on ECMO

Transfusion Guidelines for FFP in Children:

- Support during treatment of disseminated intravascular coagulation
- Reversal of warfarin in an emergency
- As an alternative, such as before an invasive procedure with active bleeding.
- Replacement therapy when specific factor concentrates are unavailable for antithrombin, protein C or S, Factor II, V, X, and XI.
- During exchange transfusion (When cryo-poor plasma is required)

Note: FFP is not indicated for volume expansion or enhancement of wound healing

Transfusion Guidelines for cryoprecipitate in Children:

- Hypofibrinogenemia or dysfibrinogenemia, or Factor XIII

    - active bleeding
    - undergoing an invasive procedure

- Bleeding episodes in small children with haemophilia A (when recombinant and plasma-derived Factor VIII products are not available)
- preparation of fibrin sealant
- Von Willebrand with

    - active bleeding
    - undergoing an invasive procedure

(Deamino-O-arginine vasopressin is contraindicated, not available, or does not elicit a response, Virus-inactivated plasma-derived Factor VIII concentrate, which contains vWF or von Willebrand recombinant concentrate, is not available)

Antepartum	Post-partum	Genetic disorders
Placenta previa (35%)	Uterine atony (70%)	von Willebrand disease
Placental abruption (35%)	Genital trauma (20%)	Hemophilia A or B carriers
Uterine rupture (1%)	Morbidly adherent placenta (10%)	Glanzmann thrombasthenia
	(Tone, Trauma, Tissue, Thrombin)	Bernard- Soulier syndrome

- 90 % of transfusion in obstetrics happens during intrapartum. 5% each happens during ante and postpartum
- Antepartum haemorrhage affects 4% of all pregnancies

Coagulation factor changes in pregnancy		
Increased	**No change**	**Decreased**
Fibrinogen	Factor II	Factor XIII
Factor VII	Factor V	Protein S
Factor VIII	Protein C	Platelet count
Factor IX		
Factor X		
Factor XII		
Von Willebrand factor		

Risk factors

Placenta previa	Placental abruption	Uterine rupture

Short cervical length
 	
Transvaginal ultrasound findings of
 	
  – Sponge-like echo (≥5 hypoechoic areas larger than 5 mm in diameter)
  – Placental lacunae
  – Lack of clear zone (space between placenta and uterus)
	≥ 35 years
	≥ 3 pregnancies
	African-American ethnicity
	Unmarried/single mother
	Smoking
	Alcohol
	Chronic hypertension
	Hyperhomocysteinemia
	Thrombophilia
	Pregestational diabetes
	Previous LSCS
	History of miscarriage/stillbirth
		Chorioamnionitis
		History of caesarean section
		History of multiple pregnancies
		H/O Pregestational diabetes
		African-American ethnicity
		H/O induction
		Advanced maternal age
		High BMI
		Eclampsia

Uterine atony	**Genital trauma**	**Placental tissue retention**
Obesity Hispanic ethnicity Preeclampsia Chorioamnionitis Hydramnios Anaemia	Nulliparity Macrosomia Precipitous delivery Instrument assisted delivery Episiotomy	Advanced maternal age Placenta previa Previous Caesarean section Previous uterine surgery Multiparity

Stanford team approach to managing patients with Morbid Adherent placenta (MAP)

- Admit at 32 weeks of gestation
- Type and screen, CBC
- PT, aPTT and Fibrinogen levels
- Plan LSCS by 34 weeks
- Prepare for a massive transfusion protocol (6 units of crossmatched PRBC, four type-specific plasma, one apheresis platelet

Massive transfusion protocol in Obstetrics:

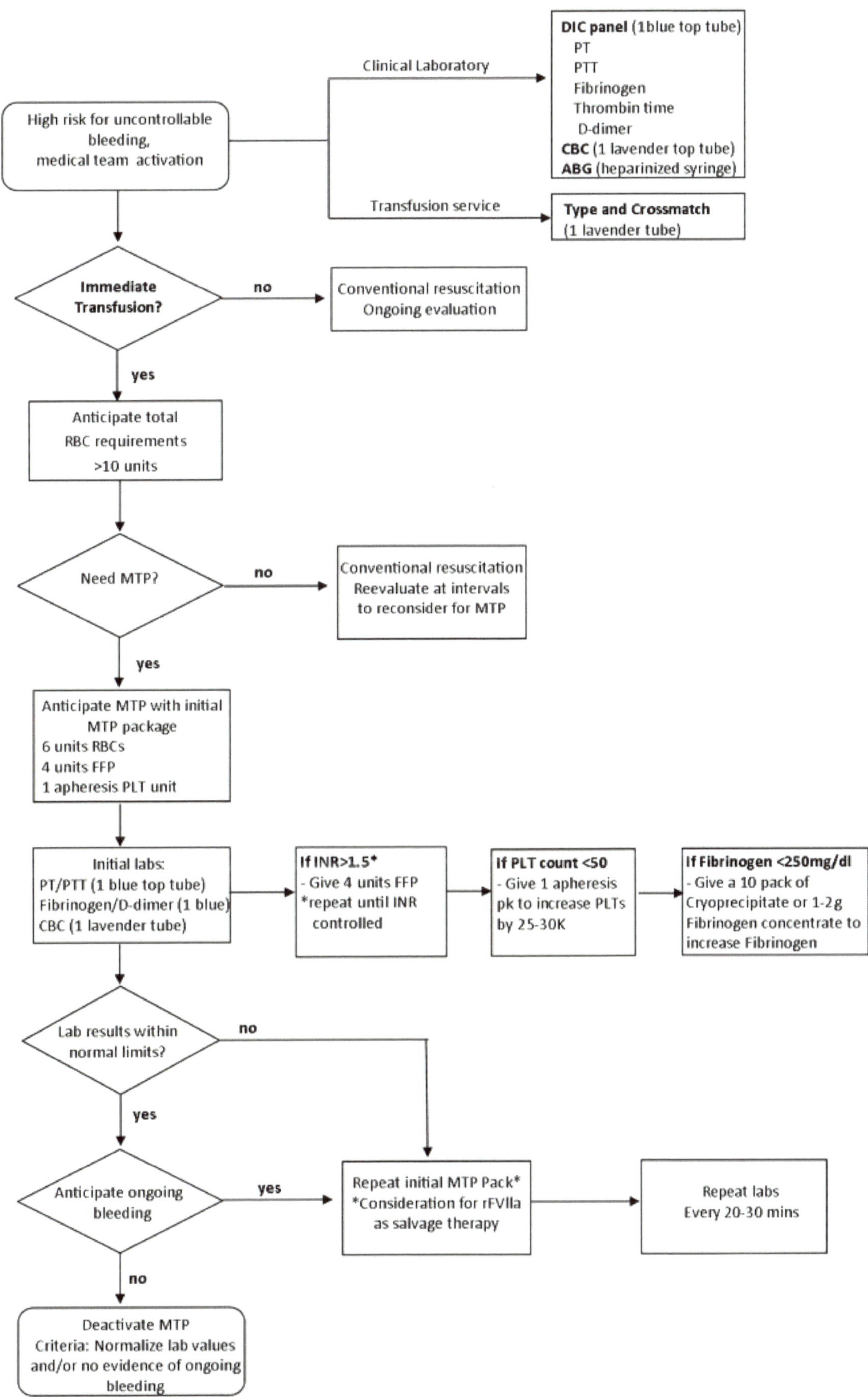

Massive transfusion protocol in Obstetrics				
	PRBCs	FFP	Platelets	Cryoprecipitate
Round 1	6 units	6 units	6 units	
Round 2	6 units	6 units	6 units	
Round 3	Tranexamic acid 1 g intravenously over 10 min			
Round 4	6 units	6 units	6 units	
After round 4, if not inactivated, the protocol will start again from round 1				

Transfusion support in HSCT

HLA matching determines: engraftment, clinical outcomes, GVHD and GVL effect (Graft versus Leukemia)

ABO incompatibility effects: increased transfusion needs (both RBCs and platelets), delayed RBC and platelet engraftment, GVHD

Epidemiological considerations:

- Less than 30% of patients have HLA-matched sibling donor
- Optimising HLA matching from available sources like matched unrelated donors, haploidentical donors or umbilical cord blood units results in ABO incompatibility in up to 50% of allogeneic HSCTs

O		Donor blood type			
		A	B	AB	
Recipient blood type	O	Identical (Compatible)	Major	Major	Major
	A	minor	Identical (Compatible)	Bidirectional (Major + Minor)	Major
	B	minor	Bidirectional (Major + Minor)	Identical (Compatible)	Major
	AB	minor	minor	minor	Identical (Compatible)

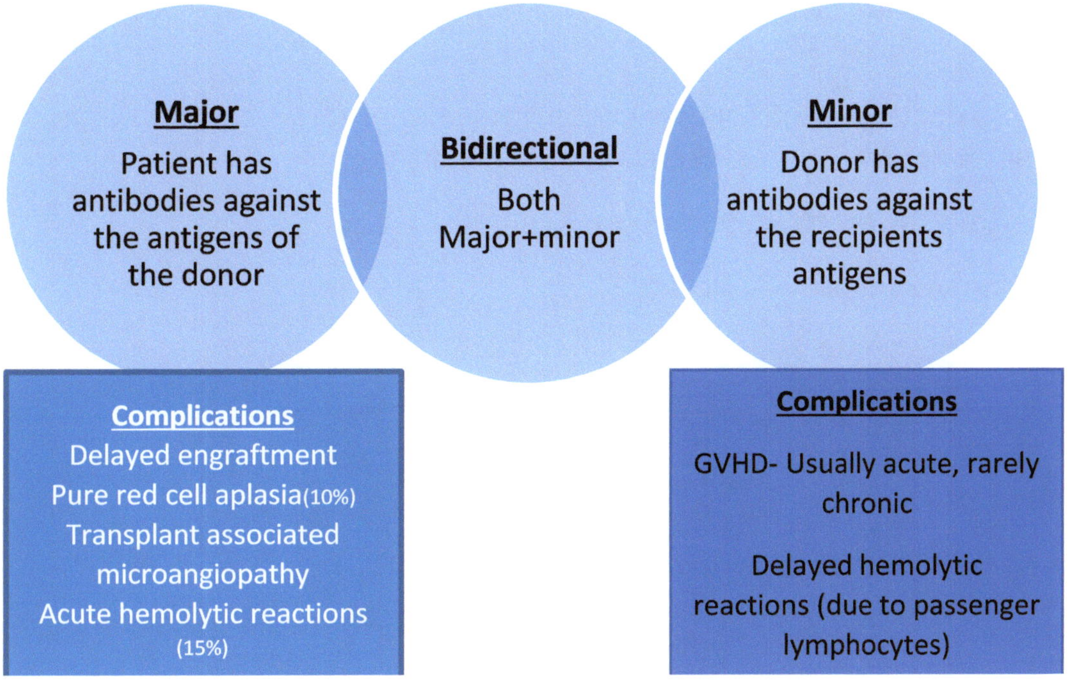

Transfusion support in HSCT patients:

Phases: Phase I: Preparative HSCT regimen

Phase II: Peri transplant

Phase III: Post-transplant (recipient antibodies and or cells detectable)

Phase IV: Post-transplant (recipient antibodies and or cells not detectable)

Incompatibility type			RBCs				Platelets & Plasma				
	Recipient	Donor	I	II	III	IV	I	II		III		IV
								1st choice	2nd choice	1st choice	2nd choice	
Major Incompatibility	O	A	O	O	O	A	O	A	AB	A	AB	A
	O	B	O	O	O	B	O	B	AB	B	AB	B
	O	AB	O	O	O	AB	O	AB	A/B	AB	A/B	AB
	A	AB	A	A	A	AB	A	AB	A	AB	A	AB
	B	AB	B	B	B	AB	B	AB	B	AB	B	AB
Minor Incompatibility	A	O	A	O	O	O	A	O	AB	A	AB	O
	B	O	B	O	O	O	B	O	AB	B	AB	O
	AB	O	AB	O	O	O	AB	O	A/B	AB	A/B	O
	AB	A	AB	A	A	A	AB	A	A	AB	A	A
	AB	B	AB	B	B	B	AB	B	B	AB	B	B
Bidirectional incompatibility	A	B	A	O	O	B	A	AB	B	AB	B	B
	B	A	B	O	O	A	B	AB	A	AB	A	A

When to officially convert the recipient's ABO group in the medical records to that of the donor graft?

- When the patient has been independent of transfusion for at least 100 days, and the donor graft's ABO group is identified on two consecutive testing

Therapeutic options for posttransplant Pure Red Cell Aplasia:

- Tapering immunosuppressive agents
- Plasma exchange
- Donor-derived lymphocyte infusions
- Erythropoietin stimulating agents – Erythropoietin, Darbepoetin
- Rituximab, Daratumumab
- Glucocorticoids

Typical workup of HSCT: Hb%, Retic counts

Anti-A and anti-B titres (IgG and IgM), weekly starting posttransplant day 4

(especially for patients with an antibody titre>128 before transplantation)

Transfusion determinants	
Patient-specific factors	Practice specific factors
ABO compatibility	Transfusion threshold
CD34+ dose	Experience of the transplant centre
Gender	Conditioning regimen
Underlying disease	
Stem cell source- Marrow, Cord, PBSC	

Threshold guidelines	
7 gm/dL	All adult patients
8 gm/dL	Those with pre-existing cardiovascular disease, risk of end-organ damage, postoperative patients

Notable points:

- Increased RBC transfusions associated with increased serum ferritin levels led to worse outcomes (reduced survival)
- More transfusions are associated with the development of higher risks of GVHD

Impact of Rh "D"

- Rh-D matching has no impact on outcomes. Grafts should have been red cell reduced
- A major mismatch can lead to the development of anti-D (Concern in females of childbearing potential)
- The donor with anti-D can lead to hemolysis (minor mismatch)

Platelet transfusion:

Factors suggested to influence platelet engraftment:

- CD34+ cell dose
- GMCSF dose
- CMV seropositivity
- HLA mismatch
- MUDs take longer than MRDs
- Conditioning regimen
- GVHD prophylaxis
    - ❖ A threshold of 10,000/µL is generally considered safe for prophylactic transfusion unless the patient is febrile
    - ❖ HSCT recipients achieve platelet independence by days 16-33
    - ❖ Irradiated blood products are to be used up to 1 year from the day of transplantation

Transfusion in Solid Organ Transplantation

Complexities are because of the following:

- These are often unplanned events because of the sudden availability of organs (In cadaveric)
- Technical expertise required
- The unique patient population involved (often end-stage organ failures)
- Regulations involved
- Bloodborne infections are also organ-transmitted, especially crucial in deceased donors

Best accepted practices:

- ➢ Blood grouping: Confirmation on two separate specimens each for recipients and donors, compatibility testing/verification. "A" group subtyping is strongly recommended
- ➢ Reduce alloimmunisation as compatible organs are difficult to find; if so: avoid unnecessary transfusions and provide leukoreduced blood products to prospective recipients.
- ➢ Irradiation of blood products is optional
- ➢ Prothrombin complex concentrates (PCC) and Fibrinogen concentrates are well tolerated in these patients with no increase in thrombotic or Ischemic events
- ➢ 1:1:2 of RBCs: platelets: plasma, especially in liver transplantation, is associated with improved outcomes
- ➢ Fresh whole blood has been preferred at times, especially for treating life-threatening haemorrhage
- ➢ Try to match the blood groups to both recipients and the donor. If not, try O RBCs and AB platelets and plasma.
- ➢ Washing of platelets in minor incompatibility has some role

For incompatible paediatric transplants:

Age group	Isohemagglutinins titres (anti-A, anti-B)
<1 year	Not mentioned
1-2 yr	≤ 16

Average blood components requirements*

Transplant	PRBCs	Platelets	Plasma
Liver	4-15		
Heart	4		
Lung(double)	4		
Lung (single)	0-2		
Kidney	0-2		
Pancreas	0-2		

*Factors determining to include preoperative anaemia, intraoperative recovery program, POCTs available

Use of autologous blood: both donor's and recipient's blood can be utilised by predeposit. Typically, autologous recovery replaces only red cells; hence other components to be replaced to avoid dilutional coagulopathy

Tackling CMV: CMV-negative donors are not a viable option; strategies include providing leukoreduced or pathogen-reduced components.

Tackling ABO/HLA incompatibilities:

Desensitisation techniques- plasmapheresis

Paired donor exchanges or complex multiple donor arrangements: willing donors and recipients swap organs in order to match compatible pairs

Conservative transfusion strategy in patients awaiting transplantation- Iron and B12 therapy, epoetin

Strategies to avoid passenger Lymphocyte syndrome:

Transfuse donor group RBCs from the beginning of the surgery

>   *Or*

Transfuse the recipient group in the initial part of the surgery and shift to the donor group by the end of the surgery

>   *Or*

Transfuse recipient group, monitor DCT postoperatively, switching to donor group if DCT turns positive due to anti-A or anti-B

"D" negative recipients: Alloimmunisation in transplant recipients is slightly lower owing to immunosuppressive/modulatory regimens

If transfused with Rh "D" positive products intraoperatively ideal time to switch back to Rh "D" negative products is 48-72 hrs post-surgery

"D" negative RBCs to be given to females of childbearing potential

Washing of the grafts has reasonably prevented clinically significant anti-D formation when transplanted with Rh "D" positive donor organ

Recipients with red cell antibodies:

Preferred option: providing antigen-negative units throughout

The second option: try to provide antigen-negative blood at the beginning and end of surgery (Alloantibody resynthesises or re-enters the intravascular space from the extravascular space)

Additional strategy: preoperative therapeutic plasma exchange (inefficacious in IgG antibodies as they are primarily extravascular)

Section IV

Applied Transfusion Medicine and Allied Specialities

LABORATORY HEMATOLOGY

– Dr. Debdatta Basu

Parameter	Normal values
RBC count	$4.2\text{-}5.0 \times 10^6\,/mm^3$ (females), $4.6\text{-}6.0 \times 10^6\,/mm^3$ (males)
Haemoglobin	12 – 15.8 g/dL (females) 13.3-16.2 g/dL (males)
WBC count	$4{,}500\text{-}11{,}000\,/mm^3$
Platelet count	$150\text{-}450 \times 10^3\,/mm^3$
MCV	79-98 fL Mean Platelet Volume: 7.4-10.4fL
MCH	26.7-31.9 pg
MCHC	32-36%
RDW	11.5-14.5% Platelet Distribution width: 9-13fL
Retic count	0.8-2.3% IPF: 3-20%
Differential Count	Neutrophils: 50-70% Lymphocytes: 25-35% Basophils: 0.4-1%
	Monocytes: 4-6% Eosinophils: 1-3% Bands: 0-5%
Hematocrit	35.4-44.4% (females) 38.8 – 46.4% (males) **Plateletcrit:** 0.108-0.282

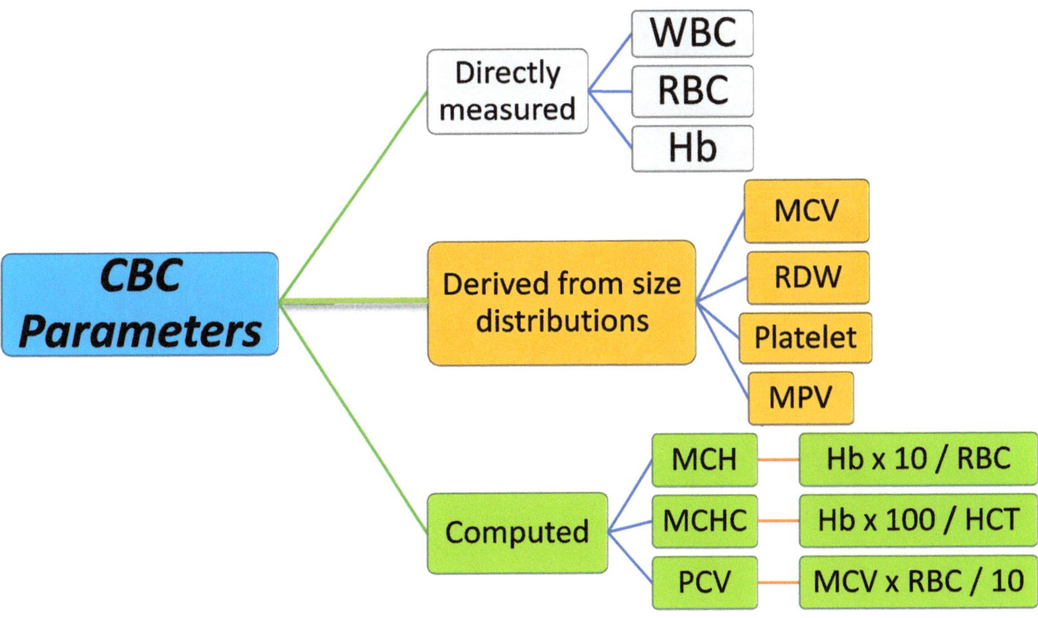

Figure 27. Derivation of various parameters in Hematology analyser

	Normal MCV	High MCV	Low MCV
Normal RDW	Anaemia of chronic disease Blood loss anaemia Hemolytic anaemia CLL,CML Hemoglobinopathies	Aplastic anaemia Preleukemia Myelodysplastic syndrome	Anaemia of chronic disease Thalassemia Intermedia
High RDW	Early Iron, B12 or Folate deficiency Sickle cell anaemia	Vitamin B12, Folate Deficiency Immune hemolytic anaemia Liver disease Cold Agglutinins Alcoholism	Iron deficiency anaemia RBC fragmentation HbH Thalassemia intermedia G6PD deficiency
Low RDW	It is rarely seen. In Thalassemia minor and aplastic anaemia		

Mentzer Index: $\dfrac{\text{MCV}}{\text{RBC Count}}$

If less than 13, Thalassemia is more likely. If >13, Iron deficiency is more likely.

Principle: In iron deficiency, the marrow cannot produce as many RBCs, and they are small (microcytic), so the RBC count and the MCV will both be low, and as a result, the index will be greater than 13. Conversely, in Thalassemia, a disorder of globin synthesis, the number of RBCs produced is as usual, but the cells are smaller and more fragile. Therefore, the RBC count is normal, but the MCV is low, so the index will be less than 13.

Combined cell index (CCI): This index is calculated by the formula:

$$\frac{\text{Red blood cell distribution width (RDW)} \times 10^4}{\text{Mean corpuscular volume (MCV)} \times \text{Mean corpuscular haemoglobin (MCH)}}$$

A cutoff of 57.3 is taken as a predictor of Iron deficiency(ferritin depletion <12µg/L)

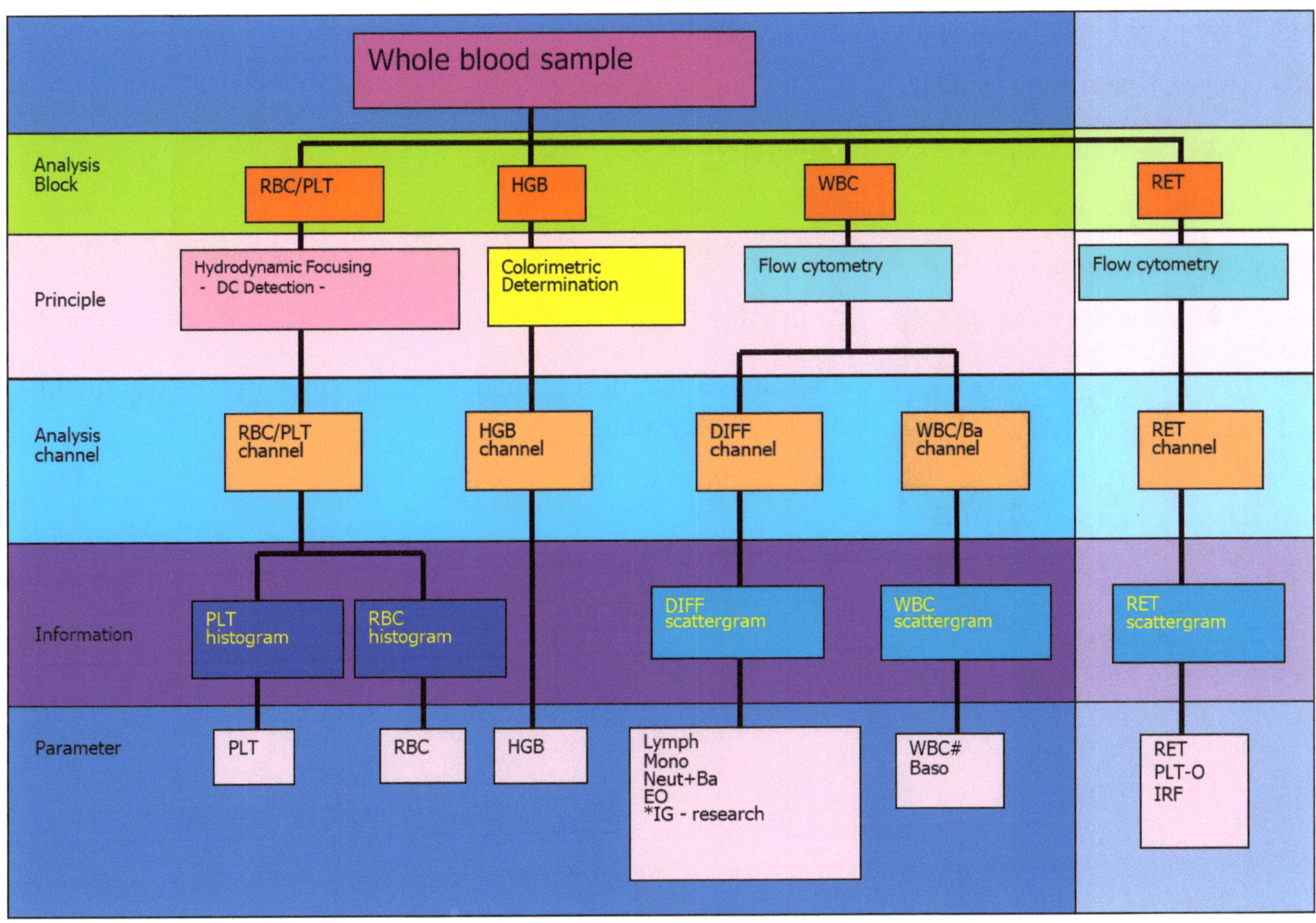

Flagging: Every instrument has its flagging system. Whenever significant abnormalities of red cells, white cells or platelets are present, these are signalled by certain "asterisks" on blood counts, histograms, or scatter plots. These abnormal results, after analysing the histograms and scatterplots, are flagged to alert the professional, which needs Manual screening of the slide by the expert to look for

- Morphological abnormalities
- Variables that are discordant

RBC flags	WBC flags	Platelet flags
nRBCs	Immature granulocytes	Platelet clumps
RBC fragments	Blasts	Giant platelets
RBC agglutination	Atypical or variant lymphocytes	Schistocytes
Dimorphic population	↑nRBCs	

Flags on calculated parameters:

RL (Lower discriminator) Flag:

LD exceeds the preset value by greater than 10%

Occurs due to platelet aggregation, RBC fragments & noise

RU (Upper Discriminator)Flag:

UD exceeds preset height by greater than 5%

Cold agglutinins are the leading cause

Multiple Peaks (MP):

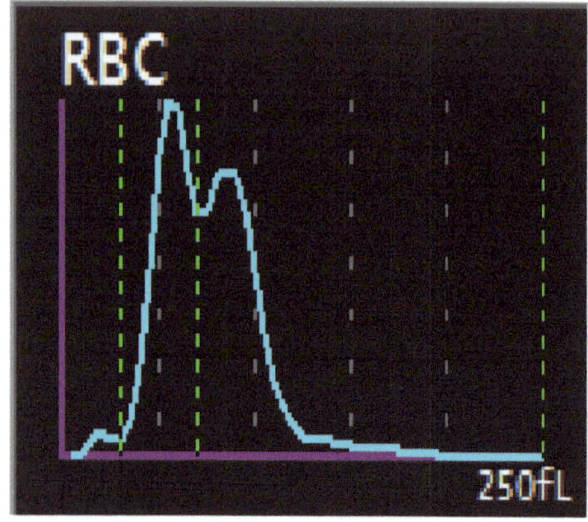

RBC: RDW-SD shows this flag

Generally seen in post-transfusion and following the treatment of iron deficiency anaemia.

Platelets:

Platelet anisocytosis

Recovery after chemotherapy

Platelet aggregation

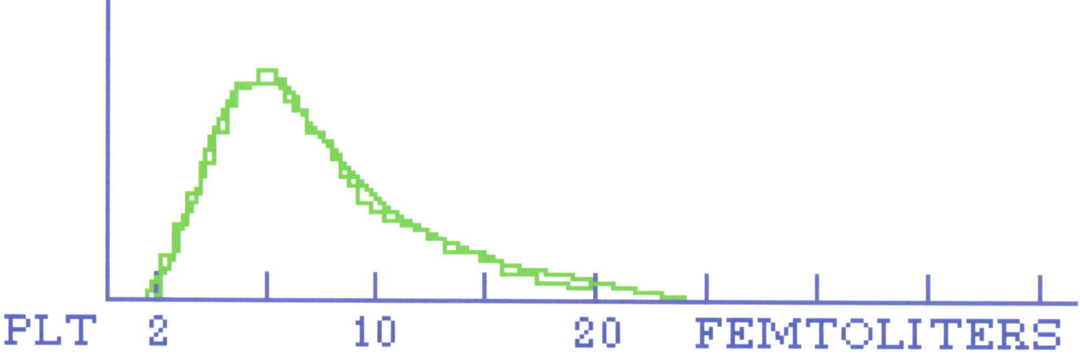

Figure 28. Platelet Histogram

Mean Platelet volume(MPV): measurement of the average size of the platelets. Normal = 7.4 – 10.4fL

MPV increases with young platelets(the younger the platelet bigger it is)

Has an inverse relationship with platelet count

Platelets are normally 1-3µm, considered large when they are 4-8 µm. They are called giant when they are equal to or larger than an RBC.

Platelets swell during the first 2 hrs in EDTA and slowly shrink back.

Platelets are large when reduced due to increased destruction and small with disorders of diminished production.

Increased MPV (Megathrombocytes)	Decreased MPV (Microthrombocytes)
ITP, TTP, DIC	
Bernard Soulier Disease	Wiskott Aldrich syndrome
May-Hegglin anomaly	TAR Syndrome (Thrombocytopenia-absent radii)
Sepsis (recovery phase)	
Heart valve prosthesis	
Sickle cell anaemia	
Myeloproliferative disorders, CML	Megaloblastic anaemia
Myelodysplasia	Aplastic anaemia, Megakaryocytic hypoplasia
Infections: dengue, malaria	Storage pool disease
Following splenectomy	Hypersplenism
Hyperthyroidism	Chemotherapy

Platelet Distribution width(PDW): compares the uniformity/heterogeneity of platelet size, analogous to RDW

If fragments from erythrocyte fragments are counted as platelets, PDW will be elevated falsely.

Increased values are observed in Essential Thrombocythemia, Aplastic anaemia, megaloblastic anaemia, CML, and Chemotherapy.

Plateletcrit: directly related to the total number of platelets and MPV. It is the volume percentage that platelets constitute on a total volume of blood. (Normal range: 0.110-0.280)

Immature platelet fraction(IPF) or Reticulated platelets: represents newly released platelets that retain residual RNA, analogous to red cell reticulocytes.

It can increase 2.5- to 4.5-folds in the clinical setting of immune thrombocytopenia (ITP, TTP etc.). It may herald the return of platelet production after chemotherapy.

Approach to a peripheral smear(PS):

Mode	Purpose
Naked eye	quality of preparation and staining
10 X (Low Power)	distribution of cells, to select area/field to study, rouleaux, agglutination, platelets, parasites
40 X (High Power)	RBC morphology, WBC - DC
100 X (Oil Immersion)	DC, RBC, WBC and platelet morphology, RBC inclusions, haemoparasites

- Take a good look at the slide with at least 10 "good" Low Power fields. If there are Fibrin strands, reject it

Reporting a smear:

Interpretation of RBC

Interpretation of WBC

Interpretation of platelets

Looking for parasites

Learning to appreciate artefacts

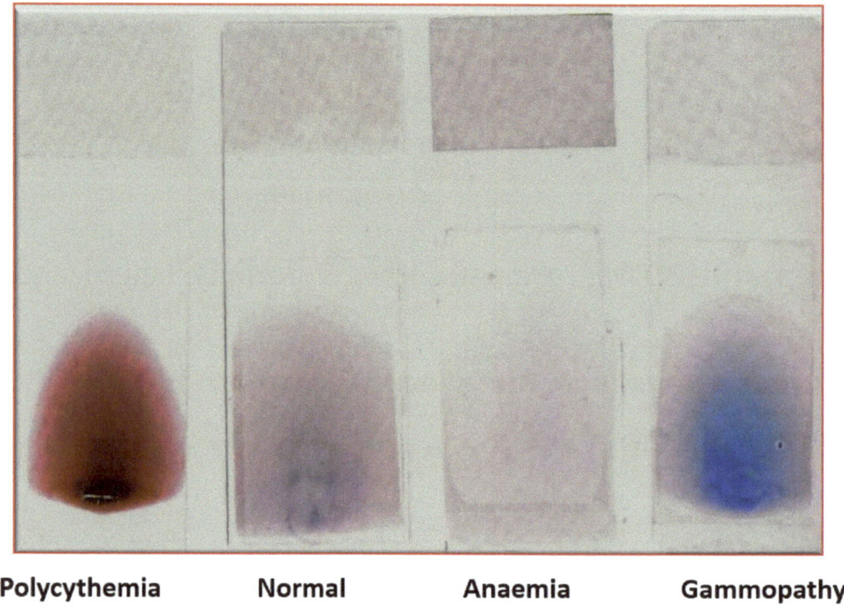

Figure 29. Significance of Observation

The best place to examine blood cell morphology is the feathery edge of the blood smear, where the red cells lie in a single layer, side by side, just touching one another without overlapping.

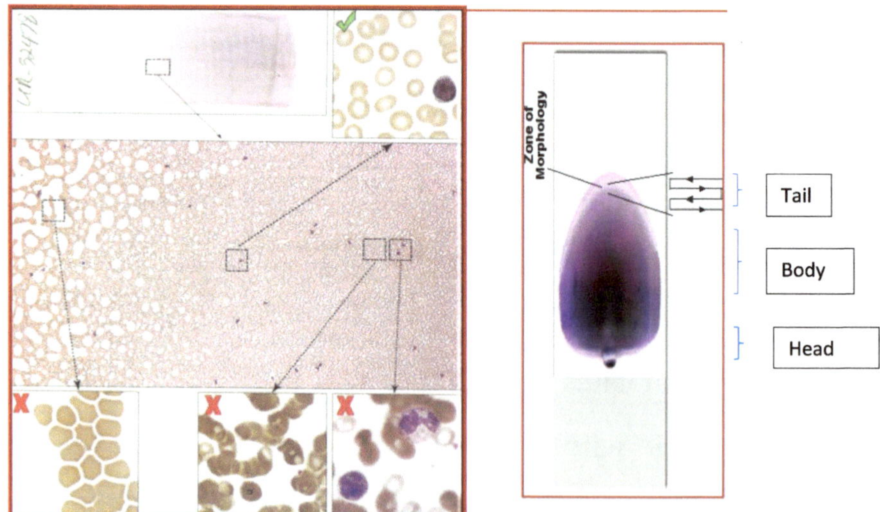

Figure 30. Parts of Peripheral smear (Showing Optimal assessment area)

Features of a well-stained PS:

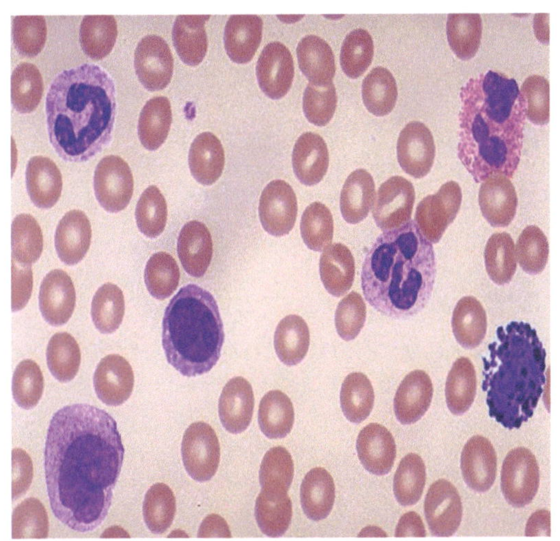

Macroscopically: colour should be pink to purple

Microscopically:

 RCS: pale orange to salmon pink - buff

 WBC: nuclei are purple to blue

  the cytoplasm is pink to tan

  granules are lilac to violet

Eosinophil: granules of orange

Basophil: granules of dark blue to black

Examining Platelets	
Size	1-2 μm
Counting	count the platelets in five to six fields(oil immersion), take an average number per field, and multiply by 20,000
Platelet to RBC ratio	1:20
Large platelets	rapid platelet turnover(younger platelets) -ITP Inherited Syndromes: Bernard Sollier Syndrome Absence of large platelets: may indicate marrow (production) related
Clumped platelets	This leads to falsely low counts in automated counters Due to anticoagulant, neutrophil fragmentation
Absence of granules	Artefact, marrow defect, Gray platelet syndrome
Increased platelet count	myeloproliferative disorder or a reaction to systemic inflammation
Examining Red Blood Cells	
Size	7-8 μm (comparable to the nucleus of a small lymphocyte)
	Variation in size is anisocytosis, and Variation in shape is poikilocytosis
Haemoglobin content	normochromic or pale in colour (hypochromic)
Distribution	clumping (called agglutination) in which the red cells pile upon one another; seen in paraproteinemias and AIHA rouleaux formation(single-row stacking) reflects abnormal serum protein levels
Examining White Blood Cells	
Size	Neutrophils 10–14 μm, Monocytes 15 to 22 μm

	Bands: immature neutrophils complete nuclear condensation and have a U-shaped nucleus. Bands reflect a left shift in neutrophil maturation to make more cells more rapidly Vacuolated neutrophils may be a sign of bacterial sepsis.
Lymphocytes	Most common in healthy individuals are small lymphocytes with a small dark nucleus and scarce cytoplasm *Reactive lymphocytes*: large lymphocytes, about the size of neutrophils, with abundant cytoplasm and a less condensed nuclear chromatin in the presence of viral infections *Large granular lymphocytes*: lymphocytes that are larger and contain blue granules in a light blue cytoplasm(about 1%) *Smudge cells:* In chronic lymphoid leukaemia, the small lymphocytes are increased in number and ruptured while making blood smear, leaving a smudge of nuclear material without a surrounding cytoplasm or cell membrane
Monocytes	The nucleus can take on a variety of shapes but usually appears to be folded; the cytoplasm is grey
Eosinophils	slightly larger than neutrophils, have bilobed nuclei and contain large red granules. (numbers are < Number of Neutrophils/30)
Basophils	large dark blue granules and may be increased as part of chronic myeloid leukaemia

RDW = (standard deviation of MCV ÷ mean MCV) × 100

Poikilocyte	Description	Image	Associated Conditions
Acanthocyte (spur cell)	Irregularly spiculated red cells with projections of varying length and dense centre due to altered cell membrane lipids		Post-splenectomy Abetalipoproteinemia, parenchymal liver disease,
Target cell (codocyte)	Target-like appearance, often hypochromic due to increased redundancy of cell membrane		Liver disease, post-splenectomy, Thalassemia, haemoglobin C disease

Stomatocyte	Mouth or cuplike deformity due to membrane defect with abnormal cation permeability		Hereditary stomatocytosis, immune hemolytic anaemia
Spherocyte	Spherical cells with a dense appearance and absent central pallor usually decreased diameter due to decreased membrane surface area		Hereditary stomatocytosis, immune hemolytic anaemia
Schistocyte (helmet cell)	Distorted, fragmented cell; two or three pointed ends due to mechanical distortion in microvasculature by fibrin strands or disruption by a prosthetic heart valve		Microangiopathic hemolytic anaemia (DIC, TTP, HUS, prosthetic heart valves, severe burns)
Bite cell (degmacyte)	A smooth semicircle is taken from one edge due to Heinz's body pitting by the spleen		Glucose-6-phosphate dehydrogenase deficiency, drug-induced oxidant hemolysis
Burr cell (echinocyte) or crenated red cell	Red cells with short, evenly spaced spicules and preserved central pallor due to altered cell membrane lipids		Artifactual seen in uremia, bleeding ulcers, gastric carcinoma

Inclusion Bodies	Description	Image	Associated Conditions
Cabot rings	Circular, blue, threadlike inclusion with dots due to Nuclear remnant		Postsplenectomy, hemolytic anaemia, megaloblastic anaemia

Howell–Jolly bodies	Small, discrete, basophilic, dense inclusions due to Nuclear remnant (DNA); usually single	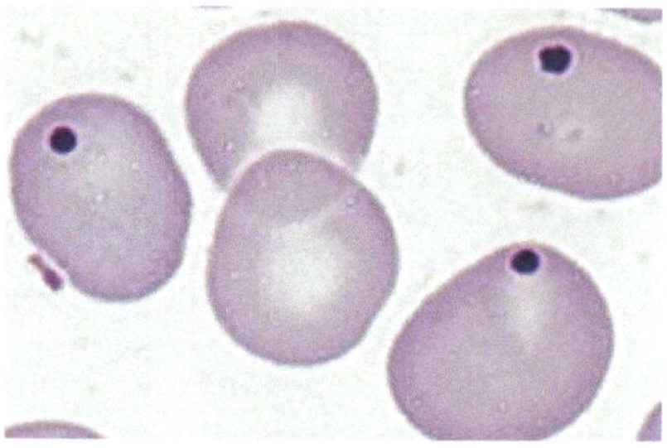	Postsplenectomy, hemolytic anaemia, megaloblastic anaemia
Basophilic stippling	Punctuate basophilic inclusions, which are precipitated ribosomes	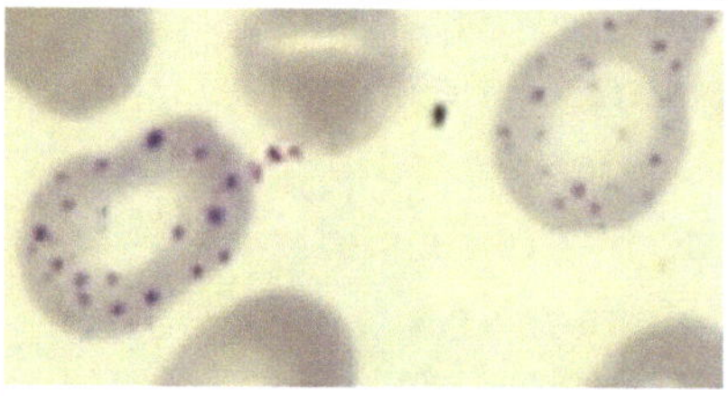	Lead poisoning, Thalassemia
Heinz bodies	clumps of damaged haemoglobin located on red blood cells	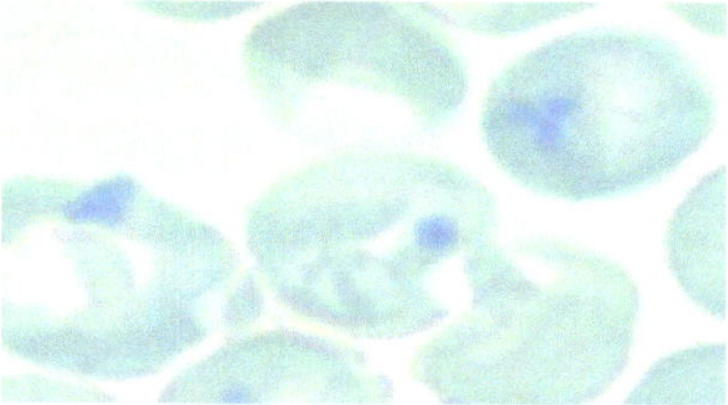	Thalassemia, hemolytic anaemia, glucose-6-phosphate dehydrogenase (G6PD) deficiency
Pappenheimer bodies	Small, dense, basophilic granules, which are Iron-containing siderosome or mitochondrial remnants	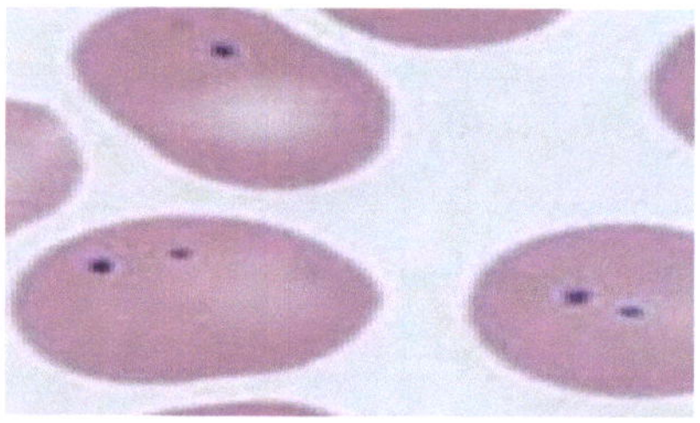	Sideroblastic anaemia, post-splenectomy
Poly chromatophilia	A greyish or blue hue is often seen in macrocytes due to Ribosomal material	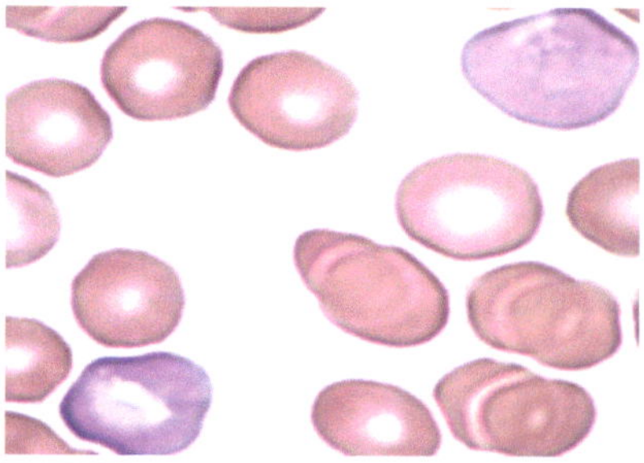	Reticulocytosis, premature marrow release of red cells
Nucleated red blood cell	nucleated RBCs that are at the orthochromatic stage of maturation	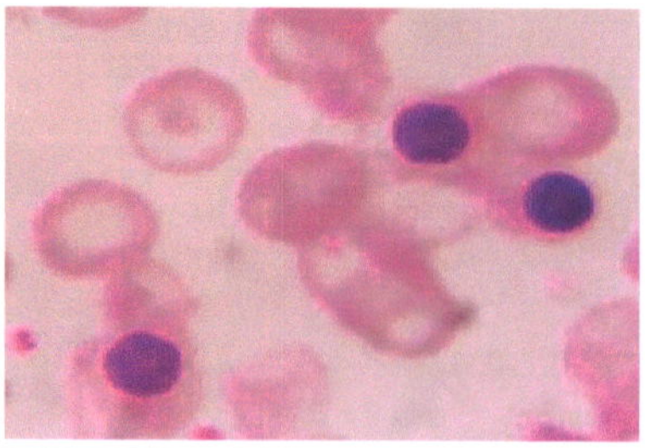	Severe anaemias

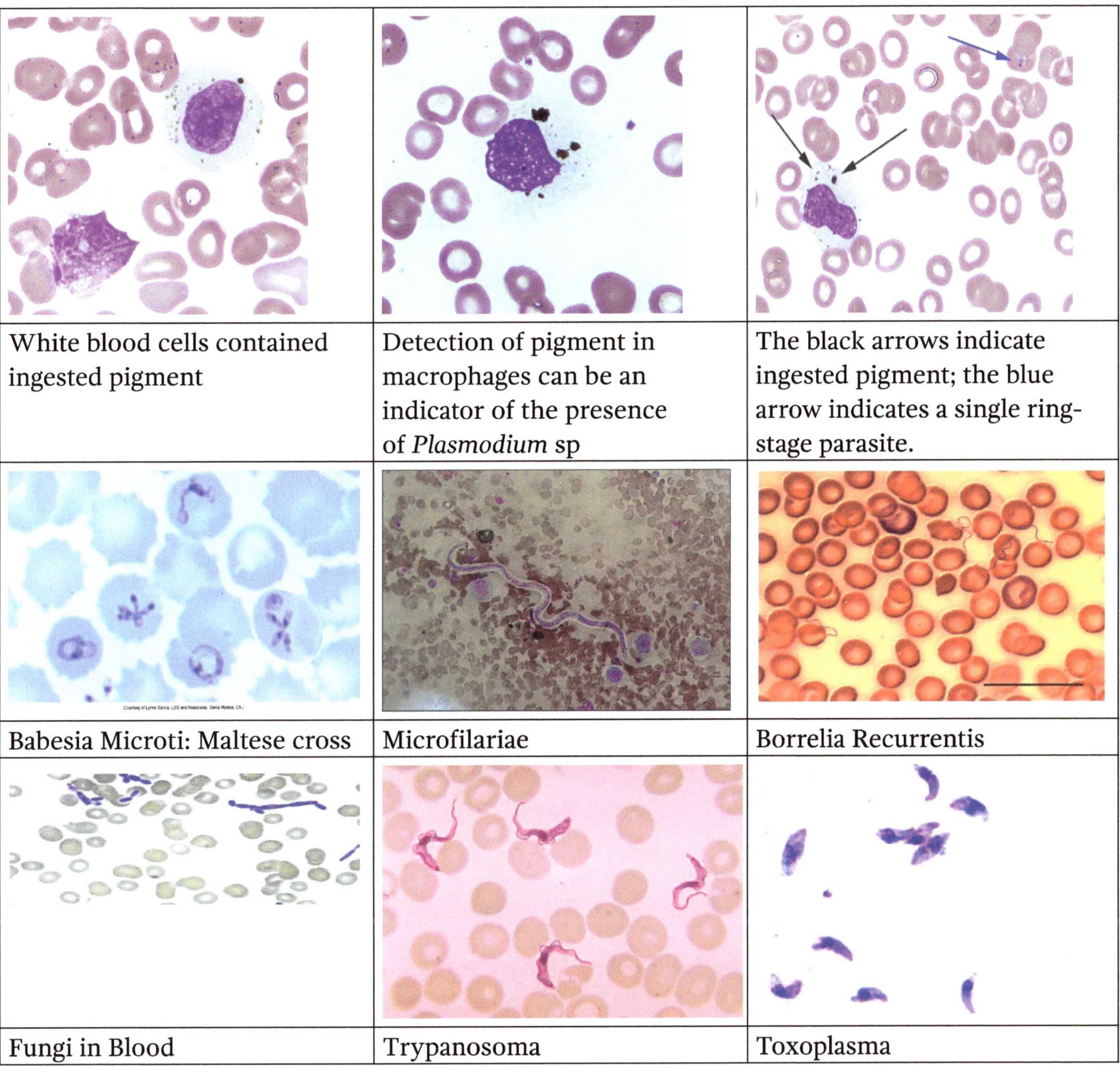

White blood cells contained ingested pigment	Detection of pigment in macrophages can be an indicator of the presence of *Plasmodium* sp	The black arrows indicate ingested pigment; the blue arrow indicates a single ring-stage parasite.
Babesia Microti: Maltese cross	Microfilariae	Borrelia Recurrentis
Fungi in Blood	Trypanosoma	Toxoplasma

HEMATOPATHOLOGY

– Dr. Srikanth U

Hematopoiesis

Hematopoiesis encompasses blood cell production from a hematopoietic stem cell (HSC). The HSC further proliferates and differentiates into lineage-committed cells called progenitor cells. Progenitor cells follow the lineage-specific pathway to differentiate into committed stem cells and morphologically recognizable bone marrow cells.

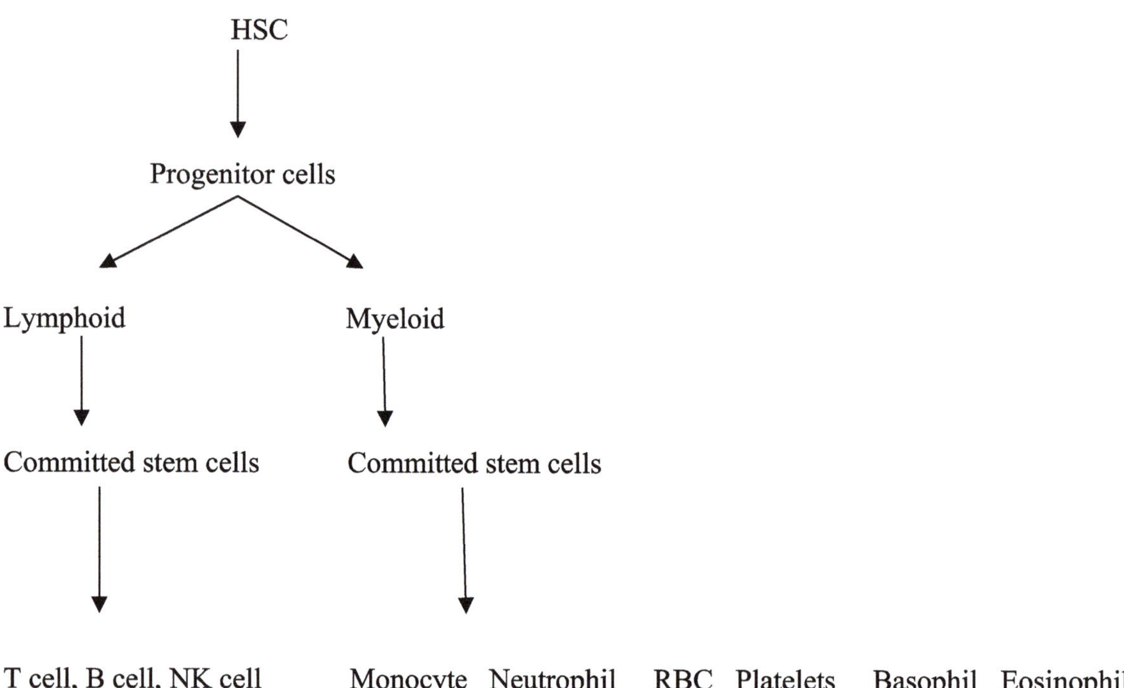

Non-hematopoietic components form the connective tissue stroma in which the hematopoietic cells are embedded. It constitutes fat cells, fibroblasts, endothelial cells, macrophages and reticulin. These components catalyze the HSC's differentiation and renewal.

Sites of hematopoiesis

Yolk sac	Till the third week of intra-uterine life
Liver	Till the third month of intra-uterine life

Bone marrow	From the fourth month of intra-uterine life and continues to be the only source of blood cells throughout life
Childhood	The entire bone marrow is hematopoietically active
Adults	Vertebrae, sternum, clavicle, ribs, pelvis, skull, proximal epiphyseal regions of femur and humerus are the only hematopoietically active sites

Bone marrow components

The bone is histologically and functionally classified into the cortex and medulla. The other scheme of classification is based on the density and the amount of interstices present. This includes the compact/dense bone (small interstices that are not visible macroscopically) and cancellous/trabecular bone (large, readily visible interstices).

The cortex is the strong, dense layer composed of mainly lamellar and some woven bone. The lamellar component consists of the Haversian systems. The medulla is a less organized cancellous bone. The cortex is covered by the periosteum.

The bone marrow comprises major hemopoietic islands of erythroid, myeloid, and megakaryocyte elements and minor components of lymphocytes, plasma cells, macrophages, osteoblasts, osteoclasts (in children) and mast cells.

Bone marrow examination

The marrow can be obtained using different needles, such as Jamshidi, Klima, Islam and Salah. Jamshidi needle is a wide bore with a bevelled cutting edge and a narrow tip. This prevents compression of the bone marrow and the formation of marrow fibrosis.

Complete marrow evaluation includes a two-step process. The first includes cytological analysis of the marrow cells using the aspirate and smears. The second step includes the needle biopsy examination allowing the histologic assessment of marrow cellularity, interstitium and accompanying diseases.

Indications for bone marrow aspirate	Indications for bone marrow biopsy
<ul><li>Red cell disorders</li><li>Leukocytic disorders</li><li>Megakaryocytic disorders</li><li>Myeloproliferative/Myelodysplastic syndromes</li><li>Iron store assessment</li><li>Infections</li><li>Metastases</li></ul>	<ul><li>Histologic assessment of marrow cellularity, marrow fibrosis, marrow architecture and vascularity</li><li>Diagnosis and staging of Hodgkin's and Non-Hodgkin's lymphoma</li><li>Diagnosis and staging of chronic lymphoproliferative disorders, metastatic carcinomas.</li><li>Investigations of pyrexia of unknown origin, multiple myeloma, leucoerythroblastic films and small round cell tumours.</li></ul>

<table><tr><td>

Sites for BMA and BMB

- Posterior superior iliac spine (most common site for aspirate and biopsy)
- Anterior superior iliac spine (second most common site for aspirate and biopsy)
- Sternum (only in age >12 years if the iliac crest is not suitable. Only aspirate can be obtained due to the high risk of causing injury to thoracic structures)
- Tibia (common site for infants)

</td></tr></table>

<table><tr><td>

Contraindications for BMA and BMB

- Severe Osteoporosis and multiple myeloma
- Coagulopathies (severe DIC, haemophilia, liver diseases)
- Skin infection and recent radiotherapy at the site of aspirate
- *Note: Isolated thrombocytopenia is not a contraindication. However, adequate post-procedure follow-up is very critical.*

</td></tr></table>

<table><tr><td>

Complications of marrow procedures

- Haemorrhage
- Infection
- Perforation (esp. in the sternal site as they pose a risk of puncture to thoracic structures)
- Pain at the procedure site

</td></tr></table>

<table><tr><td>

Marrow failure states

- Aplastic anaemia
- Fanconi anaemia
- Paroxysmal nocturnal hemoglobinuria
- Hypoplastic conditions (Myelodysplastic syndrome, acute leukaemia)

</td></tr></table>

<table><tr><td>

The BMA and BMB can be further used for the following:

- Special stains: Perl's Iron stain, Gomori's silver stain for reticulin, trichrome stain for collagen
- Fungal, AFB and bacterial cultures
- Flow cytometry, Fluorescent in situ hybridization (FISH), Cytogenetic analysis
- Molecular genetic analysis
- Immunohistochemistry (IHC)

</td></tr></table>

Examination of the bone marrow aspirate

Smears containing the aspirate should be evaluated at low, medium and high power magnification.

Low-power magnification (10x) allows estimation of the sample contents such as the spicules, detection of cellular aggregates (esp. carcinoma, metastasis) and identification of the megakaryocyte numbers.

Medium-power magnification (40x) is used to recognise segmented granulocytes, abnormal granulocyte and mononuclear cell patterns and to get an approximate myeloid to the erythroid ratio (M: E ratio).

Higher magnification using either dry (60x) or oil immersion (100x) lens allows detailed morphologic evaluation of myeloid, erythroid and megakaryocytic lineages along with an examination of the plasma cells, lymphocytes, blasts, immature precursors and non-hematopoietic elements.

Fig: Aspirate

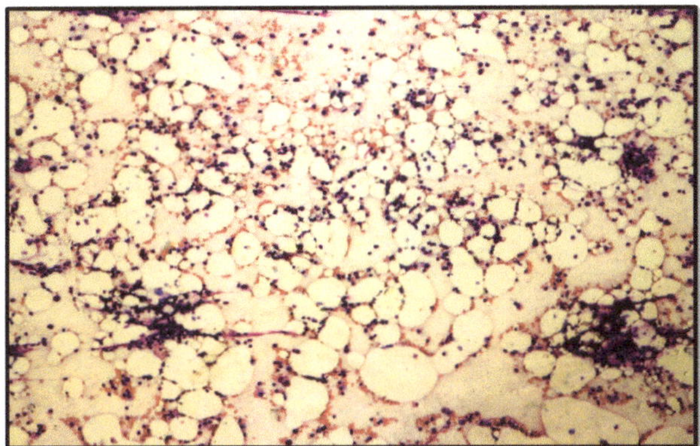

Examination of the bone marrow biopsy

Marrow interpretation should be made systemically.

Low-power magnification (10x) should be used to note the length of the biopsy specimen, overall cellular architecture and abnormalities in the bony trabeculae.

Medium-power magnification (40x) allows appreciation of the M: E ratio and megakaryocyte number.,

Higher magnification using either dry (60x) or oil immersion (100x) is used to assess the myeloid maturation, erythroid maturation and identification of small mature lymphocytes.

Differentiating cell type count of marrow	Normal approximate percentage
M:E ratio	3:1 to 15:1
Neutrophils	26-45
Metamyelocyte	3-8
Myelocyte	5-10
Myeloblast	0-2
Early normoblast	1-5
Intermediate normoblast	5-20
Late normoblast	5-20
Megakaryocyte	0-2
Lymphocytes	5-20
Monocytes	1-3
Macrophages	0-2

Cellularity of the bone marrow

The bone marrow cellularity depends on the age and site of obtaining the marrow specimen. Factors such as decalcification, paraffin-embedding and resin-embedding also influence the marrow sample assessment. Bone marrow cellularity is expressed as a percentage of the entire biopsy. This includes the fat and cellular content. The cellularity in a child is around 80%, and in an adult, it decreases to around 60%. This further decreases as age progress. Marrow cellularity is reported as normocellular, hypocellular, hypercellular or aplastic.

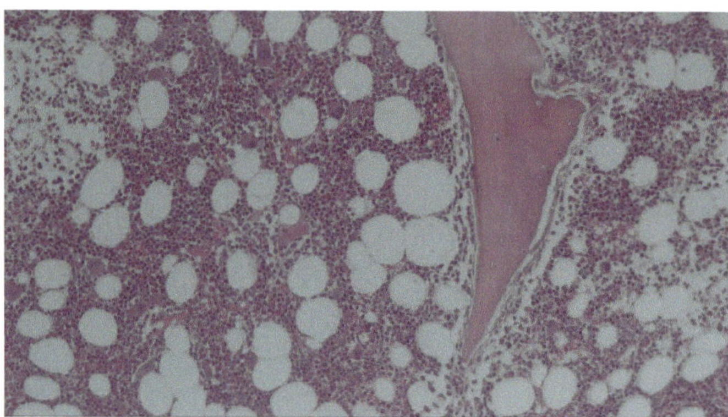

Fig: Normocellular

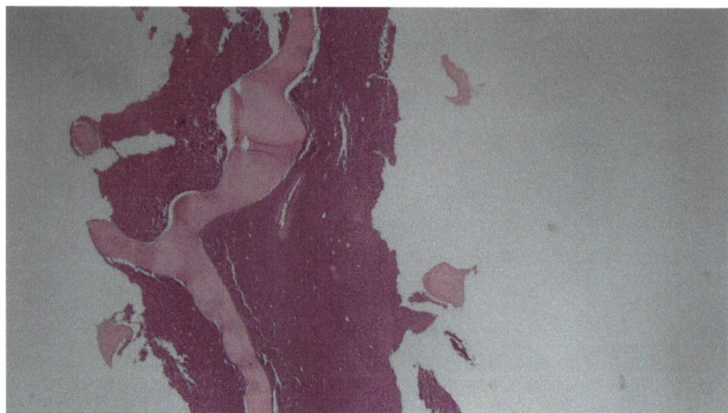

Fig: Hypercellular

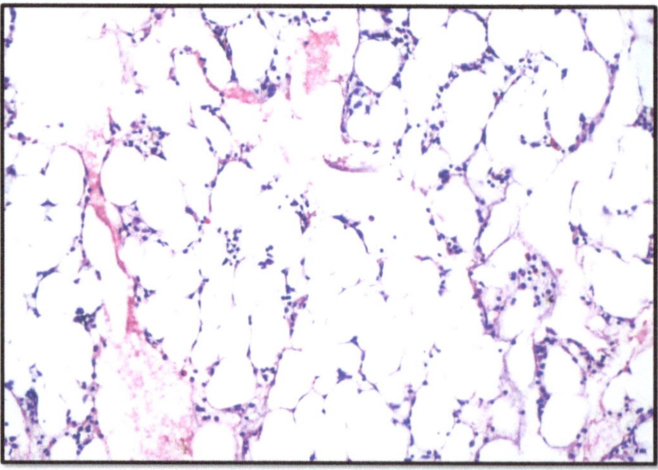

Fig: Hypocellular

M: E ratio

The M: E ratio reflects the lineage affected by either hyperplastic or hypoplastic.

Erythropoiesis

The erythroblastic lineage is usually identified as clusters of cells (islands) surrounding a macrophage. Erythropoiesis occurs close to the sinusoids.

Normoblasts are large cells with relatively scant cytoplasm and large round nuclei. The chromatin is dispersed and has small irregular nucleoli. Features used to identify erythroid cells from others are: i) they occur in clusters, ii) they adhere tightly to one another, and; iii) condensed chromatin and round nuclei.

Erythroblasts are examined for megaloblastic, micronormoblastic and dyserythropoietic forms. Cytochemical and immunohistochemical stains can confirm the identification of dyserythropoietic forms.

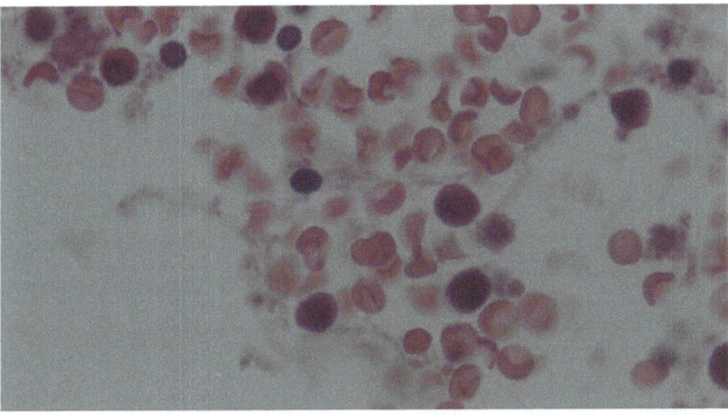

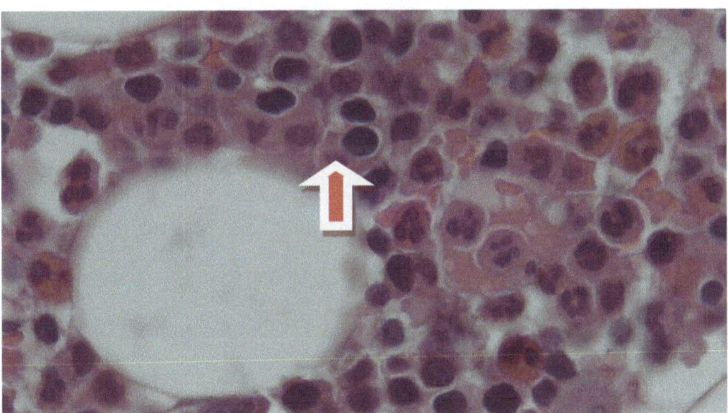

Myelopoiesis

Myeloblasts are the earliest granulocyte precursors identified and are seen in small numbers. They are found adjacent to the marrow trabeculae. They are large cells with round to oval nuclei and multiple nucleoli.

Promyelocytes are larger than myeloblasts and have strongly basophilic cytoplasm and an indented nucleus.

Myelocytes are smaller than promyelocytes. The nuclei show partial chromatin condensation and less basophilic cytoplasm than a promyelocyte.

Metamyelocytes are identified by marked U-shaped nuclear indentation

Band forms, including neutrophils, are segmented and have specific granules.

Myeloid precursors are evaluated for the blast cell number, maturation and proportion of the lineage. Maturation arrest and vacuolar cytoplasm (degenerated change) are also noted.

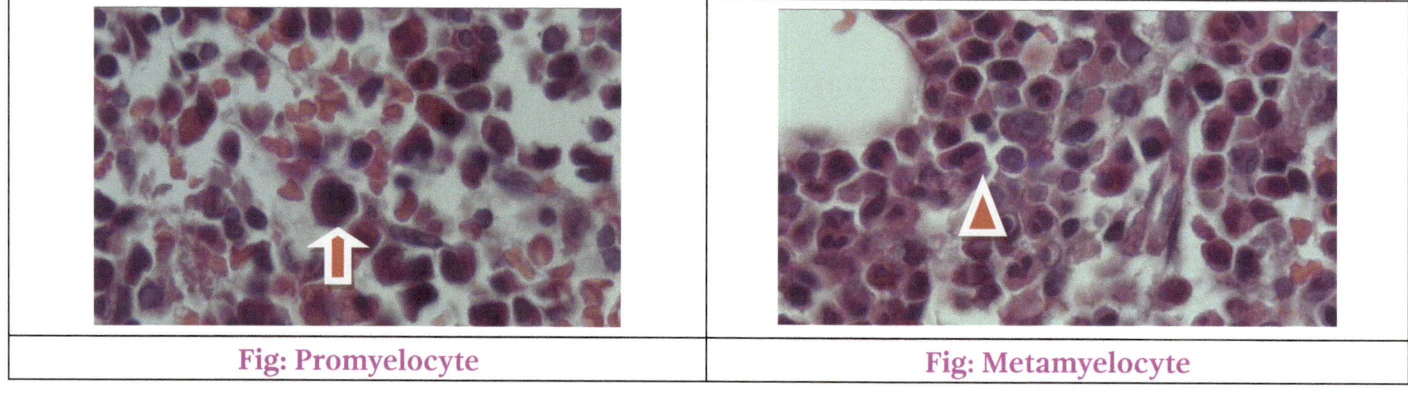

Fig: Promyelocyte

Fig: Metamyelocyte

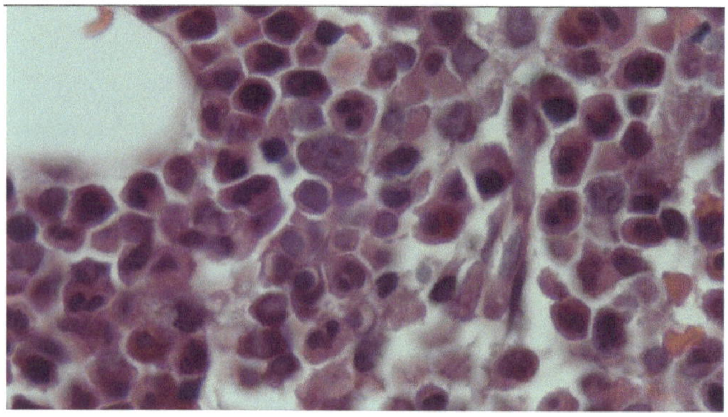

Fig: Myeloipoiesis

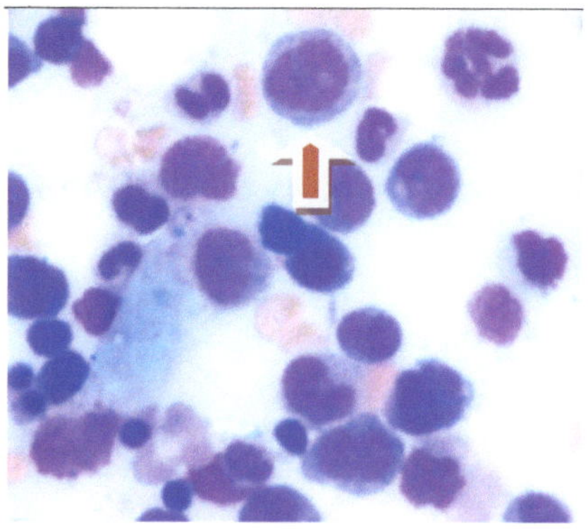

Fig: Blast

Megakaryopoiesis

Megakaryocytes are derived from a common megakaryocyte-erythroid progenitor cell. They are assessed for their numbers and dysmegakaryopoiesis. Megakaryocyte proliferation and platelet production are mainly dependent on thrombopoietin produced by the liver. Megakaryocytes may be seen engulfing other hematopoietic cells, a process called "emperipolesis".

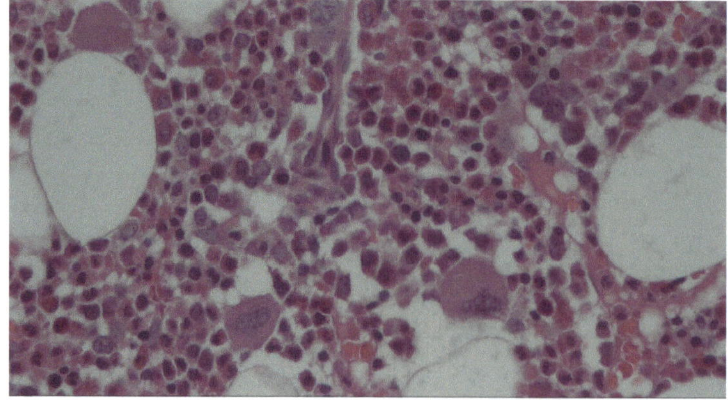

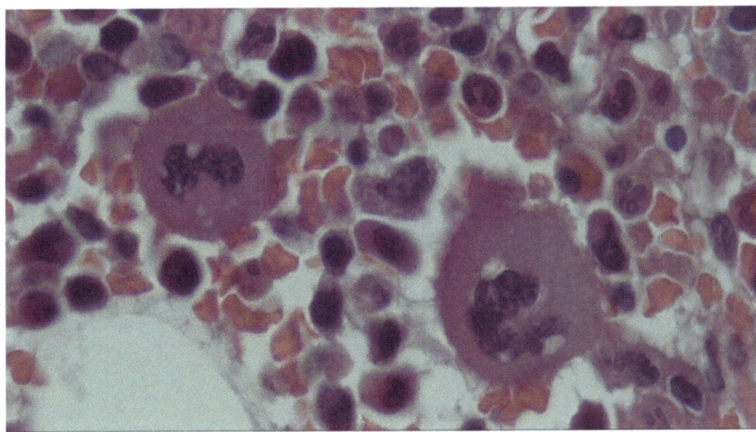

Fig: Megakaryocytes

Other cells

Lymphocyte numbers are higher in children as compared with adults. They are usually scattered in the interstitium and sometimes occur as small lymphoid follicles.

Plasma cells are scattered in the interstitium along with the lymphocytes. They are identified as oval cells with an eccentric nucleus, cartwheel or clock-face chromatin and prominent Golgi zone. Their numbers increase in chronic infections and plasma cell dyscrasia.

Mast cells are rare in normal marrow. They are difficult to be recognized on H&E stains due to unstained granules. A metachromatic stain such as Giemsa helps identify this cell. An increase in mast cells is seen in mastocytosis and aplastic anaemia.

Osteoblasts, osteoclasts, fat cells, and fibroblasts are normal elements to be noted. Abnormal cells such as granulomas, tumour cells and crystals should be examined in all the marrows.

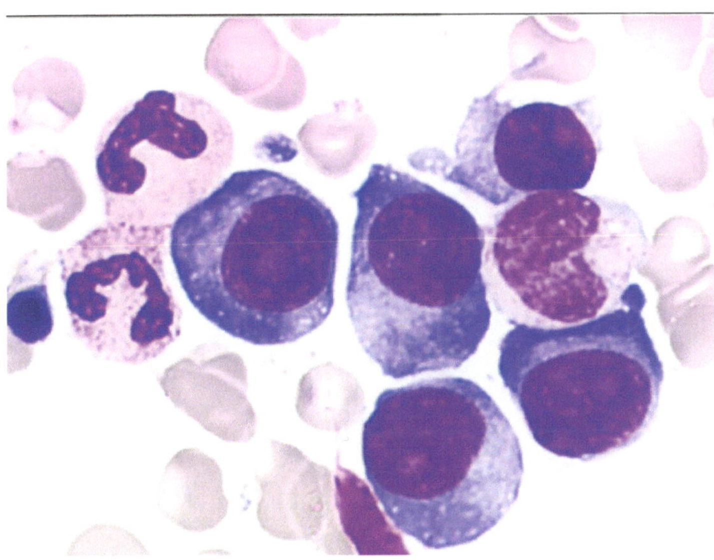

Fig: Plasma cells

Coagulation for Transfusion Medicine Residents

– Dr. Rafi M

Coagulation in Transfusion Medicine

Practitioners in transfusion medicine remain at the forefront of "therapeutic pathology," applying laboratory-based medical knowledge and expertise to diagnostic and therapeutic interventions. These interventions and expanded consultations at the laboratory coagulation and transfusion interface have led to reduced product wastage and better clinical outcomes; it can also raise the visibility of the hospital's transfusion service.

The increasing complexity of laboratory coagulation testing, the shortage of specialists in these fields, and the growing costs of hemostasis management indicate a gap in knowledge and clinical practice that transfusion medicine practitioners can fulfil. It is noteworthy that each Postgraduate has the necessary knowledge in the evaluation of bleeding disorders and the basics screening tests, and also their management

Basics of Coagulation

"Hemostasis is the physiological process that stops bleeding at the site of an injury while maintaining normal blood flow elsewhere in the circulation." It is all about the balance between coagulation and the anticoagulation system. When these system overshoots, there can be either thrombosis or haemorrhage, respectively. Hemostasis mainly consists of three phases. The vascular, Platelet & coagulation phase. (Fig1)

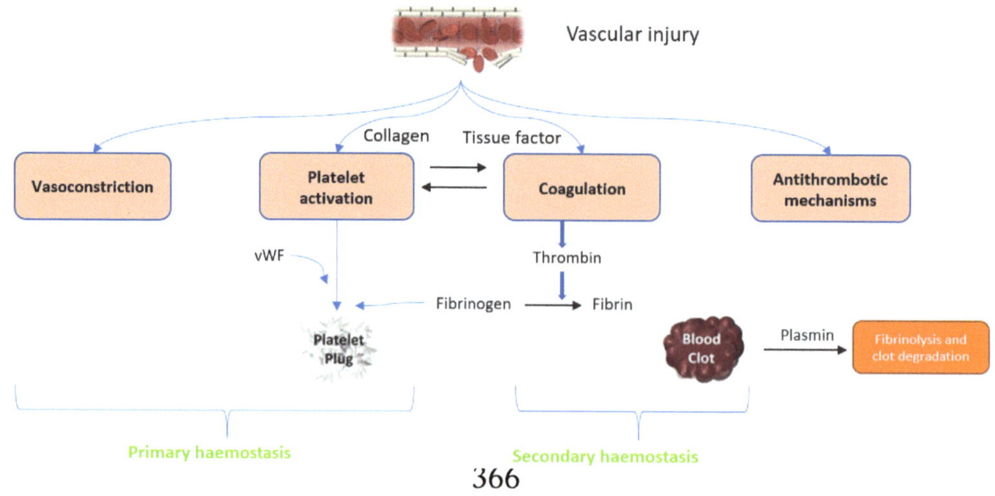

Figure 31

The vascular phase comprises certain enzymes and neural reflexes, which leads to vasoconstriction. The platelet phase can be divided into three sub-phases, The adhesion, Activation and Aggregation phases, followed by the Coagulation phase, which comprises both the intrinsic and extrinsic pathways culminating in the common pathway to form a stable soft clot, which is made stronger and transformed into the hard clot by the Factor XIII (Table 1)

Table 1

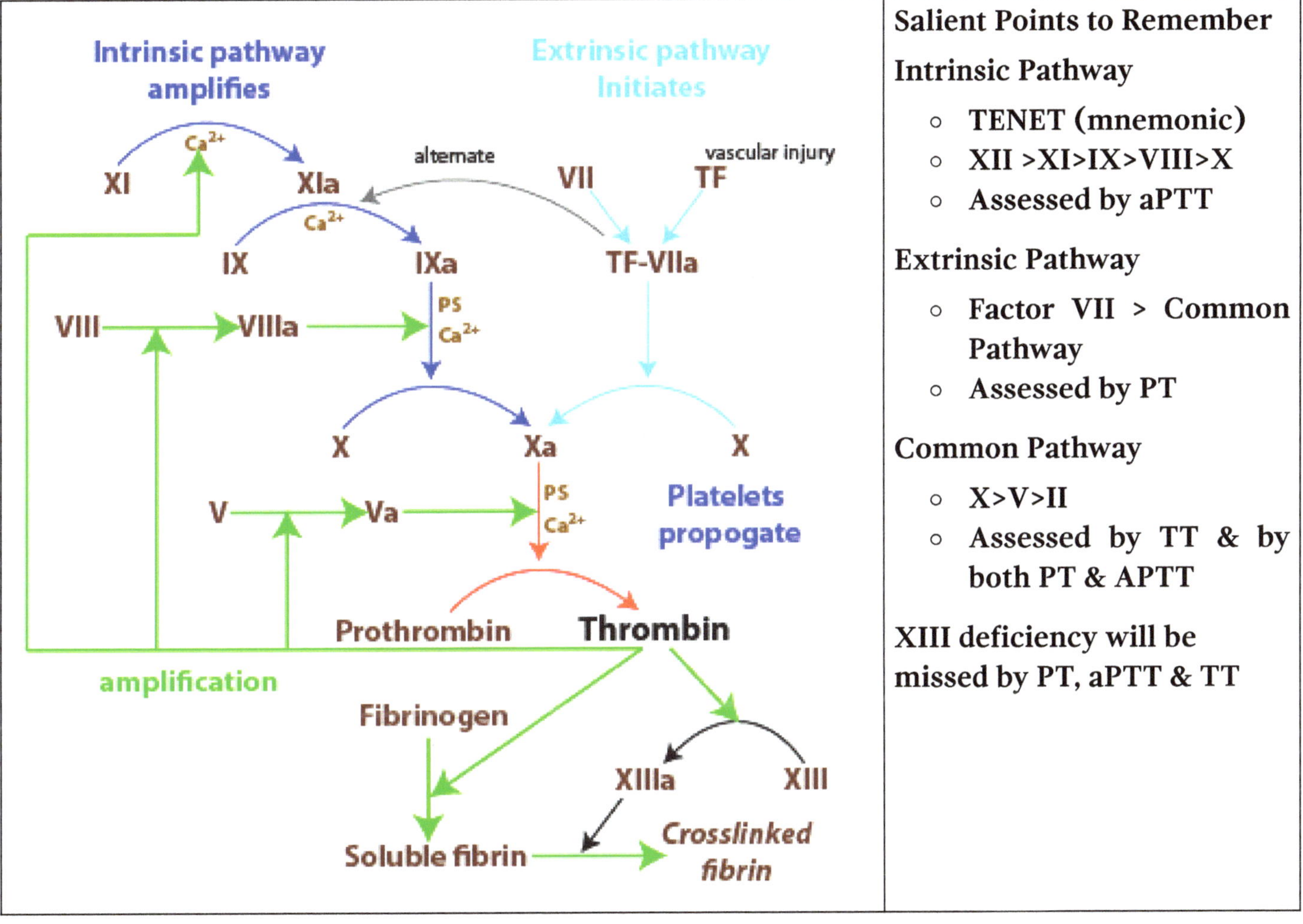

The newer revised model, known as cell-based coagulation, is shown below. In it, the Tissue factor exposed at a wound interacts with Factor VIIa and initiates clotting by two pathways: (Figure 2)

1. Activation of Factor X to Xa (i.e., the extrinsic tenase complex) and
2. Conversion of Factor IX to IXa activates factor X to Xa (i.e., the intrinsic tenase complex).
3. Thrombin also activates factor XI to XIa, leading to further generation of Factor IXa; it serves as an amplification pathway required during severe hemostatic challenges.

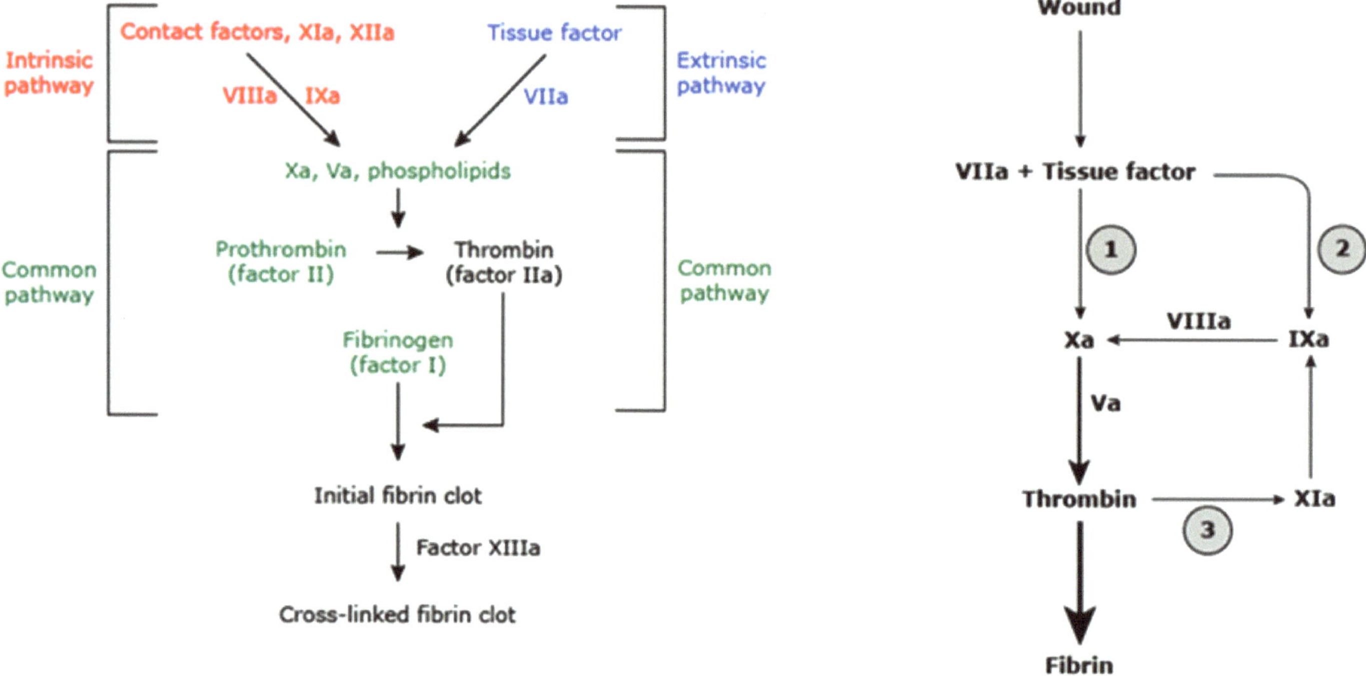

Figure 2

Any defect in the above systems will lead to bleeding and require further evaluation to be picked up, diagnosed, and managed.

Cascade model:

Utility

- Helpful in the understanding of how coagulation processes occur in plasma-based in vitro coagulation.
- Allows for clinically useful interpretation of laboratory tests for plasma coagulation abnormalities.

Deficiency:

- The cascade model suggests that the extrinsic and intrinsic pathways operate as independent and redundant pathways, while clinical manifestations of individual factor deficiencies contradict this concept.
- This model does not adequately explain the hemostatic process as it occurs in vivo.
- Deficiencies in the initial components of the intrinsic pathway (FXII, HMWK, or PK) cause marked prolongation of the aPTT, but they are not associated with a tendency for bleeding in humans. FXII is not required for normal hemostasis because some mammalian species (whales and dolphins) do not have this protein.
- The following downstream enzyme, FXI (hemophilia C) deficiency, is associated with variable hemostatic deficits in humans, with some individuals experiencing bleeding. In contrast, deficiency in either of the following downstream components of the intrinsic pathway (FVIII

and FIX) results in the severe bleeding tendencies seen with hemophilia A and B, even though these patients have an intact extrinsic pathway

- Deficiency of the primary enzyme of the extrinsic pathway (FVII) can be associated with bleeding, despite the presence of an intact intrinsic pathway
- The clinical manifestations of isolated abnormalities in either the intrinsic or extrinsic pathways argue against the idea that these enzymatic systems operate as independent generators of FXa.

Evaluation of an Abnormal Bleeding

Any person who comes with a complaint of abnormal bleeding manifestation must be evaluated in the form of a detailed history. The aetiology of bleeding can be delineated from certain pointers, as shown in Table 2

Symptoms	Coagulation disorder	Platelet disorder
Petechiae	Not common	Characteristic
Ecchymoses	Common	Common
Soft Tissue Hematoma	Characteristic	Rare
Joint Hemorrhages	Characteristic	Not usually seen
Delayed Bleeding	Common	Rare
Family History Of Bleeding	Common	Rare

The Bleeding assessment tools can be used to Objectify and score each patient as per his/her complaints. There are various tools of which the ISTH SSC BAT tool is being validated and widely used (https://bleedingscore.certe.nl/). Depending on the score, further Blood investigations, known as the screening test, must be done. Bleeding manifestations in the newborn or any spontaneous Intracranial or Life-threatening GI bleeding does not warrant a higher BAT score before further evaluation. These situations warrant evaluation by screening and confirmatory tests as per the screening results. The blood sample for these tests must be taken before any blood or factor support is given, even in an emergency, as these would interfere with the correct diagnosis.

Coagulation Testing

A detailed and meticulous history is considered the most important screening test for any bleeding disorder, especially the congenital or hereditary types. After which, objective scoring is done. If the score suggests a possibility; the first tests done are the screening tests

Screening Tests in coagulation

The screening test is a preliminary procedure to detect the most characteristic sign of a disorder that may require further confirmation. This test aims not to miss any step that would put the patient at risk of bleeding. The test should be done in a short time with comparatively little effort. It should be less expensive and very sensitive. It should serve as a selection procedure for further specific investigations

The typical screening tests are the Hess test, Bleeding Time, Platelet count, PT /INR, aPTT, Thrombin time, Fibrinogen & the Factor XIII urea clot solubility test. (Table 3)

Table 20

Phases of Coagulation	Screening Test
Vascular Phase	HESS Test
Platelet Phase	Platelet Count Bleeding Time Peripheral Smear PFA
Coagulation Phase	PT, APTT, TT FIBRINOGEN, XIII (Urea Clot Solubility)

Confirmatory tests

Based on the screening results, specific tests like Mixing studies and factor assays may have to be carried out to reach a definite diagnosis. Certain pointers from the screening tests to decide on further evaluation are shown below (Table 4)

Table 21

Pointers from Screening Tests	Further Plan
Are the Screening Tests are Normal	Consider being Normal
If isolated Bleeding Time is Prolonged	To consider Working up for Platelet Dysfunction
Bleeding Time Prolonged & Reduced Platelet Count	Workup for Platelet Dysfunction (Quantitative & Qualitative)
Isolated PT prolongation	Evaluate for extrinsic pathway Defect
Isolated aPTT prolongation	Interpretation for Intrinsic pathway defect
aPTT prolongation with BT prolonged	Evaluate for VWD, Platelet Dysfunction & Factor deficiencies
Both PT & APTT prolongation	Common Pathway defect or Multiple factor deficiency or Consumptive coagulopathy

The further plan depends on the screening tests. The usual Congenital Bleeding problem seen is Hemophilia. Haemophilia is an X-linked Congenital recessive disorder. It usually manifests in childhood with Joint bleeds and bleeding post Tooth extraction or circumcision. They usually have a typical Maternal family history. An isolated aPTT prolongation is seen in the screening test. It warrants a Mixing or Correction study

Mixing/Correction Studies

It is advised when there is PT/APTT prolongation. The procedure is to mix equal volumes of Test plasma, which gave the abnormal time, with Pooled Normal plasma (where all factors are present in normal quantity). The concept behind the mixing study is shown in (Fig 3). A factor level of 50% can give a Normal PT or aPTT screen. The possibility after a Mixing study is

- ○ Correction on Mixing, which suggests a factor deficiency
- ○ No correction: The test sample contains some Inhibitor

Note: A standard Mixing study would miss an FVIII inhibitor, which can only be picked by an incubated and fresh mixing

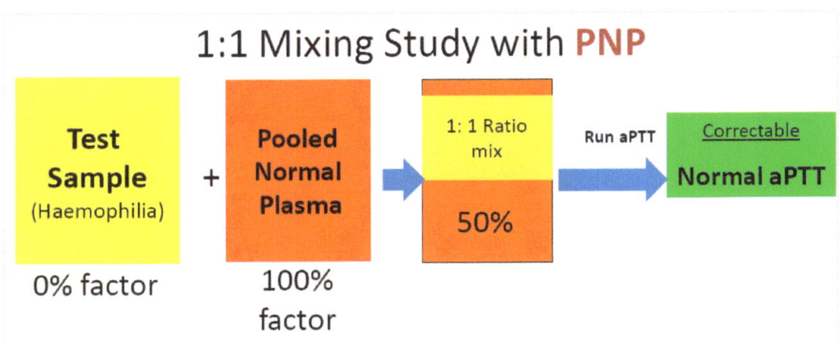

Fig 3

An algorithm based on the screening & Mixing studies is shown below in fig 4. On Correction by Mixing with PNP, further mixing studies may be done using factor-deficient plasma before the specific factor assays. (Table 5)

Table 5

Factor Deficiency evaluated by further mixing studies	
Mix with Aged Serum	**Mixing with Adsorbed Plasma**
<ul><li>Aged serum deficient in labile factors (1,2,5 &8)</li><li>Prepared by keeping serum for 48 hrs or in 37⁰c water bath for 4 hrs</li><li>If there is no resource constraint, **Factor VIII** deficient Plasma can be used</li><li>On Mixing; If aPTT is Prolonged – **Hemophilia A** is a possibility</li></ul>	<ul><li>Adsorbed plasma is deficient in Vit K-dependent clotting factors (2,7,9,10)</li><li>Prepared by using Barium sulphate/ Aluminium hydroxide for adsorbing the factors from plasma</li><li>If there is no resource constraint, **Factor IX** deficient Plasma can be used</li><li>On Mixing; if Aptt is prolonged - **Hemophilia B** is a possibility</li></ul>

All Possibilities are to be confirmed using a Factor assay. Factor VIII deficiency is seen in Hemophilia A & Factor IX deficiency is seen in Hemophilia B. Severity of the disease is established based on the factor levels. Factor levels below 1% are considered Severe, and a level between 1 to 5 % is Moderate. Any level above 5% and below 40% is usually considered mild.

A simplified version of the coagulation workup
Take a complete detailed history
Do the BAT score, after which do the tests accordingly
Complete Hemogram along with a Peripheral Smear
+
ALL NORMAL, But still Bleeding: Urea clot solubility testing: Factor XIII
BT, PT/INR, APTT, FIBRINOGEN
ALL NORMAL, REPORT AS NORMAL
THROMBOCYTOPENIA
PROLONGED PT
PROLONGED APTT
PBS
HESS TEST
INVIVO
MIXING WITH PNP
If not corrected
MIXING WITH PNP
CORRECTED
INHIBITOR SCREEN
CORRECTED
MIXING WITH ADSORBED PLASMA
MIXING WITH AGED SERUM
PROLONGED
CORRECTED
PROLONGED
SPECIFIC FACTOR ASSAY
MIXING WITH ADSORBED PLASMA
FACTOR VII DEFICIENCY
PROLONGED
AGED SERUM DEFICIENT IN:1,2,5,8
ADSORBED PLASMA DEFICIENT IN:2,7,9,10
SPECIFIC FACTOR ASSAY
FACTOR VIII/IX DEFICIENCY

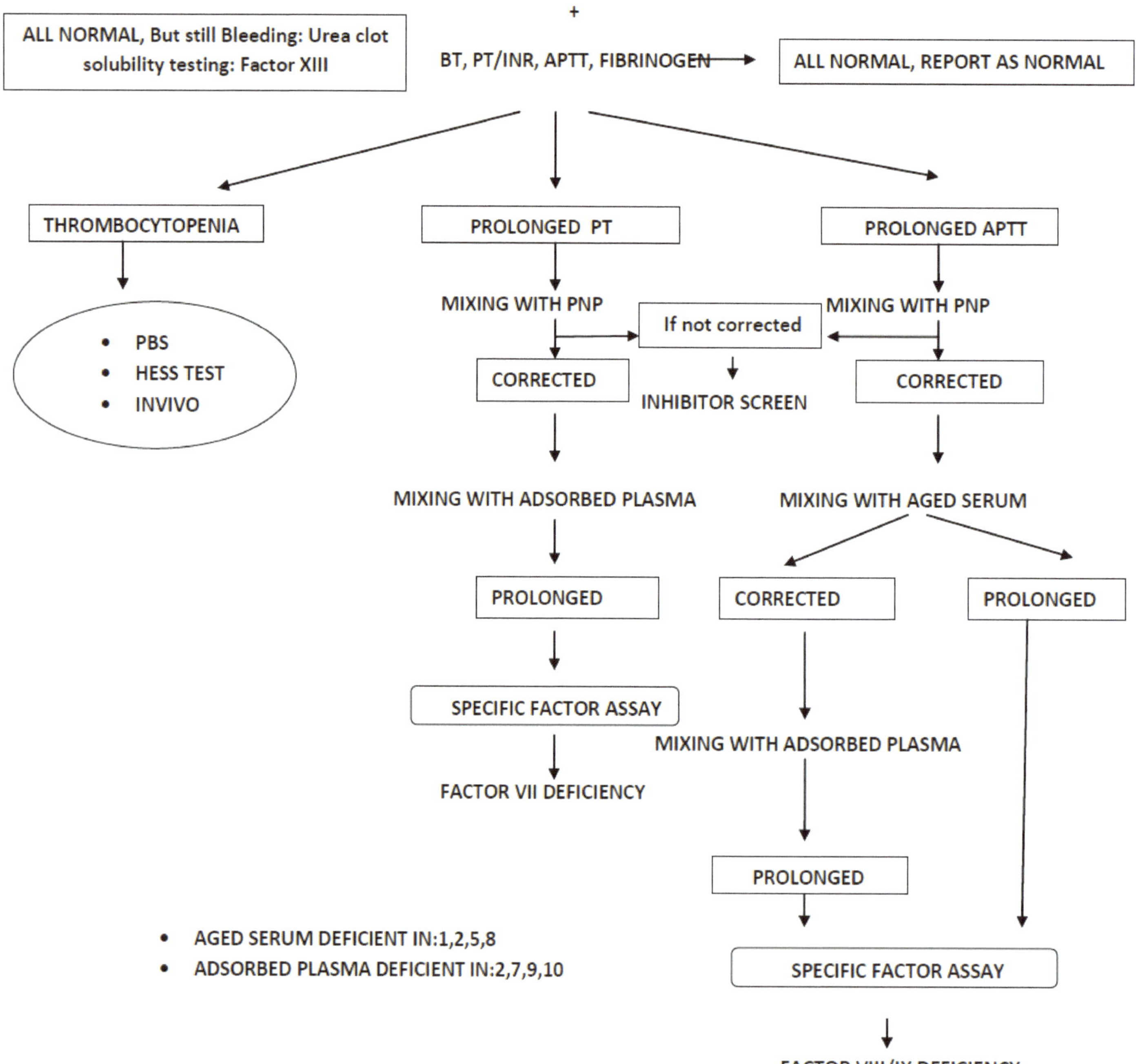

Figure 4

Applications to hemotherapy

Acquired bleeding disorder comprises a vast chunk of patients that transfusion specialists usually manage. The lab findings of most of the common disorders are shown below in Table 6

Disorder	Platelet count	PT	aPTT	TT	Fibrinogen level	Therapy Advised
Vasculopathies, connective tissue diseases, or collagen disorders affecting the skin	Normal	Normal	Normal	Normal	Normal or increased*	Pharmacotherapy
Thrombocytopenia	Decreased	Normal	Normal	Normal	Normal	Pharmacotherapy + Platelet Transfusion
Qualitative platelet abnormalities	Normal or decreased¶	Normal	Normal	Normal	Normal	Pharmacotherapy + Platelet Transfusion
Hemophilia A or B (factor VIII or IX deficiency)	Normal	Normal	Prolonged	Normal	Normal	Factor Concentrates Cryo /FFP *
von Willebrand disease	NormalΔ	Normal	Normal or prolonged◊	Normal	Normal	Factor Concentrates Cryo /FFP *
Disseminated intravascular coagulation	Decreased	Prolonged	Prolonged	Prolonged	Decreased	Platelet /Cryo/ FFP

POCT

The new tool in the armamentarium is the POCT devices in coagulation. They are used at the bedside for analysis and have a lesser TAT, facilitating earlier intervention. The Whole blood is used compared to the plasma in conventional testing; hence the in vivo coagulation is being assessed, and the interactions with platelets and RBCs are also analyzed. They have been used in various settings like trauma, Cardiac surgery, Neurosurgery, Obstetric care, and Critical care. They are also widely used in sepsis & also in transplantation surgeries.

The various POCTs available in Hemostasis measures

- o Pro thrombin time – INR
- o Activated clotting time
- o Viscoelastic tests
- o Platelet function

- D-Dimer
- Fibrinogen assays
- Modifications of thrombin time
- APTT

The most widely used ones are viscoelastic tests like TEG & ROTEM. They are Whole blood-based global hemostatic assays having a rapid turnaround time. They help in timely decision making, Mainly used for guiding transfusion support in hemorrhagic shock. The concept originated in 1948. As a POCT, coagulation initiation and amplification are more important. It also gives information about the fibrinolysis & platelet function, which is usually challenging to study using conventional methods.

The phases of coagulation that are tested using POCT in comparison to the conventional testing are shown in figure 5

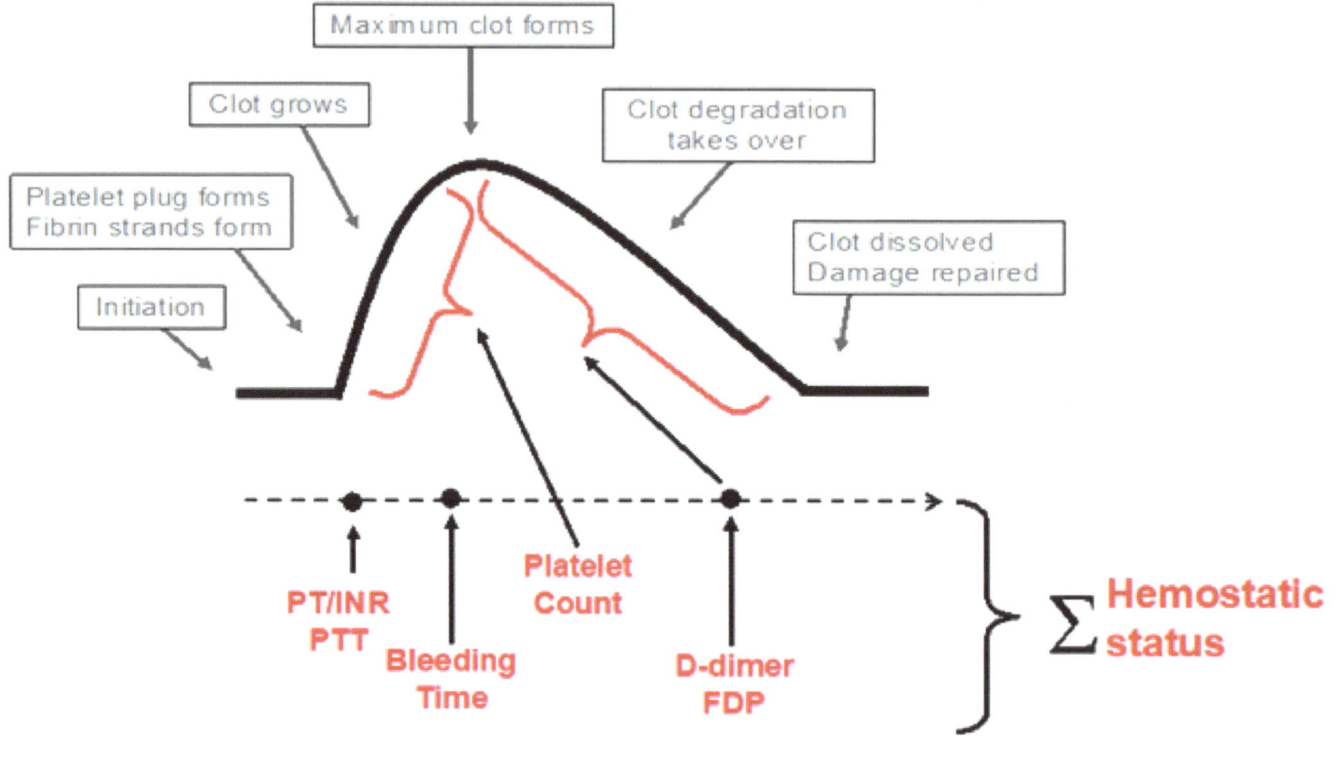

Figure 5

The TEG /TEM plot gives a Real-time display of the dynamics of clot formation and measures all the phases of hemostasis. The technical differences and the differences in the plots of TEG & ROTEM are shown below [(Table 7) & (Figure 6)]

Table 7

Characteristics	TEG	ROTEM
Pipetting	Manual	Automated
Number of samples at a time	2	4

Pin motion	Fixed	Moving (4° **75'** / **6 sec**)
Cup	Moving (4°45' / 5 mins)	Fixed
Temperature control	24-40 deg c	30-40 deg c
Temperature regulation	Heated cup	Heated metal block
Cup Interior	Smooth	Rugged
Cup material	Cryolite	Polymethyl methacrylate
Detection of the clot formation	Electromechanically	Optically

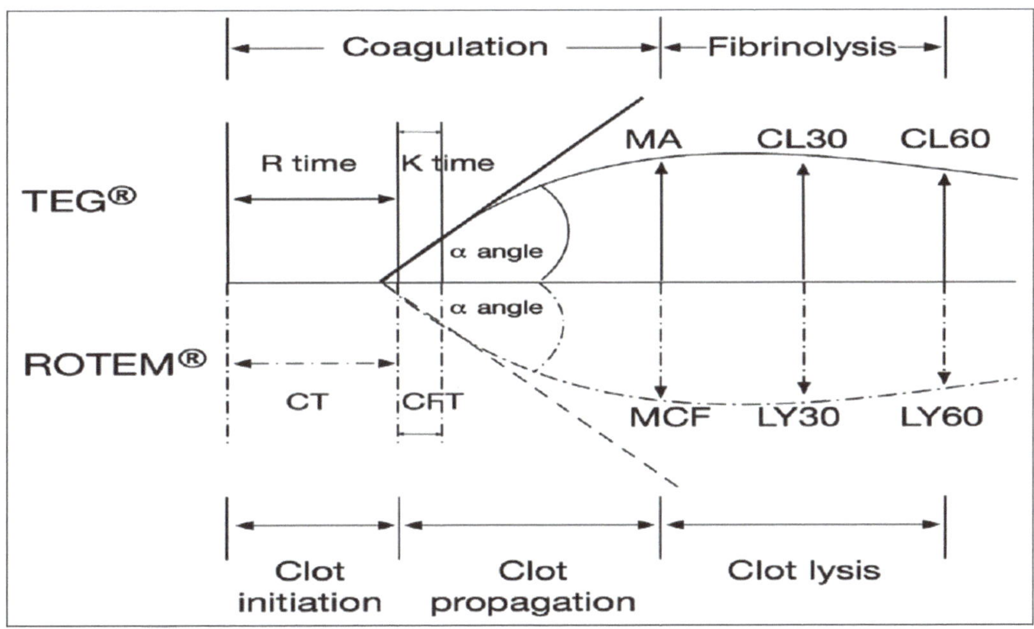

Figure 6

The utility of these POCT devices has been debated, and various international algorithms have been made. A simple algorithm is shown below (Fig 7). It is always prudent to have local algorithms when such equipment is being used at various centres

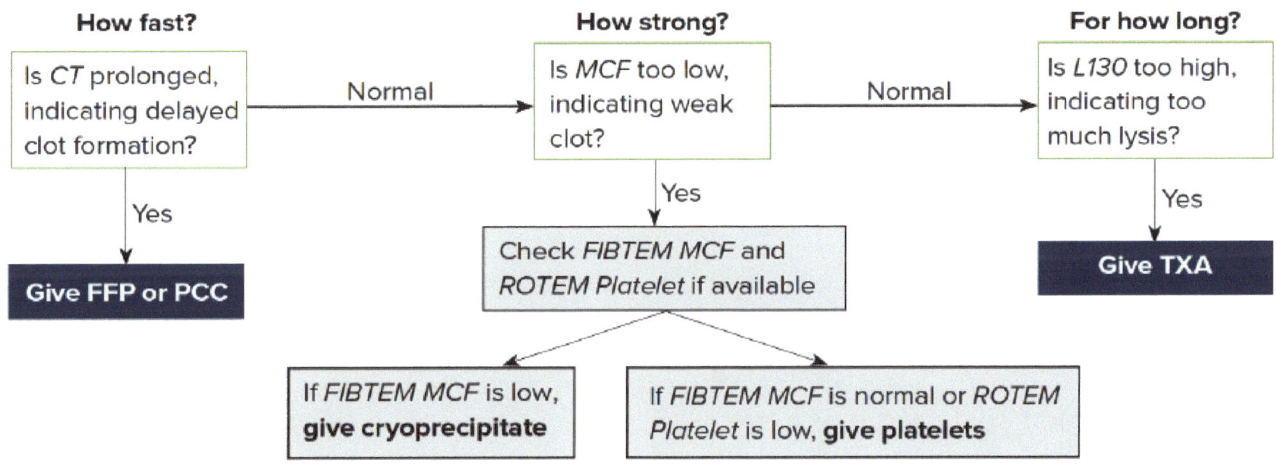

Fig 7

Component of TEG	Value	Management
Activated clotting time	>128 seconds	Predicts massive transfusion
	< 105 seconds	No transfusion
Activated clotting time	>128	RBC and FFP
K or	>2.5 minutes	Add Cryoprecipitate
α angle	<56⁰	
MA	< 55 mm	Add platelets
LY30	> 3%	Add tranexamic acid

Applications of TEG/ROTEM in Transfusion Medicine: Initiation, dosing and monitoring hemotherapy, QC for blood components, Patient blood management

Flow Cytometry in Transfusion Medicine

– Dr. Mohandoss M

PRINCIPLE:

- Flow cytometers enable the measurement of multiple characteristics of single cells within a heterogeneous population.
- Fluidic system: Presents cells in a suspension to the laser interrogation point. The interrogation point is the one at which cells pass through the laser light beam one cell at a time by a process known as 'hydrodynamic focusing'.
- Optical system: Consists of excitation and collection optics. The excitation optics are lasers with focusing lenses and prisms. The collection optics gather scattered light to specific optical detectors. Cells in suspension pass through a laser light source, and signals generated by light scattering (FSC, forward scatter and SSC, side scatter) can distinguish cells of different sizes and internal complexity or granularity, respectively. For determining the biochemical properties of a cell, cells are labelled with dyes or fluorochrome-conjugated antibodies and excited by light of a specific wavelength. The fluorochrome gains energy by absorbing light while returning to its unexcited state, and this energy released as photons of light results in fluorescence. The range of wavelength at which a fluorochrome absorbs light becomes excitation wavelength, and the fluorescence emitted becomes emission wavelength.
- Electronic system: The fluorescent signals are collected by photomultiplier tubes (PMT) with optical filters specific to wavelength range. The light signals are then processed and converted into numerical data plotted on a graphical scale such as a dot plot or histogram for analysis.
- Gating: Refers to identifying or isolating single populations of cells of interest within a heterogeneous group. By drawing a gate (or region) around the population of interest, the fluorescent properties of cells of interest alone can be displayed, making the analysis more specific.

The applications of flow cytometric analysis in transfusion medicine are

1. **Quality control of blood products**

    A. Evaluation of residual WBCs in leukodepleted blood components

    - Current guidelines require the reduction of WBCs in leukocyte-depleted blood components either by filtration or apheresis to a level below 5×10^6 WBC in at least 95% of the units tested

- Principle: Nucleic acid dye- Propidium iodide (PI) stains all nucleated cells. DNA/RNA-specific dye is excited at a particular wavelength (488nm) and emitted fluorochrome is captured. Brightly stained leukocytes are easily distinguishable from non-nucleated particles such as erythrocytes and platelets.
- Absolute number of rWBC/µl = (WBC events / Bead Events) x (Bead count per tube/ stained sample volume)

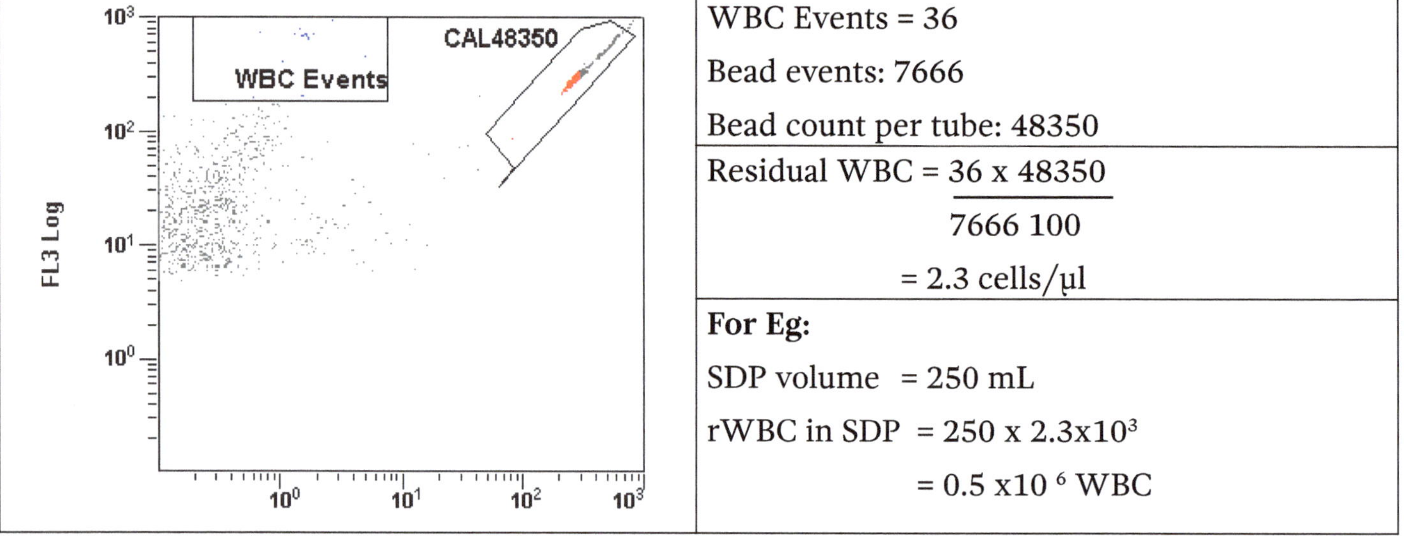

WBC Events = 36

Bead events: 7666

Bead count per tube: 48350

Residual WBC = $\dfrac{36 \times 48350}{7666 \quad 100}$

= 2.3 cells/µl

For Eg:

SDP volume = 250 mL

rWBC in SDP = $250 \times 2.3 \times 10^3$

= 0.5×10^6 WBC

Figure 1: Flow cytometric plot displaying data from Leukodepleted RBC unit. The brightly stained residual WBCs are captured in WBC events, and a known concentration of beads is added.

Functional investigations of cells/cell fractions in blood components

- The viability of cells can be estimated by nucleic acid dyes 7 Amino actinomycin D (7AAD) or Propidium Iodide (PI)
- Activation markers in blood components by expression of CD42b, CD62P (P-Selectin), as well as binding of Annexin-V, PAC-1, antifibrinogen

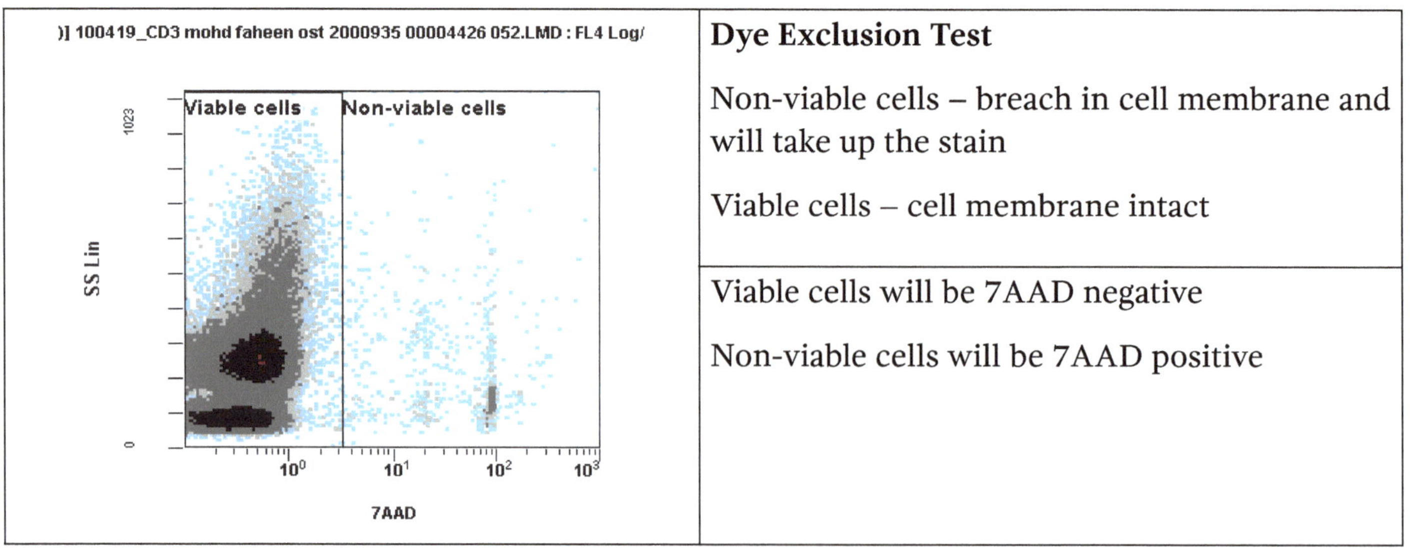

Dye Exclusion Test

Non-viable cells – breach in cell membrane and will take up the stain

Viable cells – cell membrane intact

Viable cells will be 7AAD negative

Non-viable cells will be 7AAD positive

Figure 2: Flow cytometric plot displaying data from PBSC Stem cell product. The brightly stained cells for 7AAD are non-viable, and 7AAD negative cells are viable.

B. Bacterial contaminations of blood components: Fluorescent dyes such as thiazole orange were used for staining bacterial nucleic acids to detect bacteria. The assay sensitivity is of order 10^4 cells/ml. The assay detects both- the live and the dead bacteria. BactiFlow technology helps in identifying viable bacterial cells.

- Platelet concentrates by BactiFlow technology: Testing platelets based on fluorescent labelling of viable cells. Specific enzymatic digestion of platelets (while preserving bacteria) eliminates background signals. Staining of bacteria is done using esterified fluorogenic substrates. A nonfluorescent fluorochrome passes through the cell membrane of membrane intact viable cells and has enzymatic activity. This fluorochrome is cleaved by intracellular esterases to produce fluorescence. These fluorochromes remain nonfluorescent until cleaved by functional cytoplasmatic enzymes. Thus, 2 cellular functions, esterase activity and membrane integrity are required to detect viable bacterial cell applications.
- RBC concentrates: BactiFlow was also used to detect and count bacteria based on esterase activity in viable cells in RBCs. The initial sample preparation for RBCs included RBCs' lysis, followed by the enrichment of bacteria by centrifugation. Background fluorescence of viable RBC was eliminated by enzymatic digestion and centrifugal filtration. Selective labelling of bacteria with fluorescent esterase substrate. Samples were defined negative using the BF assay if they had fewer than 500 bacteria-specific counts in the region of interest

2. Immunohematologic diagnostics

A. Red blood cell (RBC): Flow cytometry in RBC is used when an aberrant antigen's expression needs to be elucidated.

1. *Detecting and quantifying antibodies bound to RBCs* – e.g., DAT Negative AIHA. Selective quantitation of Ig subtypes is possible. However, the correlation between disease severity and RBC-bound Ig by flow cytometry is limited. Similarly, the survival of RBCs after transfusion or in patients with autoimmune hemolytic anaemia was investigated by labelling RBCs with fluorochromes and subsequent quantification by flow cytometry
2. *Quantification of antibody concentration:* Exact determination of specific antibodies, including subclass, which is more exact than agglutination titres, can be determined and applied in maternal antibody titre
3. *Detection and quantification of antigens on RBCs:* Near linear relationship of antigen density and resulting fluorescence from flow cytometry. Antigen density, dosing effect, and phenotype-related differences in antigen densities can be determined.

    3.1 Distribution of antigen densities - e.g. Rh shows a single peak while ABO antigens are wide-based peak

    3.2 Evaluate D antigen expression and antigen site density in D variants. Similarly, other minor blood group variants can be determined

3.3 In the ABO group – to determine homo and heterozygosity for alleles exhibiting the usual amount of ABH antigens, to examine changes in ABH antigen strength during storage

3.4 ABO subgroups are very distinct, and by analysing the histogram and dot plot, the genetic background can be predicted with accuracy

3.5 Resolution of Bombay and para-Bombay group discrepancies

3.6 Resolution of samples with weakened Antigen expression due to haematological malignancies or pregnancy

4. ***Estimation of Fetomaternal Hemorrhage:*** Fetomaternal haemorrhage (FMH) is the volume of foetal cells in maternal circulation. Most women will have FMH <4ml during delivery, and a dose of 500µg RhIG will be sufficient to neutralize fetal cells in maternal circulation. In RhD Negative women, it is essential to accurately estimate FMH in obstetric management of Rh D alloimmunization. Hence, foetal blood volume is determined to calculate the correct anti-D (RhIg) dosage to avoid alloimmunization for RhD from an RhD-positive foetus.

❖ Quantifying fetal cells in maternal blood by staining the HbF in fetal RBCs or labelling fetal D+RBCs. In the HbF method, the red cells are permeabilized to allow Anti HbF antibody to bind to intracellular HbF.

❖ Direct Staining: FITC or PE labelled monoclonal Anti D is used for staining fetal cells. Direct staining must always be done on the maternal sample before administering anti-D. The prophylactic anti-D received might sensitize RhD-positive fetal cells to such an extent that fluorescent-labelled Anti-D binding will be inhibited (similar to the Blocked D phenomenon). Thereby wrongly reporting as no RhD-positive cells in maternal circulation.

❖ Indirect Staining: Stained using Polyclonal or Monoclonal anti D antisera, and FITC or PE-labelled AHG reagent is used

❖ Where it is known that the mother has received anti-D, an indirect and direct flow cytometric test should be undertaken.

Controls used are

- 100% D negative cells
- 99% D negative and 1% D positive (approximating 22mL bleed)
- 99.75% D negative and 0.25% D positive (approximating 5.5mL bleed)

❖ ***Volume of fetal red cells = (Percentage foetal cells x 1800 x 1.22)mL.***

❖ Where 1800 represents maternal red cell volume and 1.22 corrects cord blood MCV

❖ Recently use of Anti-HbF in combination with an antibody towards carbonic anhydrase (CA) enzyme. The CA enzyme levels are fully expressed only after birth, so only maternal cells express CA positivity, and maternal cells containing HbF can also be distinguished from foetal cells. Similarly, a combined two-colour dual antibody method utilizing anti-HbF and anti-D has also been described

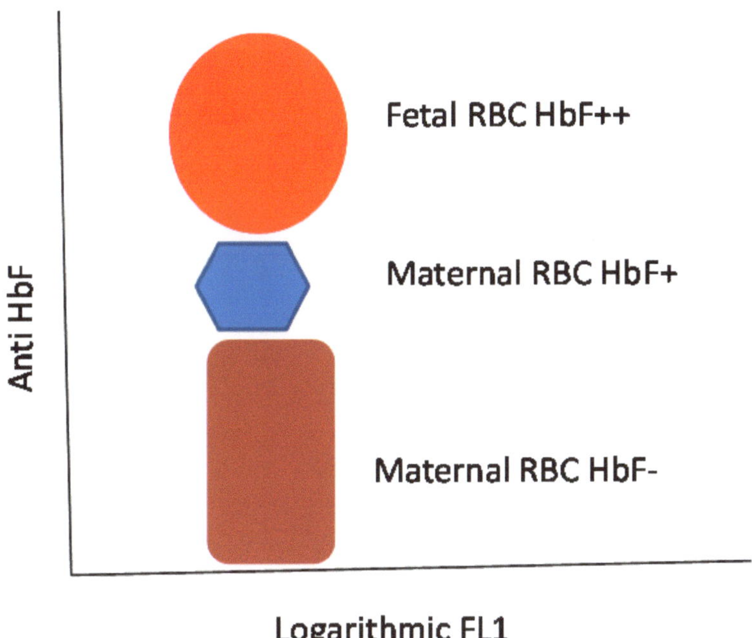

Figure 3: Diagrammatic representation of estimating Fetomaternal haemorrhage using Anti HbF

5. *Estimation of Mixed field reactions and Chimerism:* Flow cytometry will clearly show if two distinct populations are present.

   - Mixed field reactions: previous transfusions of nonidentical ABO and/or RhD blood units
   - Chimerism: two or more distinct cell populations - detect small populations of cells that are routinely used for posttreatment follow-up of leukaemia and lymphoma, minimal residual disease analysis and HLA-based chimerism analysis post-haploidentical HSCT.

6. *Genetic disorders of erythrocytes*

   - Paroxysmal nocturnal hemoglobinuria (PNH): A hematopoietic stem cell disorder characterized by partial or complete loss of GPI- anchored proteins, including complement-defence structures such as CD55 and CD59 on RBCs and WBCs.
   - For red cell analysis, CD235a and CD59 combination is used to identify Type II (partial deficiency of GPI protein) and Type III (complete deficiency of GPI protein) PNH red blood cells from normal (Type I).
   - To identify PNH clones in neutrophils, a four-colour combination using FLAER, CD24, CD15, and CD45 was used. Similarly, for detecting PNH clones in monocytes, a four-colour combination of FLAER, CD14, CD64, and CD45 is used.

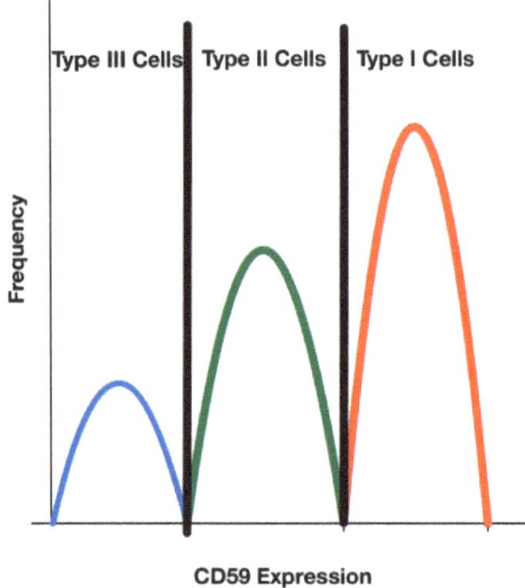

`Figure 4A: Diagrammatic representation of CD59 expression on red cells in PNH patients

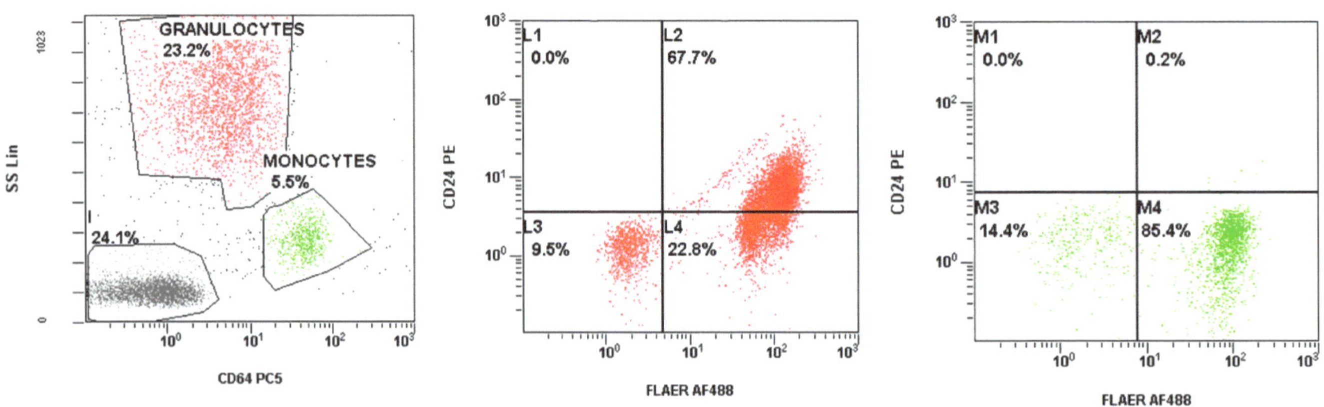

Figure 4B: Flow cytometry plots of Granulocytes and Monocytes showing PNH clones identified by a deficiency in the FLAER antibody

B. Platelet integrity and immunology

a. Detection and quantification of antibodies against platelets

b. Detection and quantification of platelet antigens

c. Platelet cross-matching: Patients with platelet refractoriness present an inadequate response to platelet transfusions. Refractoriness is usually due to alloantibodies to either human leucocyte antigens (HLA) or human platelet antigens (HPA). Flow cytometry-based platelet cross-match can be used as an alternative strategy to plate-based cross-match in identifying compatible platelet units that are likely to give an adequate posttransfusion platelet count increment where HLA-matched platelets are not available. Flow cytometry platelet immunofluorescence test (FC-PIFT) – Platelet product incubated with patient serum (5 mL) for 30 minutes at 37ºC. Positive and Negative controls are added to each batch of the test. After about three consecutive washes, cells were incubated for 50 minutes with fluorescein isothiocyanate (FITC) goat anti-human IgG [F(ab') Fragment Goat Anti-Human 2 IgG, Fc Fragment Specific) at 1:50 dilution. Samples were washed and interpreted in a flow cytometer. If the median fluorescence (MF) obtained was greater than or equal to two standard deviations (SD) above the negative MF control test was considered positive and inconclusive if MF was between one and two SD above the negative MF control.

C. Granulocyte/monocyte integrity and immunology

    a. Flow cytometry was used to identify and characterize granulocyte antigens or antibodies, e.g. in the investigation of transfusion-related acute lung injury (TRALI), in population studies or in the analysis of potential changes during pregnancy

    b. Detection of granulocyte/ monocyte function and antigens

    c. Detection of phagocytosis

3. **Hematopoietic progenitor cells**

    a. Determination and quantification of hematopoietic progenitor cells in bone marrow/ peripheral blood/cord blood using triple fluorophore gating according to the International Society of Hematotherapy and Graft Engineering (ISHAGE) guidelines. CD34 pos, 7-AAD neg, and CD45 dim cells with low side scatter fractions were defined as CD34+ cells in hematopoietic stem cell/hematopoietic progenitor cell fractions. In single-platform methodologies, a known number of well-characterized fluorescent beads are added to the analyte. They are intended to be more reliable and easier to use than Dual-platform methods, which combine data from a conventional haematology analyzer and a flow cytometer

    Single Platform: Anti-CD34 and anti-CD45 with different fluorochrome are used for CD34+ WBC identification; isoclonic antibody combined with CD45-FITC is used as a control; 7-amino-actinomycin D (7-AAD) for cell viability assessment; ammonium chloride solution for erythrocyte lysis; and fluorescent bead reference standards of precisely known concentration is used for single-platform cell counting.

    Dual platform method: The percentage of CD34+ cells was determined using double-colour immunofluorescence staining (CD45/CD34). The absolute number of CD34+ cells was obtained by the product of the percentage of CD34+ cells fraction from the flow cytometer and the nucleated cell count from the haematology analyzer.

Figure 5: Flow cytometric plots using ISHAGE Platform for CD34 Enumeration. Plot 1: To include viable cells during the assessment (7-AAD Viability Dye negative event). Plot 2: Include all CD45+ leukocytes and eliminate platelets, red blood cell debris, and aggregates. Plot 3: To include all CD34+ cells. Plot 4: To include all clustered CD45dim events. Plot 5: Finally, the cells of interest, i.e. the events fulfilling the criteria of all three gates, are then displayed on an FSC vs SSC dot plot. This is done to include clustered events with intermediate side scatter and intermediate to high forward side scatter. Plot 6: FSC vs SSC dot plot to confirm that the selected events in plot 5 fall into a generic 'lymph-blast' region. Plot 7: Known fluorescent bead standards incorporated into each sample. Plot 8: displays ungated data to verify the lower limit of CD45 expression on CD34+ events

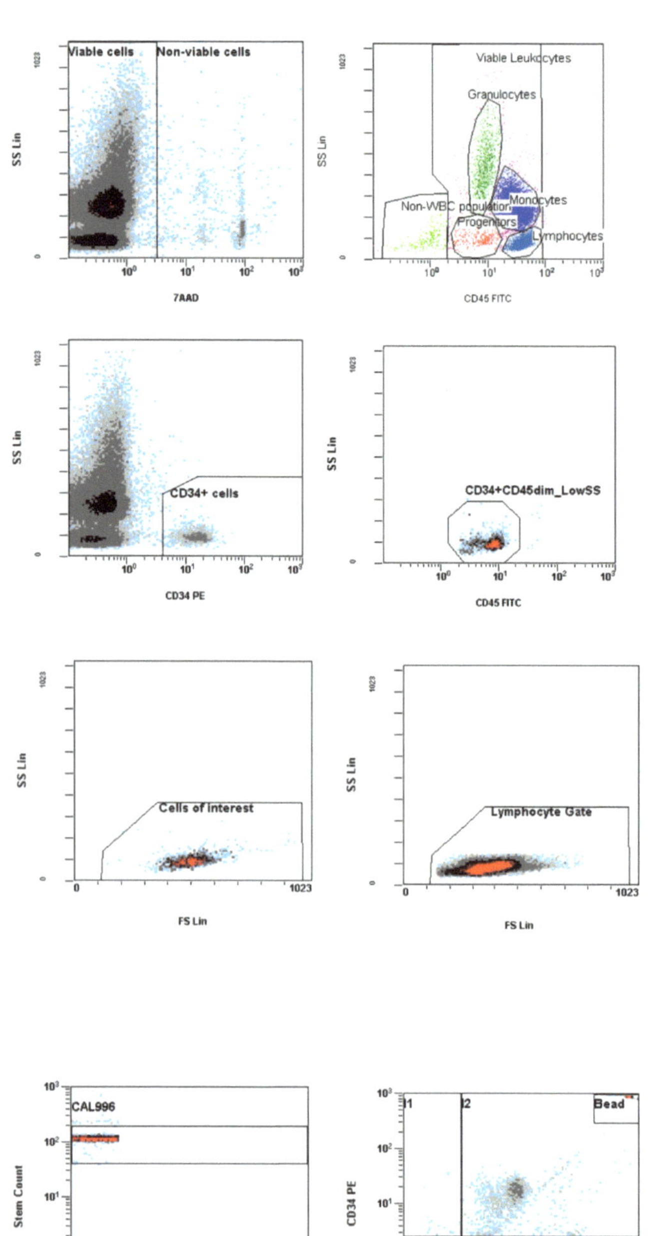

1) Events:33279; Viable cells: 96%

2) Viable Leukocytes:32869; 95.8%

3) CD34+ cells: 375; 1.09%

4) CD34+CD45dim/LowSS: 373; 1.09%

5) **Cells of interest: 372 cells/µl; 1.09%**

For Eg

PBSC Bag Volume	: 200mL
Recipient weight	: 50kg
Bag WBC count	: 328,600/µl
Dilution factor	: 10

Single Platform

CD34 count/µl = 372 x 10 (dilution)

$$= 3720$$

CD34 dose/kg = (CD34 count/1000)x Bag vol / Body weight

$$= \frac{(3720/1000) \times 200}{50}$$

$$= 14.8 \times 10^6/kg$$

Dual Platform

CD34 count % = 1.09%

CD34 dose/kg

$$= \frac{Bag\ WBC \times (\%CD34/100) \times (Bag\ vol/1000)}{Body\ weight}$$

$$= \frac{328600 \times (1.09/100) \times (200/1000)}{50}$$

$$= 14.3 \times 10^6/kg$$

b. Quantification of leukocyte subsets

c. Adoptive immunotherapy and further therapeutic applications in the analysis of

    i. Viability/apoptosis after manipulation/ cryopreservation of cells

    ii. Dendritic cells

    iii. Specificity and functionality of T cells

    iv. Natural killer (NK) cell phenotype and cytotoxicity

v. In haploidentical protocols, T cells and B cells are depleted for stem cell and NK cell enrichment performed by

1. Positive enrichment (CD34+, CD133+) of stem cells or
2. Serial CD3+ and CD19+ depletion and
3. Purification of CD56+CD3- NK cells

4. **Solid Organ Transplant**

a. Flow cytometric cross-match (FCXM):

i. Detection of circulating HLA antibodies in the serum of potential allograft recipients is an essential assessment performed before and after transplantation.

ii. If HLA antibodies are directed against the mismatched antigens of the donor, there may be severe clinical consequences.

iii. Depending upon the antibody's strength and possibly the HLA specificity, the clinical impact may range from benign to severe, constituting a contraindication for transplantation.

iv. Lymphocyte Crossmatching assesses the risk posed by the presence of donor-specific HLA antibodies (DSA).

v. Flow cytometric cross-match (FCXM) is performed by incubating donor cells with the serum from a potential recipient. If donor-specific HLA antibodies are present, they will be deposited on the surface of the target cell. Alloantibody binding is assessed by adding a fluorochrome-labelled goat, an anti-human immunoglobulin reagent.

vi. The level of measured fluorescence is then proportional to the amount of alloantibody bound to the target cell. To help differentiate the antibody class that may be binding to lymphocytes, labelled monoclonal antibodies are used to identify T-cells (CD3) or B cells (CD19 or CD 22). Potential reactivity patterns in FCXM are

T cell (CD3)	B cell (CD 19 or CD 22)	Interpretation
Negative	Negative	No HLA antibody or very low titer
Negative	Positive	Predominately Class II antibody
Negative	Weak positive	Weak Class I or II antibody
Positive	Positive	Strong Class I antibody or combination of Class I and II
Positive	Negative	Likely non-HLA reactivity

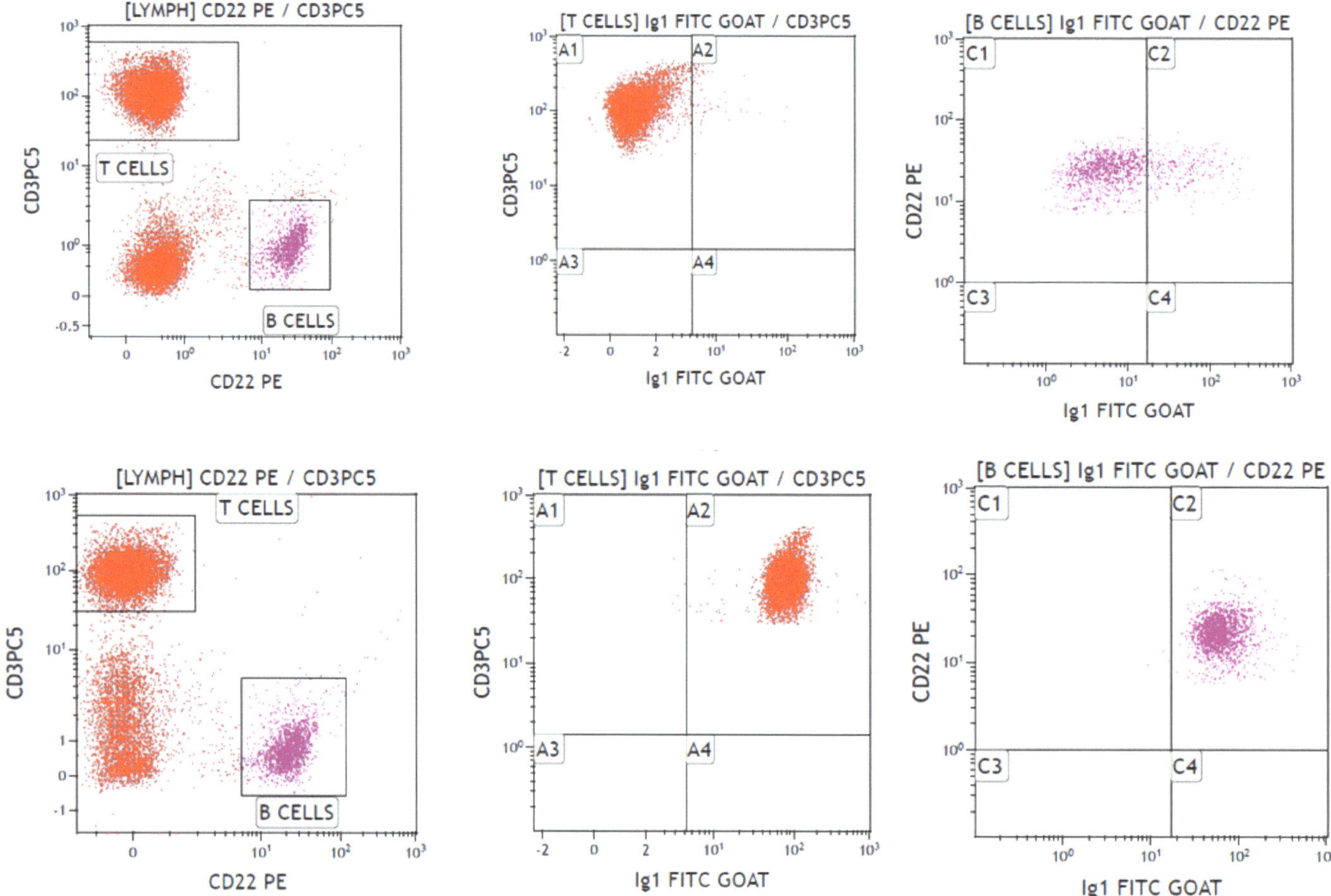

Figure 6: Plots showing flow cytometric cross-match. In the top row, the sample showed no antibodies against HLA class I and II antigens. The bottom row plot shows an antibody against both Class I and II HLA antigens.

5. **Applications in Platelet disorder**

   a. Primary platelet disorder (BernaudSoulier, Glanzmanns thrombasthenia, Storage pool disorder). CD41recognizes platelet glycoprotein GPII(αIIb); CD 61 recognizes GP IIIa(β3); CD42b reacts with GPIb on megakaryocytes and platelets; CD42a measures GPIX; CD 42d measure GPV.

      i. Normal platelets express CD41; CD 61, and CD 42b glycoproteins on the platelet surface (Figure A)

      ii. Bernard Soulier: inherited deficiency of the GPIb-IX-V complex, resulting in giant platelets. There will be normal binding of CD41 and CD 61, indicating normal GPIIb-IIIa complex, while there will be a clone of CD 42b negative cells indicating the absence of GPIb receptor in Bernaud Soulier.

      iii. Glanzmann thrombasthenia (GT) is an inherited deficiency of integrin αIIbβ3. In GT, platelets show no/reduced activity with either CD41 or CD61 and so are missing the GPIIb/IIIa complex. However, they clearly show normal activity with CD42b, i.e. normal GPIb.(Figure B)

	CD41	CD61	CD42b
Normal	Pos	Pos	Pos
BernaudSoulier	Pos	Pos	/Neg
Glanzmann Thrombasthenia	/Neg	/Neg	Pos

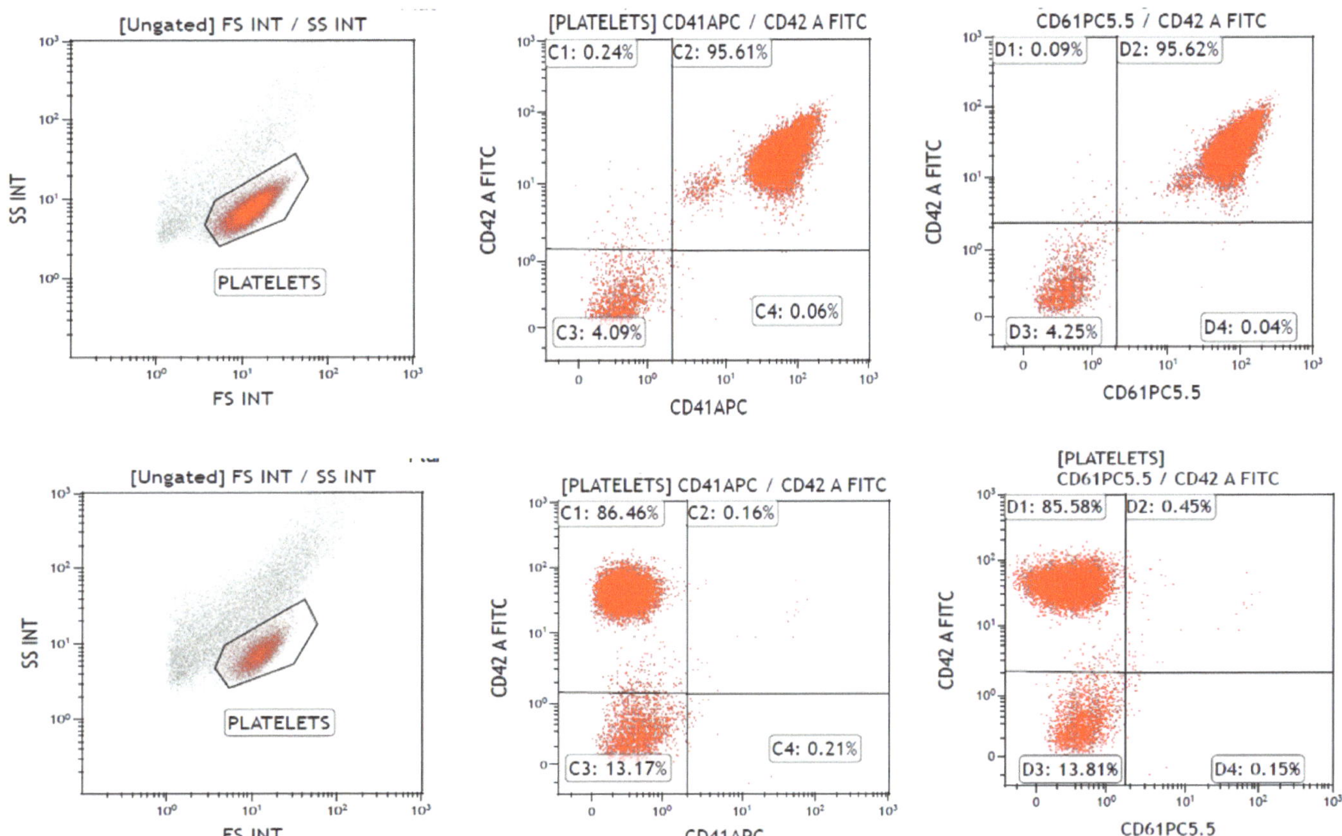

Figure 7: Flow cytometric assay on Platelet function disorder. The top row shows normal platelets

expressing CD41, CD 61 and CD 42A glycoproteins. The bottom row shows a sample from Glanzmann Thrombasthenia expressing normal expression of CD42A and absent expression for CD41 and CD 61 glycoprotein on the platelet surface.

b. Clinical disorders with Platelet dysfunction (activation or hyporeactivity) contributes to pathology (acute coronary syndrome, Cerebrovascular ischemia, Cardiopulmonary bypass)

   i. Disorders with Platelet Activation: Platelet hyperreactivity is essential in thrombotic and coronary artery disease pathogenesis. Platelet activation results in a series of changes in the platelet structure and biochemistry. These changes can be measured as markers of platelet activation by flow cytometry. Platelet-derived activation markers shed from the platelet (e.g., CD40 ligand, P-selectin, GPV) can be measured. P-selectin (CD62P) is a component of the agranule membrane and is not expressed on the resting platelets' surface. Soluble granule contents are released upon platelet activation, and P-selection is expressed on the platelet surface. P- selection specific mAbs bind only to activated platelets undergoing degranulation. Circulating degranulated platelets rapidly lose surface

P-selectin expression. Thus useful in detecting platelet activation associated with a very recent (< 5 minutes) or continuous activating stimulus but not suitable for activation as a result of an older stimulus

  ii. Disorders of Platelet hyporeactivity: Cardiopulmonary bypass causes platelet activation, and activated platelets may be lost from circulation by binding to exposed subendothelium/ adsorbed to the CPB circuit.

c. Disorders of thrombopoiesis: Measurement of reticulated platelets (measuring those containing mRNA)

d. Monitoring drug-induced platelet dysfunction both to guide therapy (clopidogrel for cardiovascular disease) or predict adverse effects (heparin-induced thrombocytopenia)

In summary, flow cytometry represents a highly innovative technique for many common diagnostic and scientific fields in transfusion medicine. It is a valuable tool in addition to serology and genomic typing in transfusion medicine.

HLA System in Transfusion Medicine

– Dr. Mohandoss M

The human leukocyte antigen (HLA) system consists of closely linked genes coded for highly polymorphic cell surface molecules. They are expressed on the surface of all nucleated cells and play a pivotal role in the fundamental necessity of the immune system to distinguish self from non-self. HLA antigens are the vehicles used to present peptides on the cell surface. The genes that code for the HLA antigens are located on the short arm of chromosome 6 (6p21.3) within a region termed the major histocompatibility complex (MHC)

Implications in Transfusion Medicine

1. Allogenic bone marrow transplantation
2. Immune-mediated platelet refractoriness – HLA antibodies directed against Class I antigens
3. Febrile non-haemolytic transfusion reactions (FNHTR) – antibodies against HLA antigens
4. Transfusion-associated acute lung injury (TRALI) - attributable to antibodies against HLA (Class I and class II) antigens
5. Transfusion-associated graft-versus-host disease (TA- GvHD) induced by the transfusion of HLA-compatible, immunologically responsive T lymphocytes
6. Haemolytic transfusion reactions by Bg system (HLA Class I on RBCs) and Chido& Rodgers system (C4 molecules coded by HLA Class III region). Red cell antibodies against these systems may cause lysis of RBC in a small proportion of antigen-positive cells.

The chapter will emphasize the basics of HLA, typing methods, and donor selection for allogeneic bone marrow transplantation and HLA-matched platelet transfusion.

Structure

Two main types of HLA genes and molecules are described, HLA class I and HLA class II. Class III genes encode proteins with a function in innate immunity (include complement components {C2, Factor B protein of alternate complement activation[Bf], C4}, TNF family, 21 hydroxylase enzyme).

HLA class I genes and molecules

*   Class I genes comprise the classical (HLA-A, -B and -C), the non-classical HLA-E, -F and -G and MHC class I chain-related MICA, MICB molecules.
*   Classical genes(A, B, C) – have major tissue distribution and are expressed on nucleated blood cells, platelets, and to a lesser extent on cells of CNS, endocrine and skeletal muscle

- HLA-E, -F & -G has a restricted tissue distribution, with HLA-G found on extravillous cytotrophoblasts of the placenta and mononuclear phagocytes.
- The function of Class I molecules is to present endogenous antigenic peptides to CD8+ T cells.
- Class I molecules (HLA-A, -B, and -C) are composed of a heavy (α) chain with three extracellular domains $\alpha 1$, $\alpha 2$, and $\alpha 3$, encoded by exons 2, 3, and 4, respectively. The heavy chain is complexed with a β – 2microglobulin light chain.
- The nucleotide substitutions within exons 2 and 3 are concentrated in hypervariable regions that define the peptide-binding groove, determining the allo-specificity of the Class I molecule.
- HLA typing in support of HSCT programs typically characterizes the Class I exon 2 and 3 sequences that encode the polymorphic $\alpha 1$ and $\alpha 2$ domains.

HLA class II genes and molecules

- HLA class II genes comprise the classical HLA-DRB1, DQB1,-DQA1,-DPA1, -DPB1 and the non-classical HLA- DMA,-DMB, -DOA and -DOB genes, which show limited polymorphism.
- HLA class II molecules are expressed on antigen-presenting cells such as B lymphocytes, monocytes and dendritic cells and were also expressed on activated T lymphocytes and activated granulocytes.
- The HLA class II expression can be induced on cells like fibroblasts and endothelial cells after activation and/or with the effect of inflammatory cytokines, such as IFNg, TNFa and IL-10.
- HLA class II molecules (DR, -DQ and -DP) present peptides derived from exogenous pathogens to CD4+ T cells. The activated CD4+ T cells promote the maturation and differentiation of cellular and humoral effectors.
- Class II molecules are heterodimeric in structure. They consist of two noncovalently bound proteins named α (product of A gene with limited diversity) and β (product of B gene with extensive diversity).
- The peptide-binding site is between the $\alpha 1$ and $\beta 1$ domains. The nucleotide substitutions of Class II B genes are located at key positions (residues) that define the peptide binding repertoire and determine the Class II allospecificity
- HLA typing of donors and recipients for HSCT targets the exon 2 DRB1 and DQB1 sequences that define the polymorphic DRβ and DQβ chains, respectively.

Soluble forms of HLA class I and II molecules can also be observed and may play a role in transfusion-related immunomodulation (TRIM) or induction of peripheral tolerance.

Homo/Heterozygous

- Most individuals are heterozygous for two different Class I and Class II alleles/antigens inherited from each parent at each HLA locus, and the two HLA antigens are co-dominantly expressed (for example, B5,10).
- When an individual inherits a paternal and maternal HLA allele having identical sequence (and therefore protein product), the term homozygous is used to describe the genotype/phenotype at that locus (for example, B5,5).

HLA Nomenclature

The naming system provides information about the antigen/locus, allele family, the amino acid difference in noncoding (silent) variation, intron variation, and level of expression.

HLA A*05:02:01:02L

HLA A- Gene or locus

(*)The asterisk represents molecular typing

(05)- Antigen; First two digit describes serologically defined antigen family (HLA-A05)

(02)- Allele; Second set of two digits describes specific amino acid coding difference that distinguishes the A*0502 sequence from other alleles within the A05 family

(01)- The third set of two digits defines synonymous (silent) substitutions in exon

(02)- The last set of two digits designates substitutions located in 3'/5' untranslated regions or introns

(L)- refers to the level of expression of the molecule, here L refers to low expression molecule

In class II genes, as both α and β chains are variable, the gene/locus must include polypeptide chains of the allele. E.g., HLA DRB1*01:01; where β1 is polypeptide chain (B1).

- LOW RESOLUTION: The lowest level specifies the HLA determinant equivalent to its serologic typing specificity or at the allele group level, for example, A*02 for A2.
- INTERMEDIATE RESOLUTION: The next step up in the level of information is usually termed "intermediate"; this refers to using DNA-based methods that can narrow down to a subset of alleles or the list of possible alleles to a few choices. For example, a sample that types as HLA-A*02 could be further characterized as encoding either A*0201 or 0205 or 0209, etc., but lacks sufficient sequence information to permit the allele to be definitively typed
- HIGH RESOLUTION: Finally, if the complete nucleotide sequence is ascertained, this level of typing is called "high resolution"; the complete allele is defined, or samples typed to the allele level and, as in the A*02 examples, would have a minimum of four digits (A*0201)

Linkage Disequilibrium

- Linkage disequilibrium, or LD, is a mathematical measurement of the "randomness" of observing two or more genetic markers together and the extent to which their co-occurrence differs from their individual frequencies within a population.
- The LD across the MHC is characterized as "long-range" (over many thousands to millions of base pairs of sequence) and "high" (two markers observed at a significantly higher frequency than would be predicted by chance alone based on their individual frequencies in the population).
- Practically, LD means that there are fewer unique combinations of HLA antigens/alleles than what would be predicted from the hundreds of known HLA alleles. A well-known example of HLA markers that exhibit strong positive LD is the HLA- A1, -B8, and -DR3 antigens. A Caucasian individual who types as A1 and B8 have a high probability of typing as DR3; A1,

B8, and DR3 are said to be in strong LD (and define a classical extended HLA haplotype, as described below).

- LD takes on significant clinical meaning when a search for potential unrelated donors is undertaken. The strong positive LD between HLA-B and -C and between HLA-DR and -DQ means that a patient and donor who are matched for HLA-A, -B, and -DR will also be matched for HLA-C and -DQ. By the same mechanism, when a patient and donor are mismatched at HLA-B or HLA-DR, they are also more likely to be mismatched at HLA-C or HLA-DQ, respectively.

Haplotypes

- HLA haplotypes are the physical linkage of two or more HLA alleles/ antigens on the same chromosome 6 strands.
- The assignment of HLA haplotypes to an individual can only be performed by typing relevant family members.
- The probability that a patient and sibling inherit the same two parental haplotypes is 25% (HLA genotypically identical) (Sibling 5 with 3). The probability that a patient and sibling inherit one identical paternal or maternal haplotype and one nonidentical (nonshared) haplotype is 50% (haploidentical) (Sibling 5 with 1, 2). The probability that a patient and sibling inherited neither shared parental haplotype is 25% (Sibling 5 with 4).

Father: A1 B7 C4 (a)   Mother: A2 B8 C5 (c)

    A10 B33 C7 (b)   A33 B40 C8 (d)

Sibling1: A1 B7 C4 (a)   Sibling2: A10 B33 C7 (b)

    A33 B40 C8 (d)   A2 B8 C5 (c)

Sibling3: A1 B7 C4 (a)   Sibling4: A10 B33 C7 (b)

    A2 B8 C5 (c)   A33 B40 C8 (d)

Sibling5(Patient): A1 B 7 C4 (a)

      A2 B8 C5 (c)

Methods of HLA Typing

SEROLOGICAL TECHNIQUE

- A broad antigen is a specificity defined by antisera reacting with an epitope common to several related HLA subtypes or splits of original specificities. E.g., B15 broad specificity with splits B62 and B63
- Complement-dependent cytotoxicity (CDC) technique has been commonly used to detect HLA antibodies.

  - Test performed by addition of well-characterized antisera of particular gene pre-poured onto Terasaki plates (60 or 72 well) and frozen at -40°C or -70°C.
  - The target cells used in the CDC assay are usually peripheral blood lymphocytes (PBLs), which can be isolated from anticoagulated whole blood by density gradient centrifugation. Patient lymphocytes to be typed are added to antisera in these plates.
  - During incubation, antibodies in antisera will bind to HLA antigens on lymphocytes and form an antigen/antibody complex.
  - The formation of the complex is detected by adding rabbit serum as a source of complement.
  - If the antigen/antibody complex is present, activation of the classical complement pathway causes the formation of lytic complement unit C7,8,9 resulting in the lysis of target cells. When no antigen/antibody complex occurs, the complement is not activated, and thus cell lysis does not occur.
  - The reactions are then fixed, stained, and read through the underside of the Terasaki tray.
  - Whether alive or dead, lymphocytes can be assessed by morphology under a phase contrast microscope or stained with eosin or trypan blue, where dead cells take up these stains through the damaged cell membrane. Using fluorescent stains such as acridine orange or ethidium bromide binds to the DNA of damaged cells and emits fluorescence.
  - Cell death is recorded as a positive reaction, and the pattern of these reactions is interpreted to assign an HLA phenotype. The scoring methods commonly used to record the percentage of dead cells

0 or blank	=	Negative
1	=	10 to 20%
2	=	20 to 40% Doubtful positive
4	=	40 to 60% Weak positive
6	=	60 to 80% Positive
8	=	80 to 100% Strong positive
X	=	Not tested or unreadable

- The major limitations of the CDC technique are that it cannot differentiate between HLA and non-HLA cytotoxic antibodies.

- Similarly, ELISA and other solid phase-based assays have been developed to perform serological typing.
- Flow cytometry techniques are used primarily to perform cross-matches before solid organ transplantation.

Molecular Techniques

The polymerase chain reaction (PCR) technique is used to amplify specific genes or DNA to identify HLA polymorphism. Molecular techniques include PCR-SSP (sequence-specific priming), PCR-SSOP (sequence-specific oligonucleotide probing) and DNA sequencing-based typing (SBT).

SSP

- Used for either low-resolution typing (Antigen level) or high-resolution (allele level typing)
- Primers are designed to a specific sequence complementary to particular HLA allele sequences in Class I and II genes (Eg: primer should differentiate HLA*03 from other alleles). The polymorphism to be detected is at the 3' end of the primer, and hence an exact match is required in order to allow the synthesis of a new strand of DNA
- The system relies on the lack of 5' to 3' exonuclease activity of Taq DNA polymerase, used in the PCR reaction.
- Using this enzyme, PCR amplification only occurs if alleles with sequences identical to those of the PCR primers used are present in the sample to be tested.
- At least 96 reactions are typically required to define HLA-A, -B, and -DRB1 alleles present at the lowest resolution. For HLA −A, B and C typing, most primer sets detect polymorphism in exons 2 and 3 of Class I genes, as these regions cover most polymorphisms. For HLA-DR, DQ and DP genes, the primer sets cover exon 2 polymorphisms, where most known sequence variations occur.
- Amplified PCR products are detected by electrophoresing the products through agarose gel containing dye such as ethidium bromide, which binds to DNA. Results are interpreted by comparing these reaction patterns either manually or with the aid of a computerized software package designed specifically for each test.
- One disadvantage of PCR-SSP is that it remains a comparatively expensive technique, consuming relatively large quantities of primers and DNA polymerase and using relatively large amounts of DNA. Typing multiple samples for HLA could also be considered a rather time-consuming procedure.

SSP result interpretation from electrophoresis: The table shows the amplification of the control gene and reactions of the patient sample for HLA A genes. The control band is present in all the lanes, and the patient's band is observed in lanes 2 and 5. The corresponding HLA allele amplicon is shown at the bottom. In this example, the possible typing of the patient is HLA*A-03, 06

Table 1: Interpretation of Sequence-specific primer technique. In the given example, the specific primers for HLA A are added to respective wells. The patient sample is compared with the control for the presence of amplification.

	Well Number											
	1	2	3	4	5	6	7	8	9	10	11	12
Control	+	+	+	+	+	+	+	+	+	+	+	+
Patient sample	-	+	-	-	+	-	-	-	-	-	-	-
HLA*A allele amplicon	01	03	04	05	06	07	08	09	10	11	12	13

SSOP:

- The technique involves the amplification of a particular HLA gene locus, e.g., HLA A or B.
- Primers are selected to amplify all known alleles of the particular HLA locus in one PCR tube.
- As discussed earlier, for HLA Class I typing, exons 2 and 3 are co-amplified as one PCR product, while for HLA Class II typing, only exon 2 is amplified. Denature PCR products to produce single-stranded amplicons
- Single-stranded PCR amplicons can hybridize with target DNA with sequence-specific oligonucleotide probes (SSOPs), which are short (15 to 21) nucleotide sequences based on the available library of HLA alleles.
- In conventional SSOP- the PCR products are membrane-bound (Eg: Nylon membrane), and the oligonucleotide probes are in a hybridization solution labelled with markers (Eg: Biotin).
- Reverse PCR-SSO methods involve immobilising oligonucleotide probes on solid phase support and hybridising the solid phase immobilized probes with liquid phase PCR products.
- Depending on the number of probes, such oligonucleotide-based approaches may define not only the broad antigen equivalent of an allele but also unique substitutions that permit definition to an intermediate (groups of alleles that share certain substitutions) or high level of resolution (the unique sequence that distinguishes one allele from another allele).
- A chemiluminescent or colourimetric reaction is used to reveal the presence of bound oligonucleotide probes.
- The pattern of positive and negative reactions are compared with the reaction pattern of known alleles and are interpreted to give HLA type with specific software
- Luminex technology uses a reverse SSO system – where polystyrene microspheres are dyed internally with red and infrared fluorophores to make 100 unique microspheres. Each microsphere is coated with different oligonucleotide probes. Test DNA is amplified and hybridized to bead sets in a PCR plate with one sample tested /well. Non-hybridized DNA is removed by washing, amplified DNA bound to microspheres is detected by fluorescent dye using flow cytometry.
- SSO is used for large sample numbers

SBT

- The gold standard for defining the complete HLA allele (high-resolution typing) is sequencing-based typing (SBT), in which each nucleotide, both invariant and variant, are genotyped.
- SBT is carried out using the PCR product as the template. The PCR amplifies a specific region of the gene/locus of interest, sequenced from both directions to generate a high-quality DNA sequence.
- Fluoroscence-based cycle sequencing requires a DNA template, sequencing primer, DNA polymerase, nucleotides (dNTPs) and dideoxynucleotides (ddNTPs). ddNTPs are labelled with one of the four specific fluorescent dyes for each nucleotide for terminating the extension.
- Thermal cycling of reactions creates and amplifies a range of extension products terminated when one of the four fluorescently labelled ddNTPs is incorporated. Each dye emits a unique wavelength when the laser is excited, and fluorescent dye on the extension product identifies 3' terminal ddNTP as A, C, G or T.
- Either Polyacrylamide gel is poured between two glass plates, or presently capillary electrophoresis is used to separate DNA sequencing products. During capillary electrophoresis, extension products of sequencing reactions enter the capillary via electrokinetic injection. Products are separated based on their total charge or size. As fragments reach the positive electrode, they pass through the laser beam path, which causes the light to be fluorescent.
- Optical detectors capture light signals, convert them to digital data, and examine them using software to align the sequences.
- The final sequences are compared with the known reference library to determine the allele combination present.
- Because SBT defines every nucleotide position, and SSOP- based methods target only those known polymorphic positions, novel alleles would escape detection and be erroneously typed in SSOP-based methods.

Table 2: HLA Typing nomenclature and Molecular methods

	Example	PCR-SSP	PCR-SSO	SBT
Low	A1, A5 or A*01, A05	Yes	Yes	Yes#
Intermediate	A*0101/0102/0104 A*0501/0502/0505	Yes	Yes	Yes#
High	A*0101 A*0501	Yes (Subtyping method)	Yes (Occasionally)	Yes

When full interpretation is not performed

G groups: Grouping alleles according to their nucleotide sequence identity in exons 2 and 3 of Class I HLA genes and exon 2 of class II HLA genes

P groups: Grouping alleles according to their amino acid sequence identity in exons 2 and 3 of Class I HLA genes and exon 2 of class II HLA genes

Hematopoietic Stem Cell Transplantation

- The principles of hematopoietic stem cell transplantation (HSCT) are the engraftment of the donor immune system into the recipient and the development of recipient tolerance towards the new immune system.
- During development, an individual's immune system develops a tolerance to self-Class I and II HLA types and is not tolerant towards HLA types in other individuals.
- There will be a brisk alloreactive immune response for receiving hematopoietic stem cells from one individual. A precise HLA typing of the donor and recipient is essential to reduce or attenuate the recipient's immune system recognition towards the graft.

Vector of Incompatibility

- Directionality or vector of HLA mismatching between the donor and recipient has clinical implications for graft failure and acute GVHD.
- Host-vs-graft (HVG): HVG vector mismatch is an HLA mismatch in which the donor (graft) antigens or alleles are not shared by the recipient (host); in this situation, residual recipient alloreactive T cells recognize the incoming donor graft as different and mount a host-anti donor response that leads to graft failure. E.g., donor alleles not present in the recipient. Recipient: HLA-B7,7; Donor: HLA-B7,8.
- Graft-vs-host (GVH): The GVH vector is in the opposite direction; in this situation, it is the presence of recipient antigens or alleles not shared by the donor that provokes donor (graft)-antihost(recipient) allorecognition, leading to GVHD. E.g., recipient alleles not present in the donor. Recipient: HLA-B7,8 Donor: HLA-B8,8
- When the donor or the recipient is homozygous at the mismatched locus, there is only one vector of incompatibility. When both the donor and the recipient are heterozygous and mismatched, then the mismatch is termed bidirectional

Best Match

A close match ensures that the patient's immune system will recognize donated cells as its own.

Match	Allele	Source
12/12	A, B, C, DRB1, DQB1, DPB1	PBSC or BM
10/10	A, B, C, DRB1, DQB1	PBSC or BM
9/10	A, B, C, DRB1, DQB1 Single Antigen/Allele mismatch	PBSC or BM
8/10	A, B, C, DRB1, DQB1 Two Antigen/Allele mismatch	PBSC or BM
8/8	A, B, C, DRB1	PBSC or BM
6/6	A, B, DRB1	Umbilical Cord Blood

Donor Selection

- Allogeneic hematopoietic stem cell transplantation (HSCT) is potentially curative for many hematologic malignancies and/or marrow failure syndromes. However, one limitation to success is identifying an adequate stem cell donor. The primary determinant of an appropriate donor is based on HLA matching.

Patient and Donor testing

- The search for a matched donor starts within a patient family with minimum HLA- A, B and DRB1 typing in low resolution.
- For selecting unrelated donors, the marrow registries require high-resolution or allele-level typing of the patient at HLA-A, B, C, DRB1 and DQB1

Related Donors

- An HLA-identical sibling remains the donor of choice for several reasons, including decreased risks of acute graft-vs-host disease (GVHD), ready availability, and a general willingness to provide additional cells if needed.
- Based on simple Mendelian genetics and current family size, less than 30% of patients will have an HLA-identical sibling donor.
- Optimal donors are 10/10 at A, B, C, DRB1, DQB1 or 6/6 matched at A, B, DRB1 subjected to extended typing
- 25% chance that two siblings inherit the same HLA phenotypes

Selection of Unrelated Donor

- When suitable family members are not available to serve as donors, then a search for a suitable unrelated donor through the worldwide network of donor registries provides a curative option

Mismatch Antigens

As the number of HLA mismatches increases, risks of graft failure, GVHD, and mortality increase. Each HLA mismatch may lower survival by 10% to 11%. The total number of HLA mismatches has additive effects

1. The risks associated with HLA mismatching are not the same for each HLA locus
2. The risks associated with HLA mismatching may be defined by the qualitative differences in the position of the mismatch within the HLA molecule and the specific amino acid substitutions
3. The similarity between the recipient and donor for extended HLA haplotypes defines the outcome

> - When only mismatched donors were available from unrelated donor searches, criteria for choosing the least risky or best-matched donors are essential.
> - Evidence from European ethnicity showed that in single-locus mismatched patients, DQB1 mismatches appear to be well tolerated compared to others
> - Mismatches in HLA A, B or C, have been shown to increase the risks of acute GVHD
> - Mismatches in A or C, or DRB1 increase the transplant-related mortality (TRM)
> - Due to strong linkage disequilibrium, where donors are mismatched for HLA-B, the matching status of HLA-C should be ensured (such that there are no B+C mismatches). Similarly, when donors are mismatched for DRB1, it is also essential to ensure HLA-DQB1 match status.

> Allele mismatches may be as detrimental as antigen mismatches, from a practical standpoint, when an unrelated donor search yields only HLA-mismatched donors, selecting an allele-mismatched donor over an antigen-mismatched donor may be considered, especially for HLA-C.

- Allele mismatch = Antigen mismatch at HLA - A and HLA -B loci
- Allele mismatch is preferred over Antigen mismatch at HLA C
- Antigen mismatch is not allowed at DRB1 loci
- Disparity preference (PBSC): DQB1 > A > B > C > DRB1

- Evidence showed a higher risk of graft failure and GVHD when the donor-recipient is mismatched at the HLA-DP gene

HLA-Mismatched Related Donor

- When no HLA-matched sibling is available, transplantation from HLA-mismatched haploidentical-related donors is an option for many patients.
- Noninherited maternal antigens (NIMAs) are the HLA antigens of the nonshared haplotype.
- From the haploidentical transplant data, experience suggests the importance of sharing maternal haplotypes between donors and recipients.
- Retrospective clinical studies have demonstrated a lower risk of both acute and chronic GVHD after transplantation from mother to child
- These observations provide a strong rationale that donor-specific suppression of T-cell responses against NIMAs is tolerizing.
- A higher risk of GVHD after transplantation from a father to a child suggests the immunizing effect of paternal antigens.
- Hence preferential selection of family members inheriting haplotypes encoding NIMAs.

Unrelated Matched Donor Process

- A formal unrelated donor search defines specific donors, their high-resolution match status, and their health status.
- Donors whose "registry level" typing suggests that they might be a good candidate for a patient are provided detailed information by their registry regarding the search and donation process and undergo a medical history.
- Donors who consent to proceed with further evaluation then undergo "confirmatory typing", in which a high-resolution definition of HLA-A, -B, -C, -DRB1, and -DQB1 is performed to ascertain the match grade.
- Suppose the confirmatory typing suggests the donor be of an appropriate match grade for the recipient. In that case, the donor is approached for a "workup," which includes a detailed information session with counselling, a medical examination, and screening for infectious disease markers.

Cord Blood

- Currently, UCB units are selected based on three loci—HLA-A and -B at low resolution and -DRB1 at high resolution (six total determinants).

- NMDP recommends a minimum of 4/6 match for HLA-A and -B antigen and -DRB1 allele to release a UCB unit for HSCT.
- Published studies have observed that survival worsens with HLA mismatch, although the degree of mismatch (1 vs 2antigen mismatch) does not matter. In contrast, data published by Gluckman et al. found no impact of HLA incompatibility at year 3 for overall survival despite higher transplant-related morbidity and lower engraftment with increasing HLA mismatch
- Cell dose has been the limiting criterion for adult recipients, and a larger cell dose may overcome the adverse effects of greater HLA mismatch. Low cell dose per kilogram recipient body weight correlates with a slower rate of engraftment, lower probability of achieving engraftment, and lower overall survival.
- Transplant centres that consider double UCB units have selection criteria that consider both the nucleated cell dose of each unit, the total cell dose(^{3}2.0 × 107 TNCs/kg) and the match-grade of each unit relative to the recipient.

Donor Factors Other than HLA

Table 3 shows additional donor factors that may increase GVHD, including

- Nulliparous female donors increased the incidence of chronic GVHD in male recipients
- Parous females increased the risk of chronic GVHD in recipients of either gender
- Chronic GVHD increases in CMV-positive donors for a CMV-negative recipient
- Previously transfused donors and
- Older donors.

Table 3: NMDP investigated donor and recipient age, race, gender, CMV serostatus, and ABO compatibility, as well as recipient disease status and donor parity on unrelated HSCT outcomes (engraftment, acute GVHD, chronic GVHD, relapse, and survival).

	Engraftment	Acute GVHD	Chronic GVHD	Relapse	Survival
Donor Age	+/-	Older donor age, along with HLA mismatch, increased risks of Grade III/IV acute GVHD	Elderly donors have an increased risk	+/-	Overall survival worsened when the donor was older
Race	+/-	+/-	+/-	+/-	+/-
Gender			Lower risk when the donor is male or nulliparous female		

CMV Serostatus	+/-		Lower risk when recipient CMV seroneg and donor CMV seroneg	+/-	+/-
ABO Compatibility	+/-	+/-	+/-	+/-	+/-

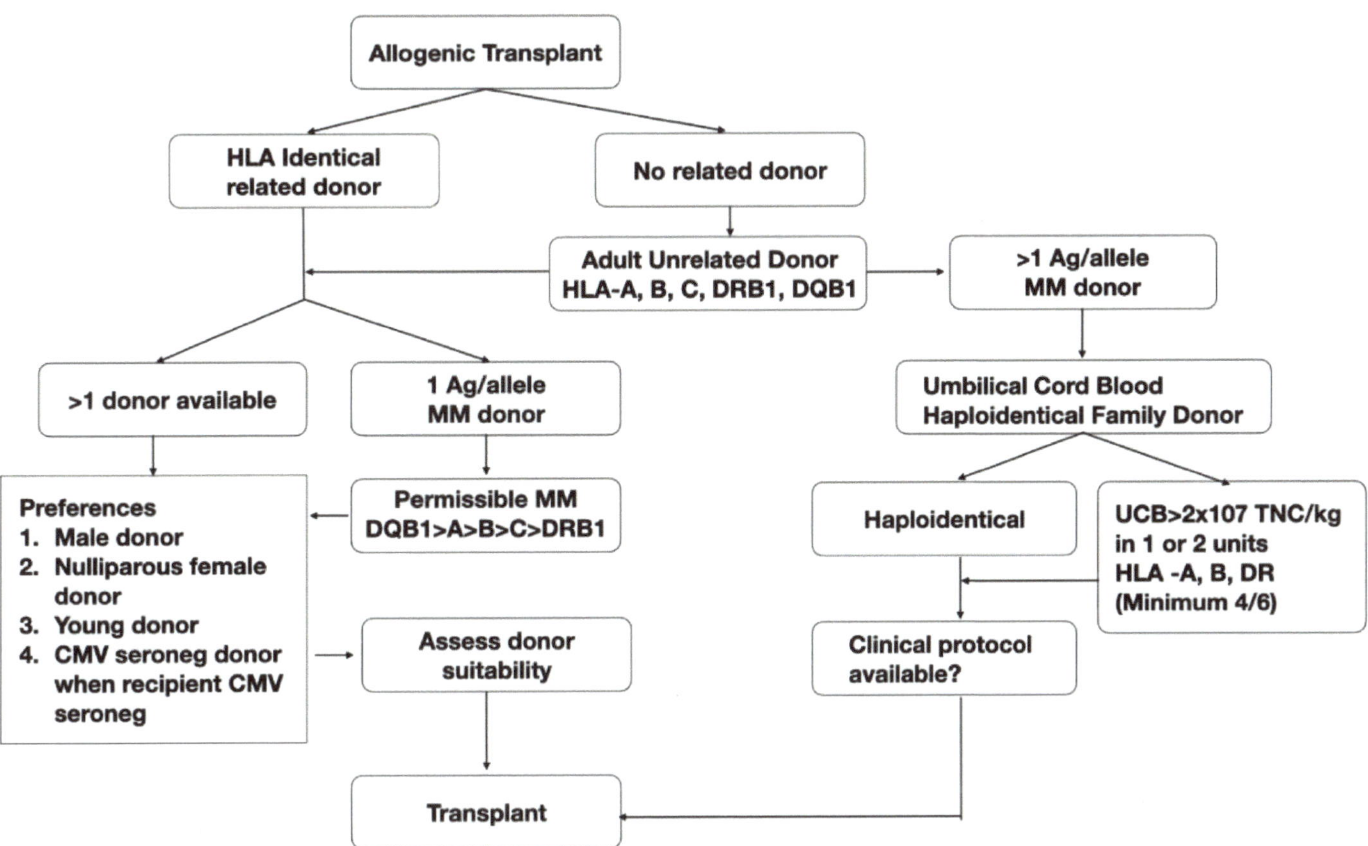

MM – Mismatch; CMV- Cytomegalovirus; UCB- Umbilical cord blood

Figure 1: Algorithm for selecting stem cell donors in an allogeneic transplant.

Example of HLA typing within a family to identify the matched related donor for the patient. Sibling 1 is a syngenic donor (twin), and sibling 4 is HLA identical donor. Gale RP et al. observed in ALL and AML that the relapse rate after syngeneic (twin) stem cell transplantation was 36 and 52% compared to 26 and 16% after HLA-identical transplantation. In other haematological diseases, syngeneic (twin) transplantation had lower non-relapse mortality than HLA identical transplantation. Sibling 4 is considered a perfect match for patients with haematological malignancies, while sibling 1 will be a preferred donor for patients with benign haematological disorders.

	Mother 32 years		Father 42 years	
	a	b	c	d
HLA-A	24:02	24:02	68:01	68:01
HLA-B	44:03	35:01	15:02	51:01
HLA-C	07:01	04:01	07:04	15:02
HLA-DRB1	07:01	11:01	12:02	15:01
HLA-DQB1	02:02	03:01	03:01	05:02

	Patient - 9 years Male		Sibling 1 -9year Male		Sibling 2 -14 year Female	
	a	c	a	c	b	c
HLA-A	24:02	68:01	24:02	68:01	24:02	68:01
HLA-B	44:03	15:02	44:03	15:02	35:01	15:02
HLA-C	07:01	07:04	07:01	07:04	04:01	07:04
HLA-DRB1	07:01	12:02	07:01	12:02	11:01	12:02
HLA-DQB1	02:02	03:01	02:02	03:01	03:01	03:01

	Sibling3 - 10 year Male		Sibling 4 -11 year Female	
	a	d	a	c
HLA-A	24:02	68:01	24:02	68:01
HLA-B	44:03	51:01	44:03	15:02
HLA-C	07:01	15:02	07:01	07:04
HLA-DRB1	07:01	15:01	07:01	12:02
HLA-DQB1	02:02	05:02	02:02	03:01

Solid Organ Transplantation

- Kidney and pancreas transplantation: In recipients with no pre-existing HLA antibodies and ABO compatibility with the donor, matching for HLA class I and Class II antigens increases the survival of grafted organs
- Early antibody-mediated rejection owing to preformed HLA-specific antibodies is considered a risk factor. Recipients need to be screened pretransplant for the presence or development of HLA-specific antibodies. If sensitization to any HLA specificities is identified, these can be highlighted as "unacceptable antigens" and avoided as mismatches with any potential donor. A prospective CDC crossmatch is also used to identify transplants with the potential for hyper-acute rejection.
- Antibody-mediated rejection due to HLA is seen in HLA-immunized recipients and re-transplantation cases.
- In heart, lung or liver transplantation, usually, ABO compatibility is ensured as it is not possible to select according to the HLA compatibility
- Heart Transplantation: more consideration is required in terms of size matching the donor and recipient. Once this is done, ABO blood group compatibility, age matching, and perhaps Cytomegalovirus (CMV) compatibility has been considered. If a centre has two potential

recipients with equal clinical suitability, there is evidence to support using HLA mismatch, with particular emphasis on HLA-DR, as a supplement to the selection process.

- Lung Transplantation: Donated lungs are allocated on the whole without consideration of HLA compatibility. Only when a potential recipient is sensitized to predefined HLA specificities is the donor HLA type used to determine suitability. HLA mismatches result in acute post-transplant complications such as rejection of long-term graft function and the development of bronchiolitis obliterans syndrome. Yet again, HLA-DR mismatch is commonly recognized as having the most significant influence
- Liver Transplantation: The influence of HLA compatibility in liver transplantation has not yet been determined.

HLA Matched Platelet Transfusion

- Pregnancy and multiple transfusions with leukocyte-containing blood components over time result in high rates of the development of HLA alloimmunization.
- Platelet refractoriness refers to persistent suboptimal increment in platelet count after platelet transfusion
- The primary cause of immune refractoriness to platelet transfusion is alloimmunization to Class I HLA antigens.
- HLA-matched platelet transfusion has become the standard of care for patients with platelet refractoriness in a well-established setting. An HLA-matched product can be requested for patients with 1hr corrected count increment (CCI) of 7.5 or less on at least two ABO-compatible platelet transfusions with HLA antibody-mediated clearance as the suspected cause, regardless of whether HLA antibodies have been detected yet.
- Antibodies to Class I and not class II HLA antigens can significantly affect the recovery and survival of transfused platelets because only class I antigens and not Class II antigens are expressed on the platelet surface. When panel reactive antibody (PRA>30%), the use of HLA is selected, and apheresis platelet is advisable.
- In HLA-matched platelet transfusion, the recipient is screened for HLA antibody with recipient and donor typed for HLA A and B antigens.
- Even if no HLA antibodies are detected, centres consider transfusing HLA- matched platelets to rule out antibodies below the detection limit or interferences with the assay used, which cause false-negative results.
- The quality of the match between recipient and donor for HLA-matched platelet transfusion is explained by Duquesnoy, as shown in Table 4.
- Most matching strategies consider grade **A, BU, and B2U** matches as equivalent according to the Duquesnoy criteria; i.e. all antigens expressed by the donor are identical to the patient, but not all patient antigens have to be expressed by the donor (i.e., the donor may be homozygous).
- Permissive mismatches were introduced to include cross-reactive groups (CREG) (Table 5)
- HLA antigens have private and public epitopes. A public epitope is shared with other HLA antigens, which serologically form a CREG. CREG, in short, describes operationally monospecific HLA antisera that react with 2 or more HLA antigens. Recipient and potential donor matched for public epitopes (CREG level), even when they are mismatched at private epitopes.

- HLA antibodies directed against a public epitope of an HLA antigen may cross-react with the other antigens of the CREG and vice versa.
- It has been further suggested that patients are often non-immunogenic and do not form antibodies against HLA antigens that share public antigens with their own HLA antigens.
- These observations suggest that the selection of platelet donors with antigens in the same CREGs as the antigens in the patient was nearly as successful in supporting alloimmune platelet refractory patients as HLA-identical transfusions.
- Having 1 CREG is considered partially compatible, 2 CREGs as less compatible and one or more mismatches (Non-CREG) is considered incompatible.
- Donors with HLA antigens from the patient's CREGs can be tried, often expanding the number of compatible platelet donors. For donor search, these antigens can be added to the permissible antigens.
- An HLA mismatch is acceptable when the donor antigen is absent in the patient but acceptable according to antibody specificity, epitope matching, cross-reactive groups, the effect of previous transfusions, or any combination of these strategies. In case of insufficient split-matched donors, partially matched products containing one or more HLA antigen mismatches are used.
- The antibody specificity prediction (ASP) method identifies the specificity of HLA antibody, and antigen-negative PLT products are provided based on the antibody specificity
- The HLA Matchmaker software tool has been used to predict HLA compatibility by identifying immunogenic epitopes represented by amino acid triplets (eplets) in antibody-accessible regions of HLA molecules

Table 4: Grading system of Duquesnoy on HLA matched platelet transfusion

Grade	Patient Typing	A1	A10	B7	B12	Compatibility
A	HLA identical – all 4 antigens match	A1	A10	B7	B12	Complete compatible
B1U	3 Ag detected – all identical	A1	A10	B7 (Homozygous)	- (Blank)	Complete compatible
B2U	2 Ag detected – both identical	A1 (Homozygous)	- (Blank)	B7 (Homozygous)	- (Blank)	Complete compatible
B1X	4 Ag detected – 3 identical and 1 cross-reactive with the recipient	A1	A28 (CREG)	B7	B12	Partial compatible
B2X	4 Ag detected – 2 identical and 2 cross-reactive with the recipient	A1	A28 (CREG)	B7	B40 (CREG)	Less compatible

B2UX	3 Ag detected – 2 identical, one blank, one cross-reactive with the recipient	A1	A28 (CREG)	B7 (Homozygous)	- (Blank)	Partial compatible
C	1 antigen mismatch, out of CREG	A1	A10	B7	B14 (Non-CREG)	Not compatible
D	≥2 Ag mismatches	A1	A2 (Non-CREG)	B7	B14 (Non-CREG)	Not compatible

Table 5: HLA Cross-reactive groups based on Rodey 1994 and Rodey GE. 2nd ed. Durango CO: De Novo; 2000. HLA Beyond Tears

CREG	antigen specificities included
1C	A1, 3, 9 (23, 24), 11, 29, 30, 31, 36, 80
10C	A10 (25, 26, 34, 66), 11, 28 (68, 69), 32, 33, 43, 74
2C	A2, 9 (23, 24), 28 (68, 69), B17 (57, 58)
5C	B5 (51, 52), 15 (62, 63, 75, 76, 77), 17 (57, 58), 18, 21 (49, 50), 35, 46, 53, 70 (71, 72), 73, 78
7C	B7, 8, 13, 22 (54, 55, 56), 27, 40 (60, 61), 41, 42, 47, 48, 59, 67, 81, 82
8C	B8, 14 (64, 65), 16 (38, 39), 18, 59, 67
12C	B12 (44, 45), 13, 21 (49, 50), 37, 40 (60, 61), 41, 47
Bw4	A23, 24, 25, 32, B13, 27, 37, 38, 44, 47, 49, 51, 52, 53, 57, 58, 59, 63, 77
Bw6	B7, 8, 18, 35, 39, 41, 42, 45, 46, 48, 50, 54, 55, 56, 60, 61, 62, 64, 65, 67, 71, 72, 73, 75, 76, 78, 81, 82

- Krueger AJ et al. compared 1hr CCIs after HLA-matched transfusions with 1hr CCIs after transfusions containing at least one HLA antigen mismatch. The 1hr CCI after an HLA-matched transfusion was 1.94 times (CI 0.74-3.15) higher than 1hr CCI after HLA-mismatched transfusions. In patients with negative HLA antibody screening tests, HLA matching did not affect 1hr CCIs. Moreover, they concluded that there is no indication of HLA-matched platelets in patients with negative antibody screens.
- A systematic review by Pavenski et al. examined the effects of HLA-matched PLT transfusion in patients with hypoproliferative thrombocytopenia. HLA-matched platelets had higher 1-hour post-transfusion count increments compared to RDP in refractory patients. The responses to HLA-matched PLTs are better in those with evidence of alloimmune refractoriness and those receiving closer HLA-matched, antigen-negative products. However, the significance of post-transfusion count increment with clinical outcomes (bleeding episodes, alloimmunization rates, refractoriness rates, post-transfusion count increment and the number of platelet units transfused) could not be determined.

- HLA matches were associated with better increments, and the degree of antigen mismatch was not associated with CCI, but CCI was associated with the number of antigens shared. HLA-matched PLTs appeared to produce better transfusion outcomes in patients with alloimmune refractoriness

Disadvantages

1. Providing HLA-matched PLTs is a costly and time and labour-intensive process
2. A vast pool of dedicated and HLA-typed platelet donors required

Alternatives

- Accepting donors with permissible mismatches based on patients' antibody reactivity patterns may be an alternative approach that may increase the donor pool.

Approach to the Laboratory Diagnosis of Thalassemia and Other Hemoglobinopathies

– Dr. Sujaya, Dr. Prabhu

Introduction:

The haemoglobin (Hb) molecule is a large tetramer composed of four polypeptide subunits. Each of these subunits contains a heme group and a globin chain. There are essentially two main types of globin chains – the alpha type (alpha [α] and zeta [ζ]) located on chromosome 16 and the non-alpha type (epsilon[ε], beta [β], gamma [γ], delta [δ]) located on chromosome 11 (figure 1). The tetramer is composed of two identical alpha chains and two identical non-alpha chains, and the composition of the globin chain determines the type of haemoglobin. Table 1 highlights the normal types of haemoglobin (Hb) according to the various developmental stages, their globin chain components, and their reference intervals.

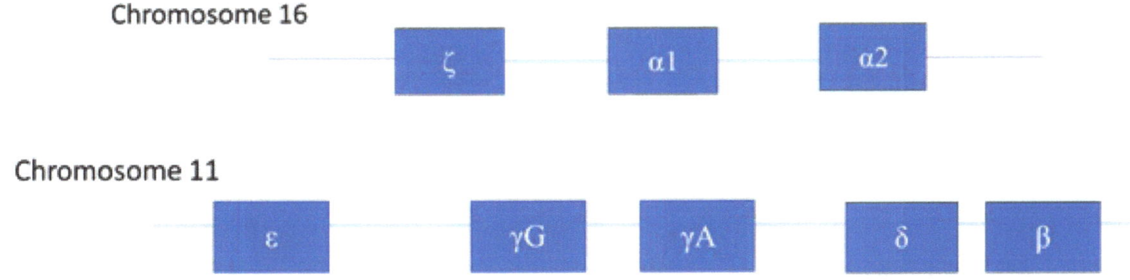

Figure 32 The genes for the globin chains

Table 1: Normal types of haemoglobin according to the developmental stage

Developmental stage	Type	Globin chains	Reference intervals
Embryonic	Gower 1	ζ2ε2	-
	Gower 2	α2ε2	-
	Portland	ζ2γ2	-
Fetal	Hb F	α2γ2	90-95% before birth; 50-80% at birth
	Hb A0	α2β2	10-40% at birth
	Hb A2	α2δ2	<1% at birth

Adult	Hb A	$\alpha2\beta2$	>95%
	Hb A2	$\alpha2\delta2$	1.5-3.5%
	Hb F	$\alpha2\gamma2$	<2%

Definitions:

Thalassemia: A quantitative globin chain abnormality where abnormal Hb results from genetic defects that affect the production and subsequently diminish the synthesis of structurally normal globin chain(s). The thalassemia syndromes are classified according to the affected globin chain. There are two major types, namely α and β-thalassemia. In β-thalassemia, various mutations diminish the synthesis of β-globin chains, whereas in α-thalassemia, inherited deletions that result in the reduced or absent synthesis of α-globin chains. Table 2-4 depicts the common mutations and major clinical phenotypes of α and β-thalassemia. The clinical severity of thalassemia depends on the degree of globin chain imbalance. The age at first presentation, transfusion dependency, ethnicity and clinical presentation determine the clinical phenotype, and they are as follows:

Table 2: Common genetic mutations in thalassemia

Mutation type	Effect on gene	Thalassemia subtype
Deletion	Loss of gene	Predominantly α-thalassemia
Promoter region	Impaired transcription	Predominantly β-thalassemia
Chain terminator region	Frameshift mutation	Predominantly β-thalassemia
	Stop codon	Predominantly β-thalassemia
Splice site region	Creates new splice site	Predominantly β-thalassemia
	Loss of splice sites	Predominantly β-thalassemia

Thalassemia trait/ minor: These cases are usually clinically asymptomatic with mild anaemia that develops during stress like pregnancy or infections.

Thalassemia intermedia: These are a very heterogeneous group of disorders with moderate clinical severity symptoms varying between thalassemia major and minor. The anaemia can intensify during stress like infections or pregnancy, and the patient may require transfusions in such scenarios.

Thalassemia major: These cases present with severe transfusion-dependent anaemia. These cases present within the first year of age. At birth, the Hb F levels are high; hence, the neonate is usually asymptomatic. After three months, the Hb F levels start reducing, and anaemia develops. The child usually manifests with hepatosplenomegaly, bone deformities of the skull and facial bones, and frontal bossing with mild jaundice. Chronic anaemia leads to cardiac failure. Endocrine abnormalities like growth retardation and diabetes mellitus due to iron deposition. The patient can have gallstones due to chronic hemolysis.

All these clinical phenotypes should be correlated with their laboratory findings. The terminologies like heterozygous or homozygous, indicative of their genotypes, are usually used in the laboratory report. In general, heterozygous thalassemia usually correlates clinically with thalassemia trait/ minor in the larger proportion of cases and with thalassemia intermedia in a smaller proportion. On the other hand, homozygous thalassemia correlates most often clinically with thalassemia major; and with thalassemia intermedia in a smaller proportion of cases.

Table 3: Three major phenotypes of β-thalassemia

Phenotype	Zygosity	Genotype	Clinical Severity
β-thalassemia major	Homozygous	β^0/β^0 and β^+/β^+	Severe
	Double heterozygous	β^0/β^+	Severe
β-thalassemia intermedia	Homozygous	β^+/β^+	Moderate
	Double heterozygous	β^0/β^+	Moderate
	Heterozygous	β^0/β	Moderate
β-thalassemia trait/ minor	Heterozygous	β^0/β or β^+/β	Mild

Table 4: Four major phenotypes of α-thalassemia

Phenotype	Zygosity	Genotype	Clinical Severity
Hydrops fetalis	Homozygous α-thalassemia	$(--/--)$ α^0/α^0	Fatal
Hb H disease	Heterozygous α-thalassemia	$(--/-\alpha)$ $\alpha^0/\alpha+$	Moderate
α-thalassemia trait/ minor	Heterozygous α-thalassemia/ Homozygous α-thalassemia	$(--/\alpha\alpha)/ (-\alpha/-\alpha)$ α^0/α or $\alpha+/\alpha+$	Mild
Silent carrier	Heterozygous α-thalassemia	$(-\alpha/\alpha\alpha)$ $\alpha+/\alpha$	Normal

Structural hemoglobinopathies: A qualitative abnormality where the mutations alter the amino acid sequences of the globin chain, altering the physiological properties of the variant Hb such as altered solubility or abnormal polymerization, thereby altering their function, as seen in Hb S.

Sickle cell trait (SCT): This terminology indicates heterozygosity for the sickle cell gene ($\beta \beta^s$).

Sickle cell anaemia (SCA): This terminology indicates homozygosity for the sickle cell gene ($\beta^s \beta^s$).

Sickle cell disease (SCD): This is a broad entity which includes all patients with clinical evidence of sickling, where a combination of sickle cell mutation and a second β-globin/ other mutation co-exists. This is referred to as the compound heterozygous state.

Thalassemic hemoglobinopathies: This group of disorder show both the features of reduced synthesis of the globin chain as well as the altered function of the Hb molecule. The classic example is Hb E.

Ethnicity:

Thomas Cooley described the first case of thalassemia in 1925 in Detroit and called it Cooley's anaemia. The term thalassemia came from the Greek word *Thalassa* which means "sea", as it was found to have originated in the Mediterranean region. The thalassemia belt extends from the

Mediterranean region through the Middle East, tropical Africa, the Indian subcontinent, and Asia and it is now recognized as one of the most common genetic disorders affecting the world's population. In India, β-thalassemia is found throughout the country, with a higher incidence in Sindhis, Punjabis, Bengalis, Gujaratis, Parsis, and Lohanas. Approximately 1–5% of people are carriers of β-thalassemia. It is estimated that around 1,00,000 and 2,00,000 individuals worldwide are born each year with severe forms of thalassemia and other hemoglobinopathies, and approximately 60,000 of those have β-thalassemia.

There are five haplotypes of HbS described in various parts of the world. Indian-Arab haplotype is the one which is prevalent in our country. SCD are most prevalent in various states in the middle belt of the country, like Gujarat, Maharashtra, Madhya Pradesh and Orissa. While evaluating these patients, the importance of a history of ethnic origin from these states cannot be overemphasized. Hb F can reach up to 10-25%, particularly in the Indian-Arab haplotype. This should be kept in mind when diagnosing homozygous Hb S.

In India, the Hb E cases are seen in eastern Bihar, West Bengal, Assam and other northeastern states.

Laboratory diagnosis:

The laboratory approach for most thalassemia and other hemoglobinopathies begins with a basic complete hemogram, peripheral smear examination and reticulocyte count. In particular, if strong clinical suspicion exists based on the patient from the thalassemia/ sickle belt and their ethnic origin, screening test and definitive diagnostic tests like Hb electrophoresis, high-performance liquid chromatography (HPLC), including family studies, a molecular analysis should be done as early as possible. It is always advocated to perform two tests based on the different principles to confirm the disease.

Complete hemogram:

Thalassemia trait/ minor cases are usually picked up incidentally during a complete blood count for unrelated symptoms. The Hb level is often normal to borderline low (usually around 10-12 gm/dl) with reduced mean corpuscular volume (MCV), mean corpuscular haemoglobin (MCH) and mean corpuscular haemoglobin concentration (MCHC) and generally increased red blood cell (RBC) counts (usually >5 million cells/cu.mm). The coefficient of variation of red cell distribution width (RDW-CV), indicative of the degree of anisocytosis, is usually less than 14% which helps us to distinguish it from iron deficiency anaemia (IDA). Nevertheless, the most prevalent and confounding factor is a nutritional deficiency in our country. Always, co-existent IDA should be kept in mind if there is reduced MCV, MCH and MCHC and increased RDW-CV often gives a clue to this diagnosis. The total white blood cell (WBC) count and platelet count are usually within normal limits.

In the case of thalassemia major, the haemoglobin is markedly reduced and can be as low as 2-3 gm/dl. MCV is usually 60-70 fL, and MCH and MCHC are also reduced. RDW-CV can be increased. Secondary folate deficiency and hemolytic crisis, particularly polychromatophils, might increase MCV, MCH and RDW-CV. The WBC count is usually spuriously increased due to nucleated RBCs. Reduced WBC count and platelet count may indicate hypersplenism.

The Hb level is usually normal to low-normal in SCT and trait of other hemoglobinopathies. Similarly, the blood counts tend to be within the normal range at birth, even in homozygous states. As Hb F is gradually replaced by Hb S, disease manifestation usually appears after six months. At the same time, the Hb level gradually decreases and is usually in the 5-12 gm/dl range. Red blood cell (RBC) count is normal in SCT, whereas it is proportionally reduced for the age and sex in SCD.

MCV, MCH, MCHC and RDW-CV are normal in SCT. However, if there is a co-existing double heterozygous state with α/ β thalassemia, Hb D[Punjab], Hb E or hereditary persistence of fetal Hb (HPFH), MCV and MCH are reduced, and RDW-CV is normal. The WBC count is normal in SCT, whereas in SCD, it is almost always increased. This is because granulocytes shift from the marginated pool to the circulating compartment. An increase in nucleated RBCs may also falsely elevate the total WBC count. This occurs in bacterial infections and vaso-occlusive crises. The platelet count is normal in SCT, whereas in SCD, it is increased, reflecting reduced splenic function. The platelet count is reduced during the vaso-occlusive crisis and bone marrow infarction.

In the case of Hb E, both in the homozygous and heterozygous state, patients are generally asymptomatic and transfusion independent and show low normal Hb, reduced MCV, MCH and normal RDW-CV. Total WBC count and platelet count are usually normal.

Peripheral smear (PS) and reticulocyte count:

Examining fresh peripheral blood samples collected in EDTA anticoagulant with a good smear preparation within 2 hr of sample collection, ideal staining technique by Romanowsky stain and PS examination by experienced hematopathologist is warranted.

In thalassemia trait/ minor cases, there are uniformly microcytic hypochromic red cells, a good number of target cells, and minimal anisocytosis (figure 2A). However, one should consider the differential possibilities such as IDA, anaemia of chronic disease, sideroblastic anaemia and lead poisoning. The only major confounding factor is the widespread occurrence of nutritional anaemia such as IDA, in which microcytic hypochromic cells are seen along with pencil cells. These differential possibilities are usually ruled out by a good clinical history and examination along with tests like serum ferritin, serum iron studies, erythrocyte sedimentation rate (ESR), C-reactive protein (CRP), bone marrow morphology with Perls' stain and serum and urinary lead levels wherever indicated.

In thalassemia intermedia and major, PS shows microcytic hypochromic RBCs, target cells, nucleated RBC, basophilic stippling and marked anisopoikilocytosis (figure 2B-D). The PS can also show the presence of nucleated RBCs. Megaloblastic anaemia should be suspected if there is a rapid decline in Hb with pancytopenia due to reduced RBC's half-life. It is important to note that overt macrocytosis may not occur in such cases. Reticulocyte count is also markedly decreased in these cases because of associated ineffective erythropoiesis.

The importance of reticulocyte preparation cannot be overemphasised. Golf ball inclusions (figure 2E) are seen in reticulocyte preparation and can be confirmed by brilliant cresyl blue stain if there is coexistent α-thalassemia (Hb H disease). Roughly 20-40% of cells might show the presence of golf-ball inclusions in Hb H disease and hydrops fetalis.

Quite often, in SCT, PS may be completely normal. The classic sickle cells are not seen, but a small number of plump cells with pointed ends is described in most cases (Figure 2F). The reticulocyte count is normal. The distinct advantage of SCT is that it gives resistance to malaria parasite infection, particularly Plasmodium falciparum, compared to subjects without hemoglobinopathies. Total WBC count and platelet count are within normal limits.

In SCA, PS is usually normal at birth; abnormalities are detectable around six months of age. By one year of age, features of hyposplenism, along with an increasing number of nRBCs, classic sickle cells, and a good number of target cells, Howell-Jolly bodies, start to appear. By adolescence and adulthood, a variable number of crescent or sickle cells ranging from very few to 30-40% is seen. In addition to these irreversibly sickled cells (figure 2G), boat-shaped cells with one or both pointed ends appear. In addition, other features suggestive of hyposplenism, such as acanthocytes, Pappenheimer bodies and occasional linear red cell fragments, are seen. Reticulocyte count appears to increase because of associated polychromasia, but absolute reticulocyte count is always reduced for the degree of anaemia.

The presence of microcytic hypochromic RBC and a good number of target cells, anisocytosis and poikilocytosis, suggest the possibility of a compound heterozygous state such as α/ β-thalassemia, Hb E and HPFH.

Various complications can be picked up from a good PS examination. Parvovirus B19 infection should be suspected if there is a sudden worsening of anaemia with a lack of polychromasia and markedly reduced reticulocyte count (<0.5%). In pulmonary infarction and hypoxia cases, 'hemighost cells' or 'blister cells' appear in the peripheral blood. These cells show Hb retracted to one-half of the cell. In splenic sequestration, there is a sudden drop in Hb and an increase in nRBCs, sickle cells, hemighost cells, platelet count and reticulocyte count. In extensive bone marrow infarction, there is a marked reduction in Hb, total WBC count and platelet count with an increase in the number of nRBCs. Differential WBC count shows neutrophilia, left shift and toxic granulation during infection and vaso-occlusive crisis. Sometimes, pneumococci can be seen inside neutrophils. An increase in lymphocytes, monocytes and platelet count suggests the possibility of hyposplenism.

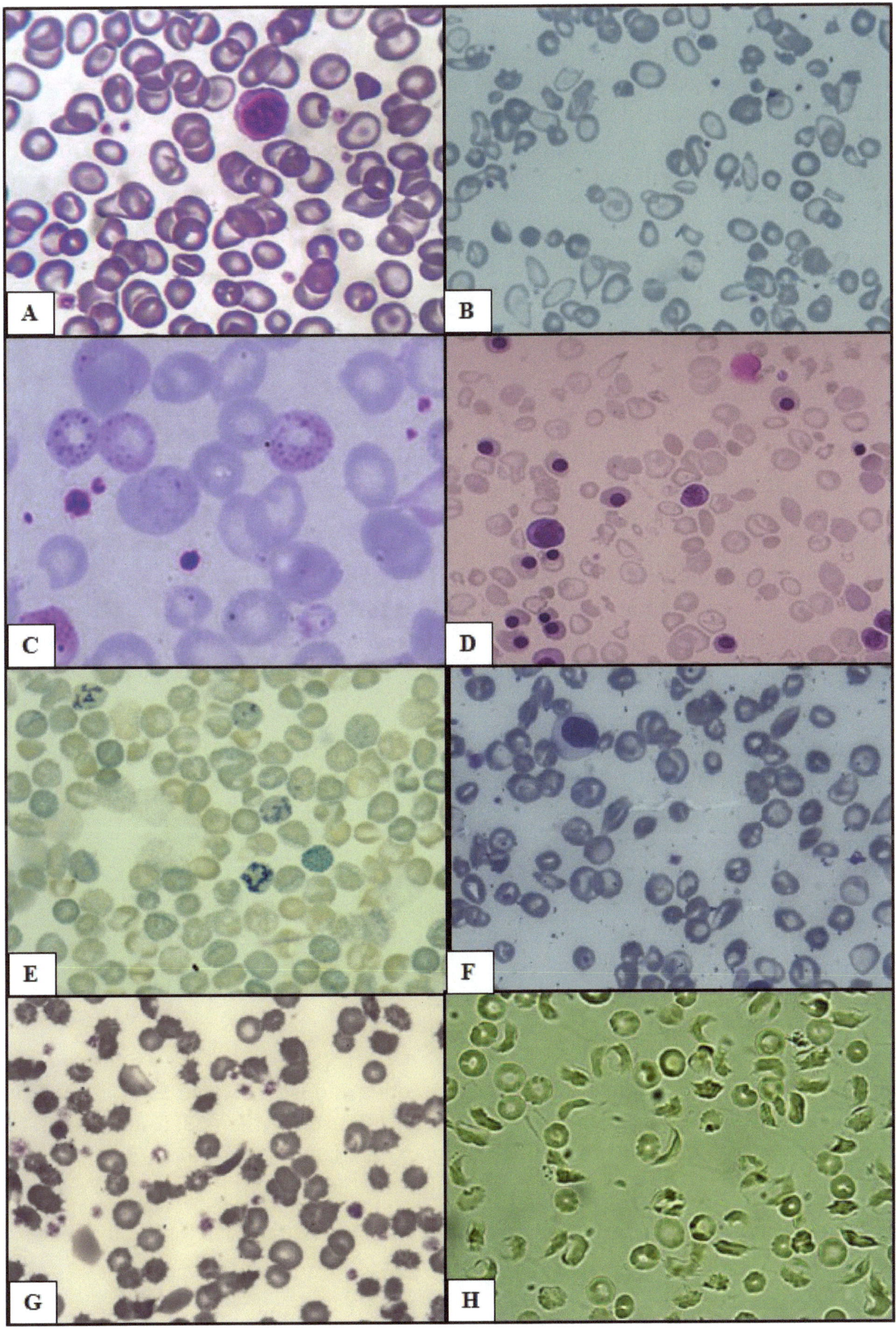

Ancillary investigations:

A liver function test (LFT) shows increased bilirubin, particularly unconjugated bilirubin, in cases of hemoglobinopathies and thalassemia. In cases with hemolysis, serum haptoglobin is usually absent, and lactate dehydrogenase (LDH) is increased. Serum ferritin is increased because of repeated blood transfusion. Ultrasound abdomen is necessary to look for the size of the spleen, infarction in the spleen, kidneys and other organs and calculi in the gall bladder.

Screening tests:

The following screening tests are useful in community field visits and outpatient department services where quick screening of cases is required. However, these are not very specific, so confirmation with other diagnostic tests is required.

NESTROFT:

It stands for 'Naked Eye Single Tube Red cell Osmotic Fragility Test'. It acts as a valuable, cost-effective screening tool and its sensitivity increases if combined with Hb A2.

Principle and procedure:

Normally, red cells suspended in the saline solution would begin to lyse at 0.4-0.5% concentration, and lysis would be complete at 0.3-0.35%. However, in the β-thalassemia trait, their osmotic resistance is altered due to the volume of the surface area of red cells. Therefore lysis might begin at a saline concentration between 0.4-0.5%, but it might not be completed even at a 0.1% solution.

Two test tubes labelled as buffered saline (2ml) and distilled water (2ml) are taken, and a drop of blood is added to each of the tubes, left undisturbed for half an hour at room temperature. Following this, the contents of both tubes are gently shaken and held against a white paper on which a thin black line is drawn.

Interpretation:

If the line is clearly visible through distilled water tube and in the buffered saline tube, it is considered negative. However, in case of a positive test, a clear supernatant and sediment at the bottom of the tube obscure the thin black line in buffered saline.

Discrimination index:

The index most commonly used is called Mentzer's index and is calculated as MCV/RBC count. If the value is less than 13, it indicates a thalassemia trait; if it is more than 13, it is usually IDA. Some other commonly used indices are the Shine-Lal index, England Fraser index, Bessman index and Sehgal index.

Two commonly used screening tests for Hb S are the sickling test and Hb S solubility test.

Sickling test:

Principle and procedure:

Add five drops of the freshly prepared reagent (sodium metabisulphite) to 1 drop of anti-coagulated blood on the slide. Apply the cover glass and seal it with petroleum jelly/ paraffin wax mixture or nail varnish to prevent the contact of environmental oxygen with the blood. Under such low oxygen tension, sodium metabisulphite acts as a reducing agent which induces sickling. Always perform the test with positive and negative controls simultaneously and look for sickling immediately and after incubation at 37°C for 24 hrs.

Interpretation:

If Hb S is present, RBCs lose their normal smooth, round shape and become sickled (Figure 2H). The sickling phenomenon occurs immediately or within 1 hr in cases of homozygotes or compound heterozygotes, whereas this process may occur after 12-24 hr in the case of the Hb S trait.

Hb S solubility test:

Principle:

Hb S is insoluble in deoxygenated state and forms crystals in a high concentration of phosphate buffers. These crystals refract light and turn the solution turbid.

Utility of screening tests:

Irrespective of the screening test results, all the cases must be confirmed by Hb electrophoresis or high-performance liquid chromatography (HPLC) as early as possible.

Disadvantages of screening tests:

1. Does not differentiate heterozygotes, compound heterozygotes or homozygotes.
2. False positive results occur in hyperleukocytosis, hyperlipidemia and paraproteinemia, whereas false negative results occur in lower haemoglobin, infants younger than six months, post-transfusion (Hb S < 20%) and use of outdated reagents.

Diagnostic tests:

The definitive diagnosis of thalassemia and other hemoglobinopathies can be confirmed by tests such as Hb electrophoresis, Hb HPLC, isoelectric focusing, and various molecular techniques.

Haemoglobin (Hb) electrophoresis:

Haemoglobin (Hb) electrophoresis is a commonly used initial test for identifying variant Hb. This technique requires high technical expertise and is labour intensive; hence nowadays being gradually replaced in most centres by automated HPLC.

Principle:

When protein molecules like Hb are applied onto the membrane and exposed to charge gradient, they tend to separate from each other and can be easily visualised using a special stain. In order to overcome the effect of plasma proteins, which tend to interfere with the interpretation of various bands, this test is best performed by using packed red cells, washed several times and red cell lysate prepared using either potassium cyanide or carbon tetrachloride or toluene. Once prepared, it should be used within one week to prevent oxidation.

Procedure:

This Hb electrophoresis can be performed on cellulose acetate at alkaline pH (8.4-8.6) or citrate agar gel at acidic pH (6.0). Agarose gel can be used for both types of electrophoresis. Depending upon the institutional protocol, both types of electrophoresis may be performed simultaneously or alkaline, followed by acid electrophoresis.

The only difference between these two types of electrophoresis is that variant Hb migrates differentially to various positions, depending upon the net charge on that particular Hb. Scanning densitometry is used to quantify different Hb. Hb A2 can also be measured directly by eluting from electrophoresis.

Interpretation of Hb electrophoresis at alkaline pH (8.4-8.6):

The relative differential mobilities of variant Hb are depicted in figure 3A and table 5. Variant Hb can have the same electrophoretic mobility. For example, Hb S and Hb D^{Punjab}, Hb A2 and Hb E cannot be separated by alkaline electrophoresis; hence further investigations are required.

Table 5: Approach to interpretation of alkaline Hb electrophoresis, their differential possibilities and further investigations required to confirm the diagnosis

Finding on cellulose acetate electrophoresis	Possible Hb variant	Further investigation required
Band in 'S' region	Hb S, D, G, Lepore	Sickling test, Hb S solubility test, acidic Hb electrophoresis, Hb HPLC
Band in 'C' region	Hb C, A2, E	Acidic Hb electrophoresis, Hb HPLC/ capillary electrophoresis
Fast moving band	Hb H	Hb H inclusion test

Interpretation of Hb electrophoresis at acidic pH (6.0):

The relative differential mobilities of variant Hb at acidic pH are depicted in figure 3B. Hb S and Hb D^{Punjab} can be differentiated; however, even with this method, Hb A2 and Hb E cannot be separated.

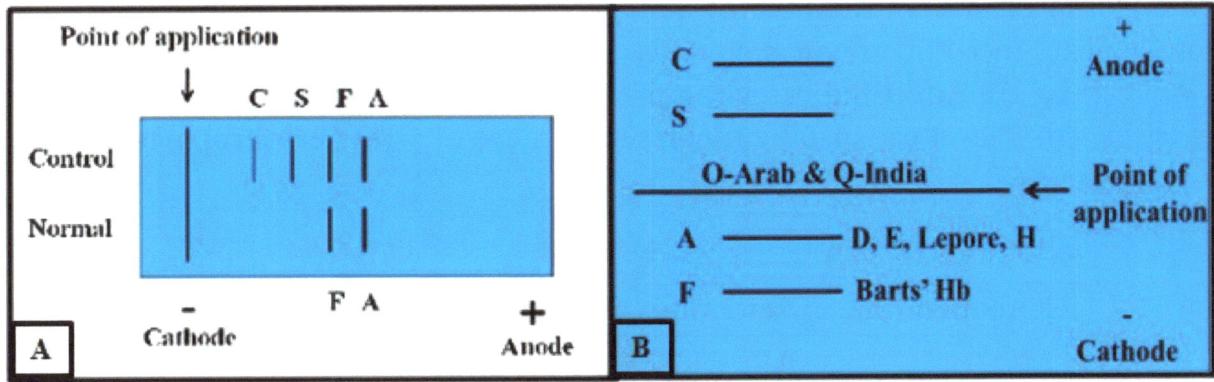

Capillary electrophoresis:

This methodology was recently introduced in India, using small sample sizes, higher voltages, and shorter running times. There are 15 different zones with different separations of Hb A0, Hb A2, Hb F and Hb S. Hb A2 will be accurately and separately quantified in a different zone apart from Hb E. Compound heterozygosity with Hb E, Hb D^{Punjab} and other variants Hb can be accurately diagnosed.

High-performance liquid chromatography (HPLC):

Principle:

It works on exchanging charged groups on the ion exchange material with charged groups on the Hb molecule. The HPLC machine has a narrow column packed with silica gels having a weak cationic charge. This helps in separating Hb variants, and the rate of elution of different Hb depends on the pH and ionic strength of the buffer.

Advantages of HPLC:

1. The test can be performed with a very tiny volume (5 µL) of blood; hence can be done even in newborn babies.
2. It is automated, less labour and time-consuming, and can be performed in batches.
3. Normal as well as variant Hb quantitation is available for all samples.

Normally in Hb HPLC, one will find Hb A0 ($\alpha2\beta2$), Hb A2 ($\alpha2\delta2$) and Hb F ($\alpha2\gamma2$). Hb A0 constitute 96-97%, Hb A2 (2-3.5%) and Hb F (<1%) of the normal Hb. If Hb A2 values range between 4% and 8%, it is indicative of heterozygous β-thalassemia (trait) because, in these cases, the synthesis of the β-globin chain is reduced and compensated by excess synthesis of the δ-globin chain. On the other hand, in the α-thalassemia trait, the synthesis of the α-globin chain is reduced; hence the levels of Hb A2 will be seen as less than 2%. Table 6 shows the retention time of normal and variant Hb in D10 HPLC machine, and figure 4 depicts the pattern in a normal individual, heterozygous β-thalassemia (trait) and α-thalassemia case.

In the case of β-thalassemia major (homozygous state) (figure 5A), the synthesis of normal Hb A0 is markedly reduced such that the levels of Hb A0 are always lesser than that of Hb F. There is marked suppression of β-globin chain synthesis which is compensated by excess synthesis of α and δ-globin chains. In the case of SCT (heterozygous state) (figure 5B), an abnormal S-window appears in HPLC tracings, and the level of Hb S will be less than Hb A0. If Hb S level is more than Hb A0, it indicates the presence of SCA (homozygous state) (figure 5C). In these cases, Hb F level can also be increased because of stress erythropoiesis or treatment with hydroxyurea.

Table 6: Retention times of normal and variant haemoglobins in D10 HPLC

Window	Retention time	Retention time range	Haemoglobins that may overlap
F	1.1	0.98 - 1.22	Okayama
P2	0.11	1.28 - 1.50	Glycosylated A
P3	1.7	1.50 - 1.90	J - Meerut
A	2.5	1.90 - 3.10	A, Glycosylated S
A2	3.6	3.30 - 3.90	A2, E, Lepore, D - Iran
D	4.1	3.90 - 4.30	D - Punjab, G - Philadelphia
S	4.5	4.30 - 4.70	S, D - Agri, A2'

Transfusion-acquired hemoglobinopathies:

This is an unusual presentation that often causes difficulty in interpreting HPLC results. Often, good clinical history, ethnic origin of the patient, the reason for which transfusion was required and repeating the HPLC after 3-4 weeks of the last transfusion are the best possible ways to identify this uncommon entity.

Role of family studies and mode of inheritance:

It is always worthwhile to screen the parents and siblings of the index case. Most thalassemia and other hemoglobinopathies are inherited in the autosomal recessive pattern. Family studies are performed with Hb electrophoresis, HPLC or molecular methods. For example, if one parent has SCA ($\beta^S \beta^S$) and the other parent has SCT ($\beta \beta^S$), there is a 50% chance of the child being born with SCA and a 50% chance of a child being born with SCT. When both parents have SCT ($\beta \beta^S$), a child has a 25% chance (1 in 4) of being born with SCA. Family studies help confirm the compound heterozygous state and screen for transplant eligibility among the family members. It is also vital for those recently transfused to rule out transfusion-acquired sickle cell disorder. One child was diagnosed with compound heterozygous Hb S-β thalassemia, with parents being heterozygous Hb S and heterozygous β-thalassemia (figure 6 A-C).

Molecular diagnosis of thalassemia and other hemoglobinopathies:

Prenatal diagnosis:

It is important to screen a couple as a part of antenatal screening for possible thalassemia traits. Parents with a heterozygous carrier and homozygous state or from high-risk ethnic groups should be offered the option of prenatal diagnosis. For prenatal diagnosis, fetal DNA samples can be obtained either by amniocentesis (at 14-20 weeks of gestation) or chorionic villous biopsy (at 8-12 weeks of gestation) if the fetus is affected, providing the option of medical termination of pregnancy (MTP) to the couples, till 20th week needs to be considered.

A variety of polymerase chain reaction (PCR) based nucleic acid assays can be performed to identify mutations in thalassemia and other hemoglobinopathies. Some tests are allele-specific oligonucleotide hybridization (ASO), dot blot and reverse dot blot assays, amplification refractory mutation system (ARMS), and direct sequencing. Considering the large number of mutations present in the human globin genes, a small panel of probes for mutations found in specific ethnic groups is initially screened. Using this approach, identification of the mutation(s) is/are usually possible. In cases where the mutation(s) are not identified, the second round of multiplex screening can be performed using a panel of rare mutations, which is successful in most of the remaining cases. Gene sequencing can be performed to identify mutations that evade both rounds of screening.

Conclusion:

To conclude, age at first presentation, transfusion dependency, ethnicity and clinical presentation give a clue to diagnosing thalassemia and other hemoglobinopathies. In all these cases, there should be a step-wise approach which starts with evaluating a complete hemogram, good PS examination, and reticulocyte count. There are many differential possibilities for microcytic hypochromic anaemias; serum ferritin, serum iron studies and other ancillary tests should be ordered to rule out these differentials. One should use screening tests judiciously and appropriate diagnostic tests such as Hb electrophoresis, HPLC, or molecular tests. Every attempt should be made to study their family members and provide the option for prenatal diagnosis to at-risk couples to prevent the birth of an affected child. The laboratory plays a great role in early identification and, thus, in preventing this major global health burden. Figure 7 highlights the step-wise laboratory approach to diagnosing thalassemia and other hemoglobinopathies.

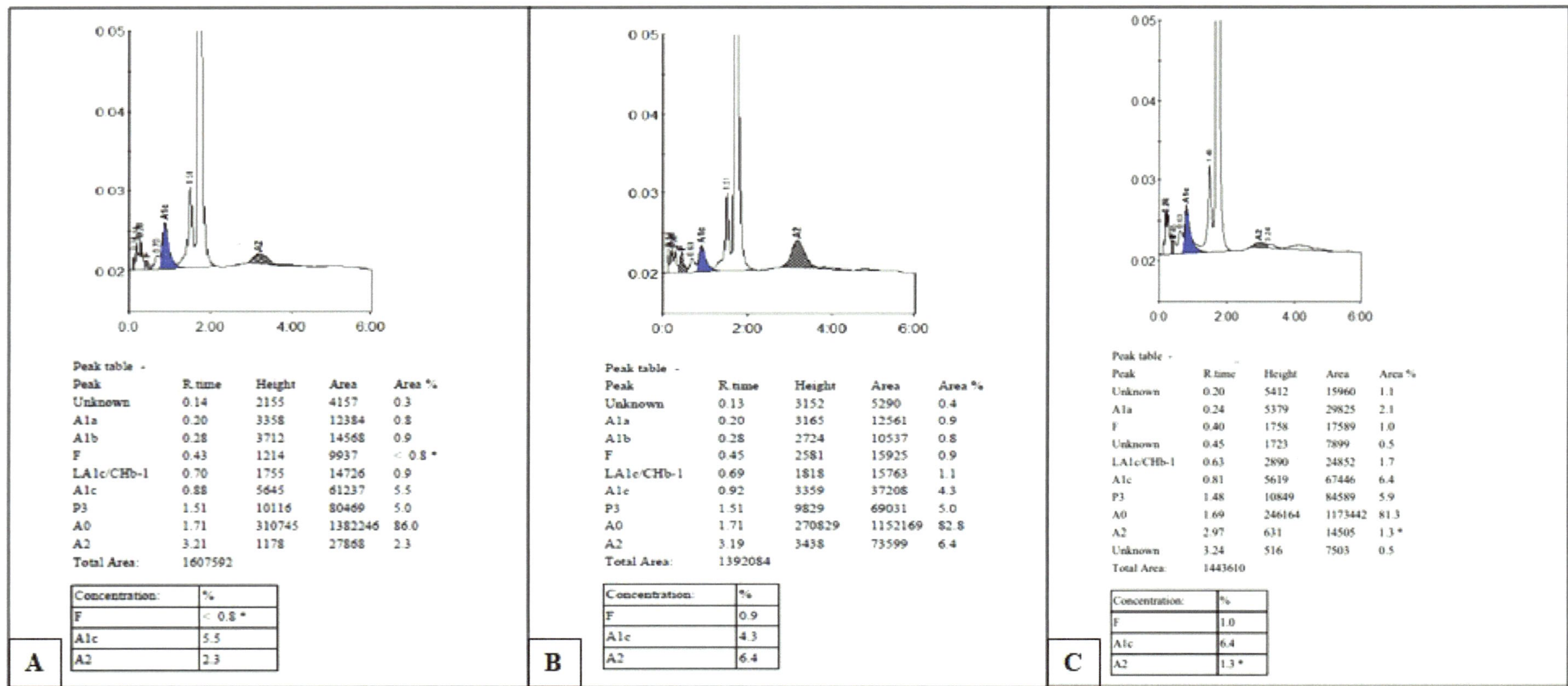

A

Peak table -

Peak	R. time	Height	Area	Area %
Unknown	0.14	2155	4157	0.3
A1a	0.20	3358	12384	0.8
A1b	0.28	3712	14568	0.9
F	0.43	1214	9937	< 0.8 *
LA1c/CHb-1	0.70	1755	14726	0.9
A1c	0.88	5645	61237	5.5
P3	1.51	10116	80469	5.0
A0	1.71	310745	1382246	86.0
A2	3.21	1178	27868	2.3
Total Area:	1607592			

Concentration:	%
F	< 0.8 *
A1c	5.5
A2	2.3

B

Peak table -

Peak	R. time	Height	Area	Area %
Unknown	0.13	3152	5290	0.4
A1a	0.20	3165	12561	0.9
A1b	0.28	2724	10537	0.8
F	0.45	2581	15925	0.9
LA1c/CHb-1	0.69	1818	15763	1.1
A1c	0.92	3359	37208	4.3
P3	1.51	9829	69031	5.0
A0	1.71	270829	1152169	82.8
A2	3.19	3438	73599	6.4
Total Area:	1392084			

Concentration:	%
F	0.9
A1c	4.3
A2	6.4

C

Peak table -

Peak	R. time	Height	Area	Area %
Unknown	0.20	5412	15960	1.1
A1a	0.24	5379	29825	2.1
F	0.40	1758	17589	1.0
Unknown	0.45	1723	7899	0.5
LA1c/CHb-1	0.63	2890	24852	1.7
A1c	0.81	5619	67446	6.4
P3	1.48	10849	84589	5.9
A0	1.69	246164	1173442	81.3
A2	2.97	631	14505	1.3 *
Unknown	3.24	516	7503	0.5
Total Area:	1443610			

Concentration:	%
F	1.0
A1c	6.4
A2	1.3 *

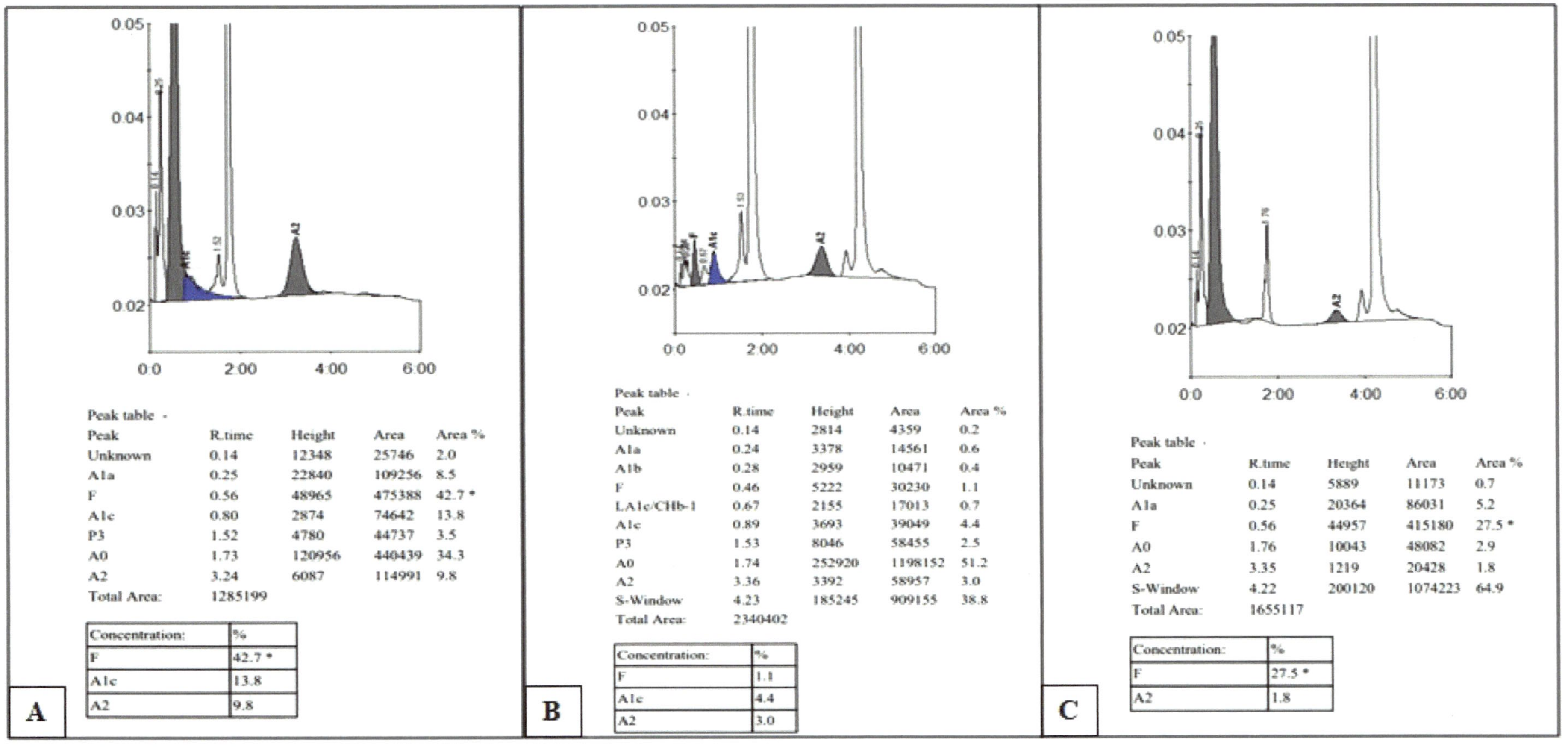

A

Peak table

Peak	R.time	Height	Area	Area %
Unknown	0.14	12348	25746	2.0
A1a	0.25	22840	109256	8.5
F	0.56	48965	475388	42.7 *
A1c	0.80	2874	74642	13.8
P3	1.52	4780	44737	3.5
A0	1.73	120956	440439	34.3
A2	3.24	6087	114991	9.8
Total Area:	1285199			

Concentration:	%
F	42.7 *
A1c	13.8
A2	9.8

B

Peak table

Peak	R.time	Height	Area	Area %
Unknown	0.14	2814	4359	0.2
A1a	0.24	3378	14561	0.6
A1b	0.28	2959	10471	0.4
F	0.46	5222	30230	1.1
LA1c/CHb-1	0.67	2155	17013	0.7
A1c	0.89	3693	39049	4.4
P3	1.53	8046	58455	2.5
A0	1.74	252920	1198152	51.2
A2	3.36	3392	58957	3.0
S-Window	4.23	185245	909155	38.8
Total Area:	2340402			

Concentration:	%
F	1.1
A1c	4.4
A2	3.0

C

Peak table

Peak	R.time	Height	Area	Area %
Unknown	0.14	5889	11173	0.7
A1a	0.25	20364	86031	5.2
F	0.56	44957	415180	27.5 *
A0	1.76	10043	48082	2.9
A2	3.35	1219	20428	1.8
S-Window	4.22	200120	1074223	64.9
Total Area:	1655117			

Concentration:	%
F	27.5 *
A2	1.8

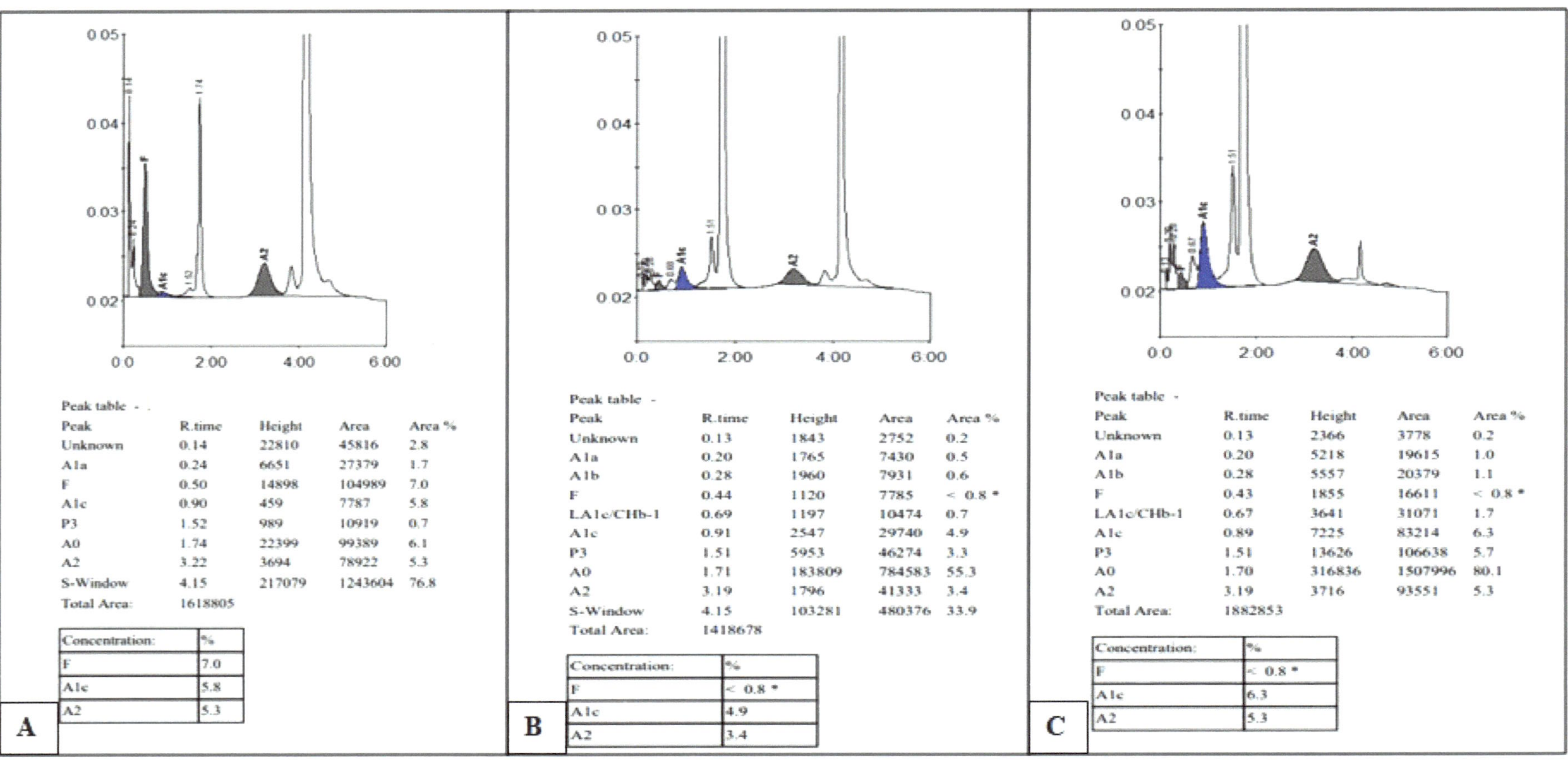

A

Peak table - .

Peak	R.time	Height	Area	Area %
Unknown	0.14	22810	45816	2.8
A1a	0.24	6651	27379	1.7
F	0.50	14898	104989	7.0
A1c	0.90	459	7787	5.8
P3	1.52	989	10919	0.7
A0	1.74	22399	99389	6.1
A2	3.22	3694	78922	5.3
S-Window	4.15	217079	1243604	76.8
Total Area:	1618805			

Concentration:	%
F	7.0
A1c	5.8
A2	5.3

B

Peak table -

Peak	R.time	Height	Area	Area %
Unknown	0.13	1843	2752	0.2
A1a	0.20	1765	7430	0.5
A1b	0.28	1960	7931	0.6
F	0.44	1120	7785	< 0.8 *
LA1c/CHb-1	0.69	1197	10474	0.7
A1c	0.91	2547	29740	4.9
P3	1.51	5953	46274	3.3
A0	1.71	183809	784583	55.3
A2	3.19	1796	41333	3.4
S-Window	4.15	103281	480376	33.9
Total Area:	1418678			

Concentration:	%
F	< 0.8 *
A1c	4.9
A2	3.4

C

Peak table -

Peak	R.time	Height	Area	Area %
Unknown	0.13	2366	3778	0.2
A1a	0.20	5218	19615	1.0
A1b	0.28	5557	20379	1.1
F	0.43	1855	16611	< 0.8 *
LA1c/CHb-1	0.67	3641	31071	1.7
A1c	0.89	7225	83214	6.3
P3	1.51	13626	106638	5.7
A0	1.70	316836	1507996	80.1
A2	3.19	3716	93551	5.3
Total Area:	1882853			

Concentration:	%
F	< 0.8 *
A1c	6.3
A2	5.3

Figure 7: Flow chart approach to the laboratory diagnosis of thalassemia and other hemoglobinopathies

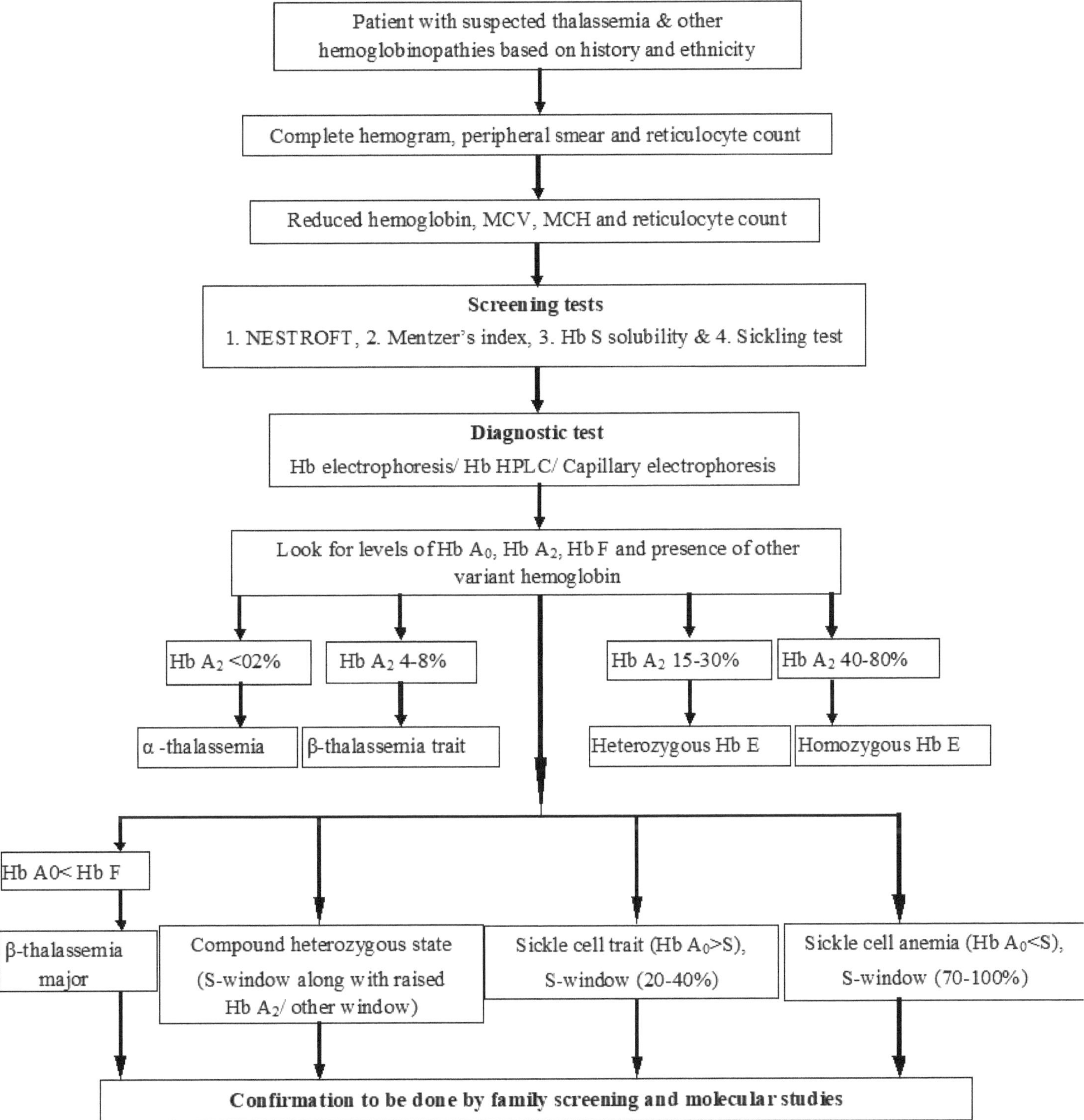

TRANSFUSION SUPPORT IN HEMOGLOBINOPATHIES

– Dr. Dibyajyoti

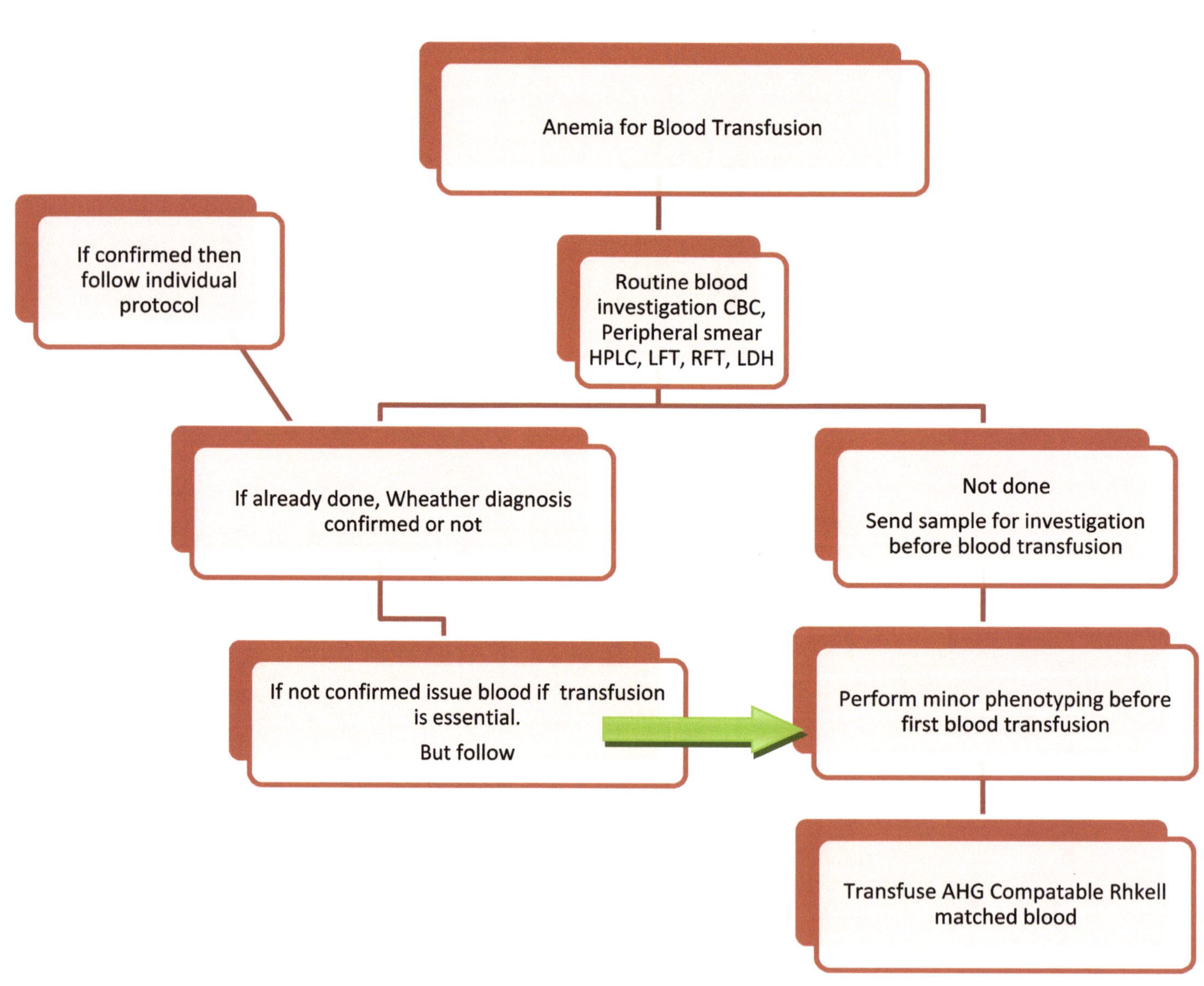

Transfusion Support in Thalassemic Patients

- Thalassemia Major patients usually present early and are transfusion-dependent. Patients with β Thalassemia trait (Thalassemia minor) have elevated haemoglobin A2 on haemoglobin electrophoresis, mild anaemia, and microcytosis. Thalassemia carriers are asymptomatic & usually have no hematologic abnormalities. They do not require red cell transfusion.
- Patients with β Thalassemia intermedia present late with variable anaemia levels and are of the Non-Transfusion-Dependent-Thalassemia (NTDT) phenotype. Due to the severity of their anaemia or disease complications, some patients will go on to chronic transfusions.
- The mainstay of treatment is blood transfusion and iron chelation. The transfusion goal for Thalassemia patients should be between 9 and 10g/dl. To achieve this goal, we require monthly transfusions in infants and young children, with transfusions every three weeks in adolescent and adult patients. Post transfusion, haemoglobin should be 12–13g/dl.
- Splenomegaly can lead to hypersplenism with an increase in blood requirement. If the annual blood requirement is over 200ml/kg/year, splenectomy should be considered. Splenectomy usually reduces the annual red cell requirement. Before the splenectomy, patients should be fully immunised.
- Leukoreduced products are indicated for all Thalassemia patients, but they always do not need irradiated blood products. Radiation damages the red cell membrane and shortens red cell survival. The only indication for irradiation is for immune-suppressed patients or who will possibly have a progenitor cell transplant.
- Saline-washed Red cells are not required unless the recipient had urticaria or other transfusion reaction that washed units could avoid.
- Cytomegalovirus (CMV) infections should be prevented in patients who are likely to receive a progenitor cell transplant and pregnant women. Leukocyte-reduced blood products are CMV free and thus should be used to prevent CMV infections.
- Transfusion should be by PRBC (packed Red Blood Cell), not whole blood units. The volume of transfusion should be calculated for pediatric patients.
- Red cell units can be "split" by the blood bank to conserve the blood supply. Transfusion in patients with anaemia may lead to a mild volume overload that most patients tolerate, but it can lead to cardiac overload in older patients or those with cardiomyopathy that requires monitoring. Diuretics should be considered if the transfused volume exceeds 20ml/kg.
- For Thalassemia patients, the age of beginning transfusion influences the rate of alloimmunisation. Children beginning transfusion early (<one year of age) have less alloimmunisation (11% vs 30%).

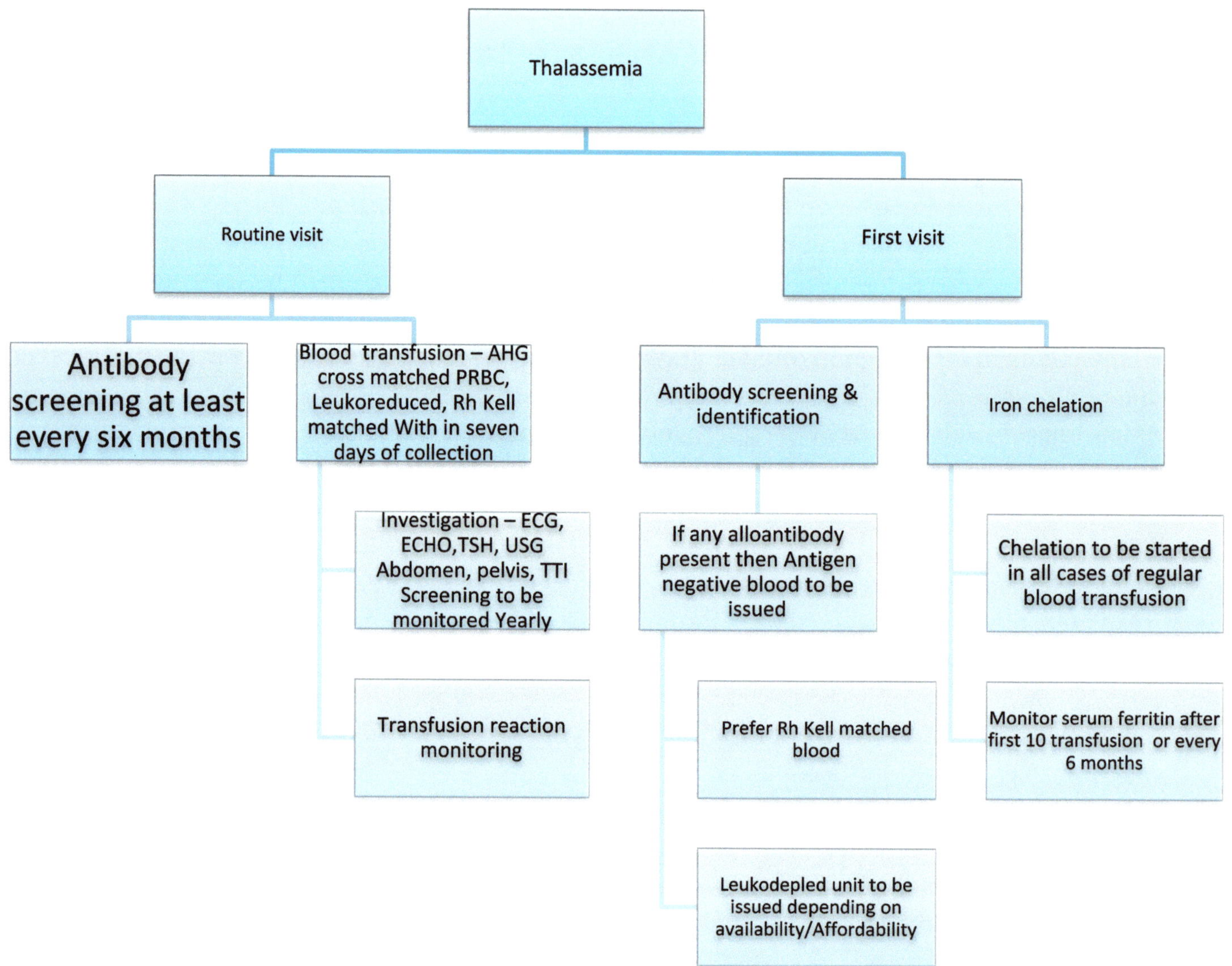

- Alloimmunisation is an immune response to foreign antigens after exposure to genetically different cells or tissues. Consequences of alloimmunisation are Difficulty obtaining compatible blood, increased frequency of transfusion, acute or delayed hemolytic transfusion reactions and hemolytic disease of the newborn.
- The common antigens causing red cell alloimmunisation are D, E, e, C, c, K, k, Jka, Jkb, Fya, Fyb, S, s, M, N, P, Le a, and Le b. Whenever any alloantibody is detected, corresponding antigen-negative blood should be provided to patients.
- Indirect Coombs test, Antibody screening panel (2 cells, 3 cells, 4 cell panels) & antibody detection panels (11cell, 16 cell panels) are commonly used to detect alloantibodies.
- It is advisable to perform an extended RBC phenotype (ABO, Rh, Kell, Kidd, Duffy, Lewis, MNS) of all Thalassemic patients before administering a first blood transfusion. Antibody screening is to be performed regularly to detect culprit alloantibodies if present—proper counselling to all alloantibody-positive patients is required to get antigen-negative blood transfusion only. Phenotype-matched blood (at least Rh & Kell) should be administered whenever possible.

Transfusion support in Sickle cell disease(HbSS).

Blood transfusion does more than raise the haemoglobin (Hb) level for oxygen delivery. Transfusion also lowers the percentage of sickle Hb (HbS) and increases Hb oxygen saturation, decreasing the propensity for vaso occlusion.

MECHANISMS

1. Dilution of HbS-containing red blood cells (RBCs) via the addition of HbA-containing cells from the blood of normal donors
2. Suppression of erythropoietin release caused by the rise in Hb, thereby reducing the production of new HbS-containing cells
3. The decrease in the percentage of HbS-containing cells due to the longer circulating lifespan of HbA-containing cells
4. Increase in Hb oxygen saturation levels by approximately 1 to 6 percent, which increases oxygen delivery to the tissues

WHEN TO TRANSFUSE?

- Acute symptomatic anaemia (e.g., the onset of heart failure, dyspnea, hypotension, marked Fatigue). A progressive trend for a decreasing Hgb over several days without a compensatory increase in reticulocyte count.
- A drop in baseline reticulocyte count (i.e., relative reticulocytopenia) with symptoms of acute hemodynamic compromise (increased pulse, decreased oxygen saturation, change in mental status, poor perfusion, orthostatic blood pressure changes).
- Haemoglobin is at least 2 g/dL below their baseline, with acute clinical symptoms, signs of hemodynamic compromise, or increased respiratory effort or oxygen requirement to keep the oxygen saturation above 92 percent.

SCD PATIENTS WITH DHTR

- Patients present most commonly 7–10 days after transfusion with a triad of fever, jaundice and anaemia, which may be accompanied by sickling pain with laboratory evidence of haemolysis and reduced survival of the transfused red cells (including a fall in %HbA). Positive DAT and new alloantibodies are identified in the patient's plasma or red cell eluate. Reticulocytosis is a common finding.
- Unless anaemia is severe, transfusion should be avoided. Alloantibody identification may be cumbersome. If the new alloantibody's identity cannot be determined, the provision of extended antigen-matched blood should be considered.

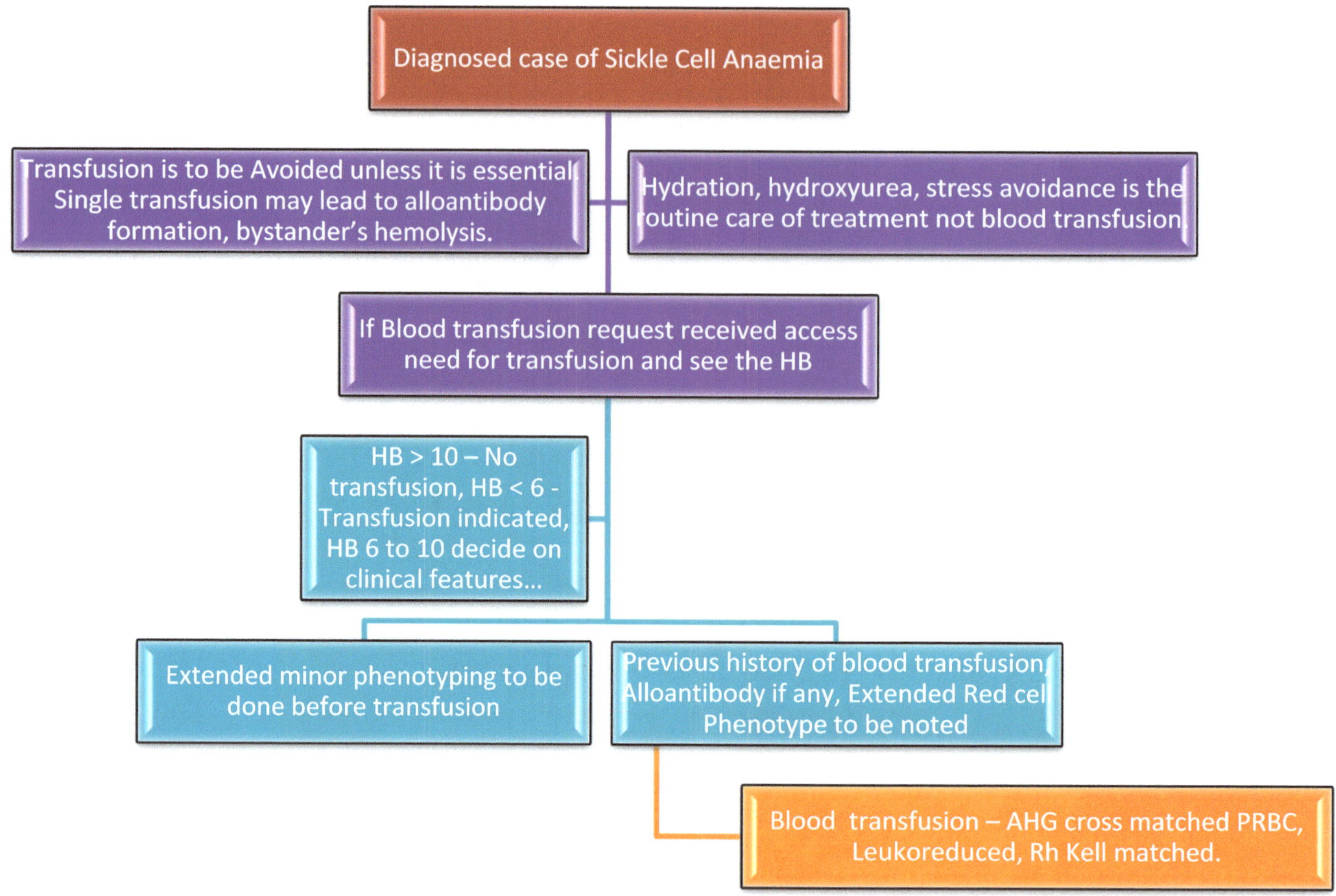

Patient Needing Transfusion with Ongoing Hyper Hemolysis Syndrome

- Hyperhemolysis is a subtype of delayed hemolytic transfusion reaction, which can potentially cause life-threatening acute anaemia. The presenting features are characteristically severe sickle pain, fever and hemoglobinuria. There is the destruction of both donor and autologous red cells. Post-transfusion Hb is lower than before transfusion.
- %HbA decreases or becomes absent. HbS and HbA are detected in the serial analysis of urine by HPLC.
- The DAT is often negative. New red cell alloantibodies are usually not detected in the serological investigation. However, new alloantibodies are usually identified in DAT-positive cases, although their appearance may be delayed.
- A fall in the absolute reticulocyte count is seen (compared to the patient's usual level)
- Hyperhemolysis can induce multi-organ failure (MOF) and death, most likely because of damage to the underlying vasculature by released free haemoglobin (Hb) and heme.
- Additional transfusion, even with antigen-matched crossmatch-compatible units, may lead to further hemolysis and a protracted course or even death, But it must not be withheld in patients with life-threatening anaemia.
- Management is dependent on the severity of anaemia and the speed of hemolysis. In mild cases, further transfusion should be avoided. Early intravenous immunoglobulin (IVIG) administration and steroids may correct the anaemia and resolve hemolysis in severe cases.

- In rapid, severe hemolysis, further transfusion may be required to prevent death from anaemia; this should be given with IVIG and steroid cover. IVIg therapy is often used for the prevention of antibody-mediated immune destruction.
- Recurrence of hyperhemolysis may be prevented by administering IVIG and methylprednisolone before subsequent transfusions. Eculizumab, an inhibitor of the C5-convertase, will be administered at the start of hyperhemolysis to prevent irreversible MOF.
- Additional transfusions with profound anaemia and organ hypoxia, further transfusions may be unavoidable. If transfusion is indicated, extended matching in addition to rituximab prophylaxis for patients with existing antibodies is recommended

Pregnant patients with SCD

The prophylactic transfusion should be considered for women with :

1. h/o previous or current medical, obstetric or fetal problems related to SCD
2. Previously on hydroxyurea because of severe disease.
3. Multiple pregnancies.
4. Long-term transfusions for stroke prevention or amelioration of severe sickle complications should continue with regular transfusions throughout pregnancy.
5. Worsening anaemia or those with acute SCD complications (acute chest syndrome, stroke etc.)

Acute Chest Syndrome

- It accounts for about 25% of hospital admissions and is a leading cause of death in sickle cell disease. For patients with acute chest syndrome and severe anaemia, a simple transfusion may be sufficient to increase oxygenation and reduce the risk of more severe disease.
- Hyperviscosity and hypervolemia can complicate simple transfusion. Patients who present with elevated haemoglobin (8g/dl or higher) should receive an exchange transfusion as the initial therapy. Hydroxyurea should be considered for all patients who have had an episode of acute chest syndrome,

Red Cell Antigen Profiling

- Extended red cell antigen profile by genotype or serology over only ABO/RhD typing for all patients with SCD (all genotypes) at the earliest opportunity (optimally before the first transfusion)
- An extended red cell antigen profile includes C/c, E/e, K, Jka/Jkb, Fya/Fyb, M/N, and S/s at a minimum. Serologic phenotyping may be inaccurate if the patient has been transfused in the last 3 months. Genotyping is preferred over serologic phenotyping as it provides additional antigen information and increased accuracy.
- Prophylactic red cell antigen matching for Rh and K antigens over only ABO/RhD is done for patients with SCD receiving transfusions. Extended red cell antigen matching (Jka/Jkb, Fya/Fyb, S/s) may further protect from alloimmunisation.
- SCD at risk for hyperviscosity (i.e., with Hb above 10 g/dL and HbS>50%). Minimise simple blood transfusion therapy use in individuals with a Hb>10 g/dL and an HbS>50% of total Hb.

Other Hemoglobinopathies

1. **HbE disease (HbEE)**

   - HPLC - HbE >95% HbA2 ≈ 2.5% HbF <3%
   - Hb - 10 to 14 g/dL, High RBC count, MCH 20 pg, MCV 65 fl
   - Clinical feature - Mild anaemia and hemolysis may be caused by infections/ medical drugs
   - Transfusion requirement – Rare, If required, Thalassemia protocol is to be followed.

2. **HbE Heterozygosity (HbAE)**

   - HPLC - HbE 25 to 30%
   - Hb – Normal or hypochromic
   - Clinical feature - Mild anaemia.
   - Transfusion requirement – Rare, If required, Thalassemia protocol is to be followed.

3. **HbE β+-thalassemia**

   - HPLC - HbE + HbA2 = 25 to 80%, HbF = 6 to 50% HbA = 5 to 60%
   - Hb - Hb low to a varying degree, Hypochromia, Microcytosis
   - Clinical feature - Variable, intermediate, hypochromic anaemia
   - Transfusion requirement – Less often, If required, Thalassemia protocol to be followed.

4. **Sickle-cell β+-thalassemia (HbS β+-thalassemia)**

   - HPLC - HbS >55%, HbF >20%, HbA2 >3.5%
   - Hb - Hb 9 to 12 g/dL Hypochromia, microcytosis
   - Clinical feature - Variable, mild sickle-cell disease
   - Transfusion requirement – If required, the Thalassemia protocol is to be followed.

5. **HbS Heterozygosity (HbAS)**

   - HPLC – HbS = 35 to 40% HbA2 ≥ 3.5%
   - Hb - Normal
   - Clinical feature - No apparent illness
   - Transfusion requirement – Rare, If required, Sickle cell protocol is to be followed.

6. **HbSC disease (HbSC)**

   - HPLC - HbS ≈ 50%, HbC ≈ 50%, HbF <5%
   - Hb 10 to 13 g/Dl, Target cells, MCV <75 fl
   - Clinical feature - Weak symptoms of sickle-cell disease, chronic hemolytic anaemia
   - Transfusion requirement – Rare, If required, Sickle cell protocol is to be followed.

7. **Heterozygous β-thalassemia (β-thalassemia minor)**

   - HPLC - HbA2 >3.2%, HbF 0.5 to 6%
   - Hb 9 to 13 g/Dl, MCV 55 to 75 fl, MCH 19 to 25 pg
   - Clinical feature - Mild anaemia
   - Transfusion requirement – If required, the Thalassemia protocol is to be followed.

Myelodysplastic Syndromes:

The role of therapy in lower-risk MDS should focus on improving symptoms and minimising transfusion needs. Patients receive red cell transfusions if haemoglobin is less than 8 g/dL or if the patient has symptomatic anaemia. Platelets are transfused if the platelet count is less than 10 k/μL or the patient has active bleeding. These parameters can change based on geographical distribution and practice patterns. There has also been a question about the need for irradiated blood products, particularly for patients that could be potential candidates for SCT. This is not the standard practice. Finally, some centres support white cell transfusions as an early intervention for patients with neutropenic fever or resistant infections. These are considered experimental at this point.

Aplastic anaemias:

Patients with symptomatic anaemia and/or thrombocytopenia associated with wet purpura or bleeding require immediate blood transfusions. All transfusions in patients with suspected aplastic anaemia should be irradiated to prevent transfusion-associated graft-versus-host disease (GVHD). If the patient is a potential BMT candidate and is cytomegalovirus (CMV)-negative or the CMV status is unknown, CMV transmission should be avoided by either leukoreduction or using CMV-negative products. Blood donation from family members should be avoided to prevent alloimmunisation, which could complicate future BMT. After stabilising the patient, blood products should be used judiciously to prevent cardiopulmonary compromise and reduce the risk of haemorrhage; a platelet goal of 10 000/μL will suffice for most patients, although some patients will tolerate even lower platelet goals without bleeding or petechiae. Granulocyte transfusions are not of benefit to patients with aplastic anaemia.

Paroxysmal Nocturnal Haemoglobinuria

Blood transfusions may be required for the treatment of anaemia. The recommendation that blood be given in the form of saline-washed or frozen-thawed, deglycerolized red cells to avert a hemolytic episode due to complement within the accompanying plasma has been questioned. However, hemofiltration is recommended to prevent transfusion reactions resulting from the interaction between donor leukocytes and recipient antibodies. Transfused red cell survival is normal in patients with PNH, and transfusion to near-normal haemoglobin levels can produce short-lived "remissions." Clinical improvement may result from a temporary decrease in the production of abnormal cells with a consequent reduction in hemolysis and other disease-associated epiphenomena. Iatrogenic hemochromatosis can occur from chronic transfusions, but this process will be delayed because of iron loss from hemoglobinuria and hemosiderinuria. Iron overload in patients with classic PNH is rare. Nevertheless, iron overload remains a concern in patients who require chronic transfusion when the anaemia is primarily a consequence of marrow failure rather than hemolysis.

Sideroblastic Anemia

Transfusion of packed red cells is necessary for patients with symptomatic anaemia, but it should be kept to a minimum because it accelerates iron overload.

Most, if not all, patients with uncomplicated SA have high levels of endogenous erythropoietin, and it would appear unlikely that additional administration of the hormone would be beneficial.

G6PD deficiency anaemia

Exchange transfusion during the first week of life is often required to prevent bilirubin encephalopathy. Beyond the newborn period, anaemia rarely is of such severity as to require regular blood transfusions. However, transfusions may be lifesaving during aplastic crises, and transfusions can also be needed for increased hemolysis induced by viral triggers.

Pyruvate Kinase Deficiency anaemia

During the first years of life, severe anaemia is managed with red cell transfusions. Maintenance of the haemoglobin concentration above 8 g/dL permits normal growth and development. However, the decision for transfusion therapy must relate to patient tolerance of anaemia rather than an arbitrary level of haemoglobin. Because of increased red cell 2,3-DPG content, patients may tolerate moderately severe anaemia with few symptoms. Splenectomy partially ameliorates anaemia in many patients and can be beneficial in decreasing the transfusion burden.

Section V

Management of Blood Transfusion Services

BIOMEDICAL WASTE MANAGEMENT

3 "R" s of waste minimisation – Reduce, Reuse, Recycle

Introduction

Knowledge and awareness of rules/guidelines for personal and biological safety are essential to creating a safe, organised, collaborative and productive lab environment. Constant surveillance for hazardous materials and practices is a must. It also requires the identification of potential hazards and preventing or managing them properly without compromising safety. The lab is responsible for documenting waste management procedures, applying random checks at critical areas, and maintaining a contract with a biomedical waste collection agency. Lab personnel must verify and monitor good housekeeping in the entire system and deal with waste collecting agencies for disposal and contract.

- "Bio-medical waste means any waste generated during the diagnosis, treatment or immunisation of human beings or animals or research activities pertaining to or in the production or testing of biological or health camps."

  It includes sharps, non-sharps, blood, body parts, chemicals, pharmaceuticals, medical devices and radioactive materials

Any waste generated will become highly hazardous if it is not segregated at the source itself. Waste should be managed following established blood centre policy. Handling of bio-hazardous waste is controlled through a notification issued by the Ministry of Environment and Forests, Government of India; hence any lapse on the part of concerned staff may attract severe penalties for the institution. Thus, bio-waste must be handled without adversely affecting health and the environment.

A few critical steps include a safe or secure location for handling bio-waste, colour coding, pre-treatment like disinfection or sterilisation on-site, provision of immunisation (HBV and Tetanus), training of all staff involved in the process, establishing a bar-code system for containers, conducting regular health checkups, maintaining records of accidents and remedial action, incineration, autoclaving etc.

Bio-waste must be segregated into containers or bags, and untreated ones should not be mixed with other wastes. Containers or bags must be labelled as a biohazard and better be bar-coded. Untreated waste shall not be stored for more than 48 hours in the vicinity. If it becomes necessary to store the waste beyond such a period, the authorised person must take permission from the prescribed authority. After that, it may be stored at 2-80C with strict measures to avoid adverse effects on human health or the environment.

Lab supplies that come into contact with media, cultures, reagents, or potentially hazardous material should not be left on the benchtop. Place used/contaminated lab supplies in proper waste containers. Waste should not be disposed of in any other container, and the container must be closed when it is 3/4th filled.

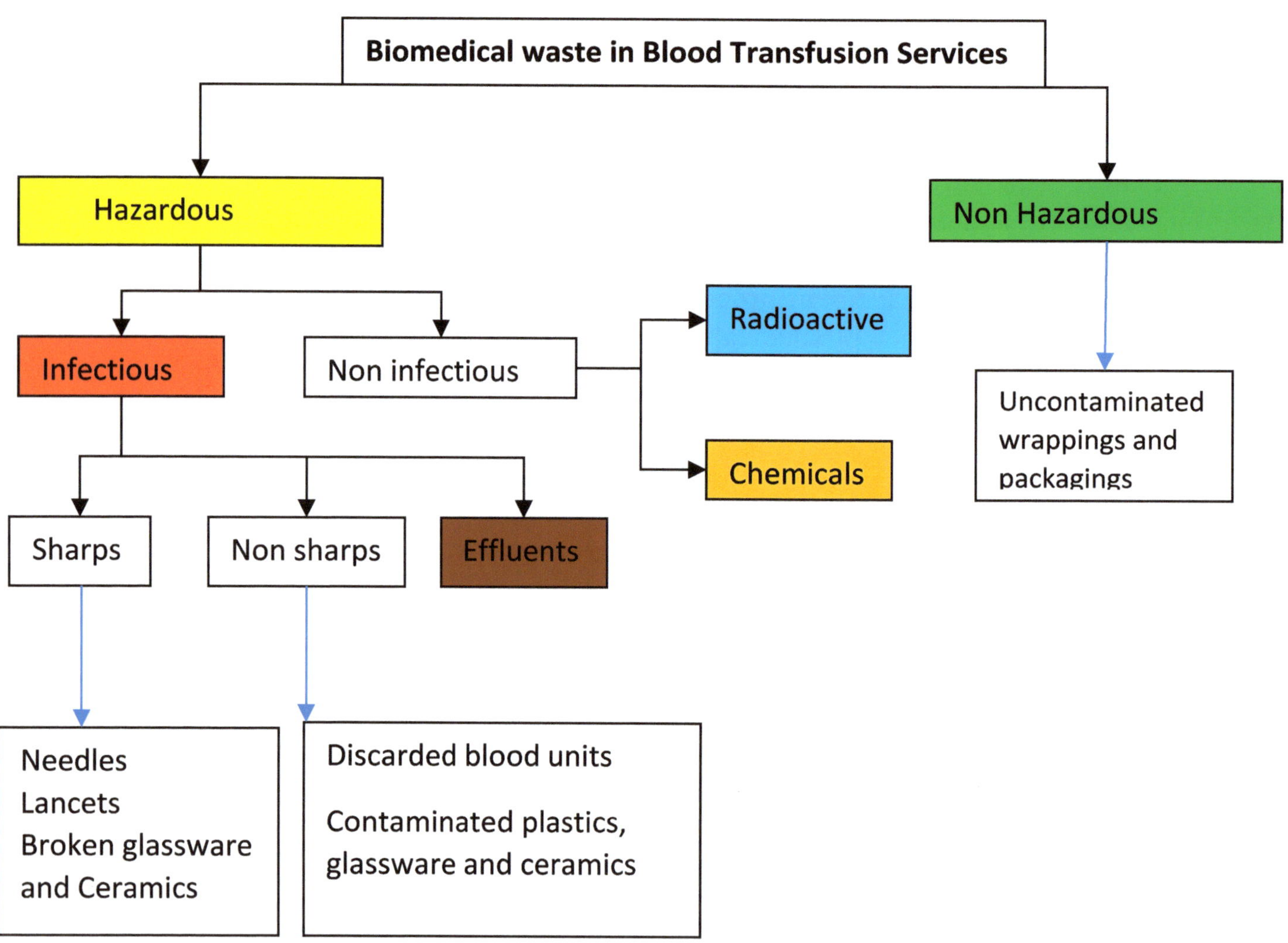

Sharps must be disposed of at the site of generation. If policy permits, burn the syringe needle with a needle destroyer at the point of use before disposal. Otherwise, discard needles in puncture-proof rigid containers after disinfection in 0.5-1% fresh sodium hypochlorite solution. Place the disposable glass in a special bin for disposal without further handling. Put other discarded materials in robust plastic bags, which should then be sealed and handed over to the waste collection agency for disposal. Broken glass or sharps should be removed with a dustpan to avoid sharps injury.

Place reusable glassware and plastic items in a bucket containing 1 % hypochlorite. Leave it for at least 30 minutes. Then the items are washed and dried. Soak pipettes in 1 % hypochlorite for 30-60 minutes. Liquid waste containers attached to laboratory equipment are cleaned daily and filled with 50ml of 1% Hypochlorite solution before starting the machine. The accumulated waste is disposed of the next day.

Known HIV-positive samples must be lined up separated from routine testing samples, and all consumables used for testing those samples should be discarded in a 5% hypochlorite solution.

Transportation of bio-waste has three steps;

    a. internal transport,
    b. temporary holding and
    c. external transport.

For internal transport, dedicated wheelbarrow, trolleys, or carts must be driven through specific routes to reduce the passage of loaded carts through wards and other clean areas. Carts should be easy to load, unload and clean and have no sharp edges that could damage waste bags or containers. Carts and recyclable containers used repeatedly for transport should be disinfected after each use.

The designated on-site storage facility shall be located within the premises close to the treatment, away from food storage/preparation areas, large enough to contain all the hazardous waste with spare capacity, totally enclosed and secured from unauthorised access, inaccessible to animals, insects or birds, easy to clean and disinfect and have an impermeable hard-standing base, adequate water supply, drainage and ventilation. This waste should not be stored for more than 48 hours and should be packaged securely before the subsequent transport. The universal biological hazard symbol should be affixed on the storage area, vehicles, doors, and waste containers.

All bags that must be sent to external (off-site) transportation must be labelled as prescribed. The waste producer is responsible for properly packaging and labelling the containers. Each transport must be documented appropriately, and all vehicles must carry a consignment note (if possible, GPS tracking) from the point of collection to the treatment facility. Vehicles used to collect bio-waste should not be used for any other purpose. The system must be easy to load, unload, clean and fully enclosed to prevent spillage.

Section	Sharps	Non-Sharps	Effluents
Screening and Donation area	· Broken slides and glassware, ampoules, tubes, slides · Lancets and needles · Cuvettes · Pipettes · Tiles · Micro-capillary tubes · Broken test tubes and glass slides · Needles from blood collection bags and other used needles · Scissors	·Glassware · Filter paper strips for haemoglobin estimation · Gauze and swabs · Gloves · Blood units	Used copper sulphate solution, disinfectants
Refreshment room		· Phlebotomy dressings, including plaster, bandages and swabs	
Pretransfusion Laboratory	·Broken glassware and ampoules · Test tubes and slides · Pipette tips	·Blood sample tubes · Column agglutination cards · Gloves · Micro-plates · Used test kit materials	· Liquids from cell washers · Blood and serum samples · Red cell suspensions for blood group serology testing
Component laboratory	· Wafers for sterile connecting devices	· Blood units that are: – ruptured; – expired; – seroreactive; or – unsuitable due to other causes · Gloves · Transfer bags and accessories for component preparation · Segments from blood bag tubing · Leukoreduction filters	
Transfusion area/daycare	· Blood administration sets, intravenous sets and other disposable needles · Used syringes	· Leukoreduction filters · Used blood bags	

Category	Type of Waste	Type of Bag or Container to be used	Treatment and Disposal options
Yellow	Soiled waste Expired or Discarded Medicines Chemical Waste Bloodstained linen waste Microbiology and Biotechnology waste	Yellow coloured non-chlorinated plastic bags Containers	Incineration or Plasma Pyrolysis or deep burial
Red	Contaminated recyclable waste	Red coloured non-chlorinated plastic bags or containers	Autoclaving or micro-waving/ hydroclaving followed by shredding or mutilation
White (translucent)	Sharp and metallic waste	Puncture-proof, Leakproof, tamper-proof containers	Autoclaving or Dry Heat Sterilisation followed by shredding or mutilation, or encapsulation in a metal container or cement concrete
Blue	Glassware	Cardboard boxes with blue coloured marking	Disinfection, autoclaving, microwaving or hydroclaving
Black	General waste		General waste disposal, recycling

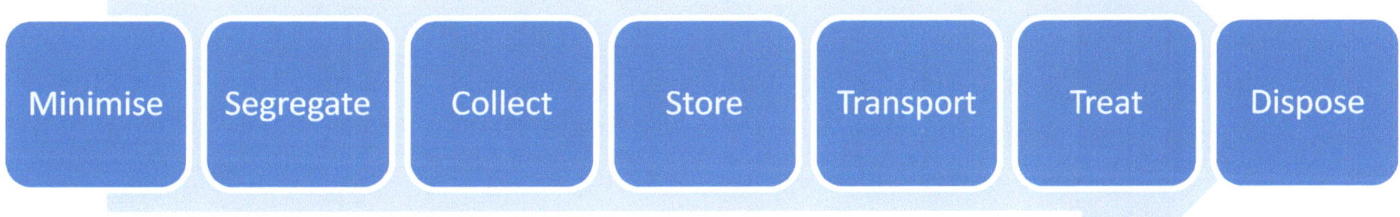

Figure 34. Steps in Biomedical waste management

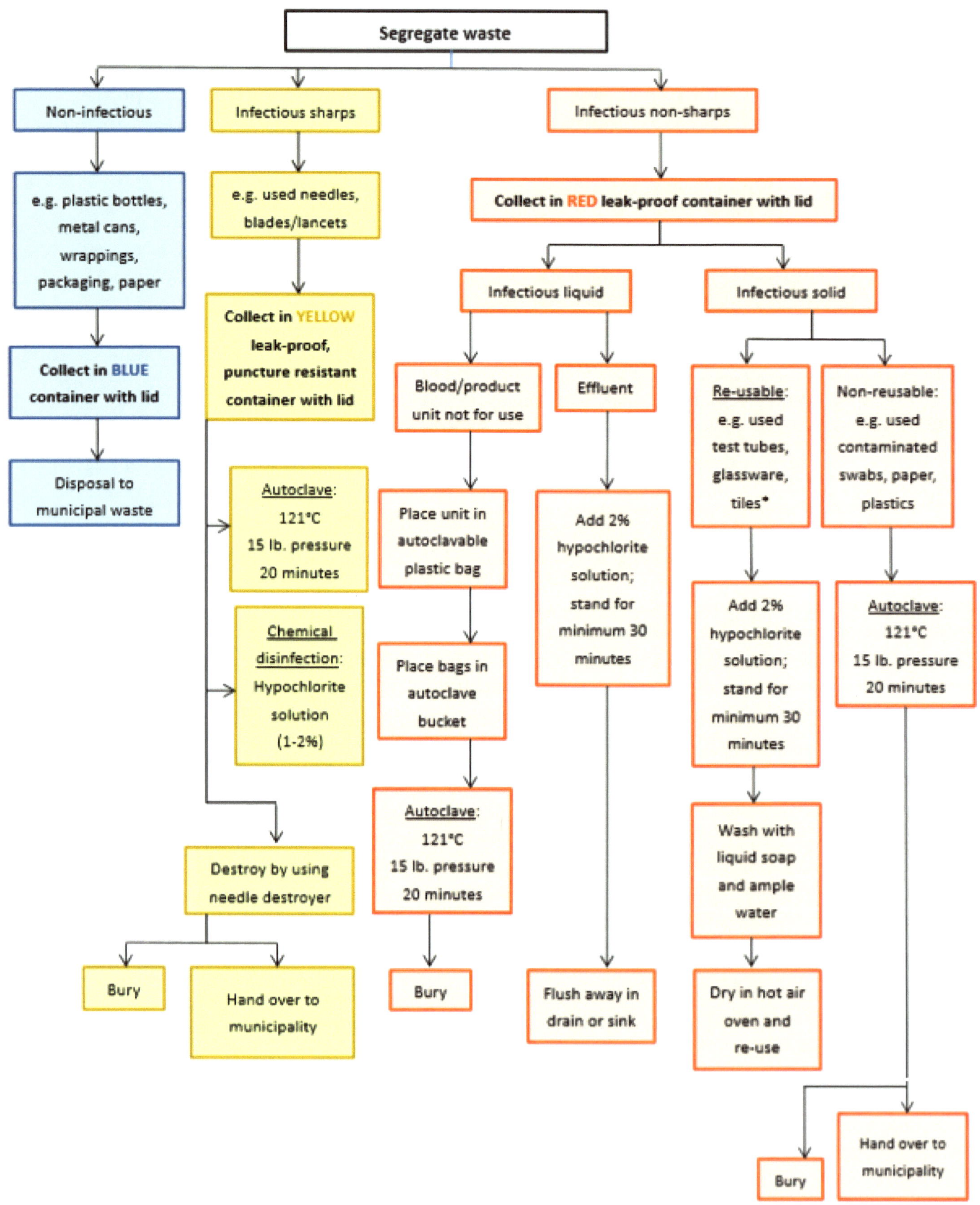
Segregate waste
Non-infectious
Infectious sharps
Infectious non-sharps
e.g. plastic bottles, metal cans, wrappings, packaging, paper
e.g. used needles, blades/lancets
Collect in RED leak-proof container with lid
Collect in BLUE container with lid
Collect in YELLOW leak-proof, puncture resistant container with lid
Infectious liquid
Infectious solid
Disposal to municipal waste
Autoclave: 121°C 15 lb. pressure 20 minutes
Blood/product unit not for use
Effluent
Re-usable: e.g. used test tubes, glassware, tiles*
Non-reusable: e.g. used contaminated swabs, paper, plastics
Chemical disinfection: Hypochlorite solution (1-2%)
Place unit in autoclavable plastic bag
Add 2% hypochlorite solution; stand for minimum 30 minutes
Add 2% hypochlorite solution; stand for minimum 30 minutes
Autoclave: 121°C 15 lb. pressure 20 minutes
Place bags in autoclave bucket
Destroy by using needle destroyer
Autoclave: 121°C 15 lb. pressure 20 minutes
Wash with liquid soap and ample water
Bury
Hand over to municipality
Bury
Flush away in drain or sink
Dry in hot air oven and re-use
Bury
Hand over to municipality

SPILL MANAGEMENT

Spills: are defined as flow, move, fall, or spread **over the** edge **or** outside the limits **of something**

Cleaning, disinfection and management of spill

The laboratory unit should be cleaned following the established blood centre policy. The unit should have its dedicated cleaning equipment to prevent the possible contamination of other areas.

Disinfection means reducing the number of pathogenic microbes so that the material, object, or surface becomes safe for handling. Glassware, instruments, etc., should be washed or sterilised within the unit following the relevant infection control standards and manufacturers' instructions. For disinfection of glassware, discard it in plastic bins containing 1% sodium hypochlorite (10,000 ppm chlorine). Disinfected blood/fluids can be washed down with running tap water. Disinfected glassware is treated in chromic acid and dried in a hot air oven.

Spillage of blood and blood products is an occupational hazard for personnel. Immediately the spill must be cleaned with standard precautions. After a spill, place an absorbent sheet or gauze over the spill, pour concentrated sodium hypochlorite solution (4%) and let it stand for a minimum contact time of 30 minutes before wiping it with gloved hands. Later, using gloves, wipe clean the spilt sample and place the waste in the yellow bag or bin. Mop clean the area again with a 1% hypochlorite solution.

- Evaluate the spill.
- Wear appropriate protective clothing and gloves. If sharp objects are involved, gloves must be puncture resistant, and a broom or other instrument should be used during clean-up to avoid injury.
- Remove clothing if it is contaminated.
- Evacuate the area for 30 minutes if an aerosol has been created.
- Post warnings to keep the area clear.

Confining the spill:

Remove sharp and broken material, glass by forceps

Remove visible organic matter with absorbent material (Paper towel)

Soaking up excess liquid using absorbent granules

Small spills: (up to 10 cm in diameter)

- Select appropriate PPE
- Wipe up the spill with an absorbent material
- Place the contaminated absorbent material into an impervious container or disposal bag
- Clean the area with a warm detergent solution using a disposable cloth or sponge
- Wipe the area with sodium hypochlorite and allow it to dry
- Perform hand hygiene

Large spills: (more than 10 cm in diameter)

- Select appropriate PPE
- Cover the area with an absorbent clumping agent
- Use a disposable scrapper and pan to scoop up absorbent material and any unabsorbed blood
- Wipe up the spill with absorbent material
- Place contaminated absorbent material into an impervious container or disposal bag
- Mop the area with a detergent solution
- Allow adequate contact time with the disinfectant.
- Discard contaminated materials safely per biohazard guidelines. All blood-contaminated items must be autoclaved or incinerated.
- Wipe the area with sodium hypochlorite and allow it to dry
- Wipe up residual disinfectant if necessary.
- Perform hand hygiene

If the spill occurs in the centrifuge, turn the power off immediately and leave the cover on for 30 minutes. The use of overwraps helps prevent aerosolisation and contain the spill. Use absorbent material to mop up most of the liquid contents. Clean the spill area with detergent.

Spill Kit		
▪ Scoop and scraper	Single-use gloves	Protective apron
Surgical mask	Goggles	Absorbent Agent
▪ Waste bags and ties	Detergent	

Personal protection

All staff must undergo pre-employment, annual health checks, incident or illness records maintenance and infection control training for occupational health and safety. Protection against personal injury is essential for all workers at risk. Protective clothing includes helmets, with or without visors, face masks, eye protectors (safety goggles), gowns, leg protectors or industrial boots and disposable gloves (medical staff) or heavy-duty gloves (waste workers) etc.

If an injury happens, without any panic, rinse the site with soap and water. Mop with disinfectant and cover the site with a transparent bandage. In case of an accidental needle injury, the doctor of the attached hospital should be contacted for post-exposure prophylaxis. If not immunised earlier, Hepatitis B vaccination must be taken as per the schedule. If immunised, after titer checks, do vaccinate accordingly. Take prophylactic medication for HIV, as suggested by the clinician. Reporting and communicating any untoward incident must be done according to institutional policy.

Needle-stick injury:

- Strictly avoiding re-capping of needles is an important step.
- If a needle-stick injury is sustained, for example, on the hand:

- Remove the glove immediately
- Wash the hands thoroughly with soap under running water for a lengthy period
- Encourage bleeding from the wound, but do not apply excessive pressure
- Immediately inform the supervisor or manager

- In the case of a needle-stick injury with the potential to infect with HIV, follow the guidelines for the management of PEP (Post-exposure prophylaxis)

Aseptic techniques

Asepsis or sterility is a central concept in any laboratory, and asepsis aims to promote practices preventing contamination of lab supplies, equipment and individuals. The aseptic technique requires constant attention. Strict adherence to these practices is the key to the integrity of tests performed in the lab. The point that has to be remembered is that bacteria are ubiquitous in the environment, surfaces and bodies. Handling lab materials sensibly and avoiding unnecessary motions or contact with contaminated objects or surfaces should be practised.

Electrical safety:
<ul><li>Report faulty connections, frayed electrical cords, damaged switches and other potential hazards should be promptly and get them repaired</li><li>Please refrain from using any faulty equipment until it has been repaired. (label them and remove them from the working area.</li><li>Reduce the use of Extension cords as much as possible. Get the permanent wiring done as early as possible</li><li>Secure the wires. Never allow loose trailing wires either on the ground or elsewhere</li><li>Ensure your hands are absolutely dry when handling electrical equipments, switches, plugs etc.</li><li>Do not meddle/adjust wires when they are plugged in</li><li>Avoid plugging too many electrical items into the same circuit (overloaded circuits constitute a fire hazard)</li><li>All personnel should be trained on the primary management/intervention of electric shock.</li></ul>

Disinfection and Sterilisation:

Germicide: It is the agent that destroys germs. It includes both antiseptics and disinfectants. The type of microorganism is identified from the prefix (e.g., virucide, fungicide, bactericide, sporicide, and tuberculocidal).

Antisepsis: Antisepsis is the process of removal of germs from the skin. When related to the patient's skin, it means disinfection of living tissue or skin. It reduces or removes transient microbes from the skin related to the health care worker.

Decontamination and cleaning: Decontamination removes pathogens from objects to be safe to handle. Cleaning removes visible soil (e.g., organic and inorganic materials) from surfaces and objects. Technically, it achieves a minimum reduction of ≥ 1 log CFU of microorganisms.

Disinfection is eliminating vegetative forms of microorganisms except for bacterial spores from inanimate objects. Technically, this method reduces$\geq10^3$ log CFU of microorganisms by this method without spores.

Levels of disinfection:			
	Can	**Cannot**	**Examples**
High-level Disinfectant	Used for a shorter duration and able to kill 10^6 log microorganisms	Spores	glutaraldehyde ($\geq$2.0%), hydrogen peroxide (7.5%), hypochlorite (650–675 ppm), and hypochlorous acid (400–450 ppm).
Intermediate level Disinfectant	Mycobacterium tuberculosis and noncritical items contaminated with blood/body fluids.		
Low-level Disinfectant	vegetative form of bacteria, a few fungi, and some enveloped viruses from the noncritical items		3% hydrogen peroxide, quaternary ammonium compound, diluted glutaraldehyde, phenolics

Sterilisation: Sterilisation is defined as the complete elimination or destruction of all forms of microbial life (i.e., both vegetative and spore forms), carried out by various physical and chemical methods. Technically, a reduction of$\geq10^6$ log colony forming units (CFU) of the most resistant spores is achieved at half a regular cycle.

Irradiation and Radiation Protection

Chapter 31

– Dr. Udaykrishna

On November 8, 1895, Wilhelm Conrad Rontgen: path-breaking discovery of X- rays.

Shortly After Rontgen's discovery, on March 1, 1896, Becquerel confirmed his suspicion of radioactivity using uranium crystals.

Marie Curie, along with Pierre Curie, coined the term Radioactivity. Consequently, Polonium and Radium were discovered by the couple.

The radioactivity unit was called Curie and defined as the emanation in equilibrium with 1 g of radium. However, in 1975, the International Commission on Radiation Units and Measurements replaced the Curie with the Becquerel.

The ICRU definition of Radiation Quantities and units

1. **Exposure:**

The quantity exposure (X) is the quotient of the absolute value of the total charge of the ions of either sign produced by radiation in the air by the mass of the air when all the charges produced in the air are completely stopped in the air, i.e., the state of electronic equilibrium exists.

$X = \Delta Q / \Delta m$ air

The quantity exposure is defined only for X and gamma rays, and it is a measure of the ionisation of air.

The exposure is measured in R (Roentgen)

2. **Absorbed Dose:**

The quantity absorbed dose (D) is the quotient of the mean energy imparted to matter of a unit mass by ionising radiation.

$D = \Delta E / \Delta m$ med

The SI unit of the absorbed dose is joule/Kg. The special name of the unit of absorbed dose is Gy.

3. Equivalent Dose:

The equivalent dose (H) is a quantity derived from the absorbed dose and takes care of the type of radiation and its energy for the difference of biological effects imparted by the radiation (harm to the body tissues).

H= D x wR

W R takes care of differences in the biological effectiveness of different types of ionising radiation. The unit of equivalent dose is Joule/Kg, and its special name is Sievert (Sv).

4. Radioactivity:

The spontaneous emission of radiation from the nucleus of an unstable atom, wherein the unstable atom disintegrates into a comparatively stable atom (either a different atom or the same atom in a lower energy state).

The number of disintegrations the radioactive substance undergoes per unit of time is known as activity (A) of the radioactive substance.

A= λN

The SI unit of activity is Bq (1 disintegration per second), and the special unit is Ci.

QUANTITY	EXPOSURE (X)	DOSE (D)	EQUIVALENT DOSE(H)	ACTIVITY (A)
DEFINITION	X= ΔQ/Δm air	D= ΔE/ Δm med	H= DwR	A= λN
SI UNIT	C/Kg air	GRAY (Gy) J/Kg	SEIVERT (Sv)	BECQUEREL (Bq)s^{-1}
OLD UNIT	Roentgen (R)	Rad (100 ergs/g)	Rem	Curie
CONVERSION FACTOR	1 R= 2.58 x 10^{-4}C/kg	1 Gy= 100 rad	1 Sv= 100 rem	1 Bq= 1 Ci/ 3.7 X 10^{10}

ΔQ is the charge of either sign collected;

Δm air: mass of air;

ΔE: absorbed energy;

Δm med: mass of medium;

W_R: radiation weighing factor;

λ: decay constant;

N: number of radioactive atoms;

STP: standard temperature (273.2 K) and standard pressure (101.3 kPa)

The discovery of X-rays marked the beginning of numerous experiments worldwide. Considering the dangers of radioactivity and radiation, the International X-ray and Radium Protection Committee was organised in 1928 and was renamed the International Commission of Radiological Protection in 1950. (ICRP).

Risks with radiation exposure can only be restricted and cannot be eliminated due to the:

- Natural availability of Radioactive Sources.
- Increasing Manufacturing of Artificial Radioactive Sources.
- Essential Necessity of these sources in healthcare, industries and agriculture.

Deterministic effects:

These effects occur at relatively large doses and are sure to occur if the dose exceeds a threshold level. The severity of a deterministic effect in exposed individuals increases as the dose increases above the threshold.

Examples:

Skin Erythema: 2-5 Gy

Irreversible Skin Damage: 20-40 Gy

Sterility: 2-3 Gy.

Stochastic effects:

Delayed effects of radiation exposure can also induce malignancies and hereditary effects, expressed after a latency period and are called stochastic effects and occur without a threshold level:

- The probability of occurrence is higher for higher doses.
- The severity of the cancer is independent of dose.

Examples:

Cancer induction

Radiation-induced genetic effects.

Radiation Protection Quantities:

5. **Effective Dose:**

Effective dose (E) is a quantity for radiation protection. Different tissues have a different probability for stochastic effects of radiation. Effective dose incorporates tissue weighting factor for differences in biological effectiveness of different tissues for ionising radiation.

$E = H \times W_T$

W T is Tissue Weighing Factor

The effective dose has the same unit as the equivalent dose.

6. Organ dose:

Organ dose is the mean dose in a specified tissue or organ in the human body.

D T = 1/ mT ∫m T D d m = ε T/m T

mT - the mass of the organ or tissue under consideration

ε T is the total energy imparted by radiation to that tissue or organ.

7. Committed Dose:

When radionuclides are taken into the body, the resulting dose is received throughout the period they remain in the body. The total dose delivered during this period is the committed dose. It is defined as the specified time integral of the rate of receipt of the dose.

Summary of annual dose limits according to BSS schedule II and ICRP report 60

	Effective dose (whole-body) (mSv)	Equivalent dose (eye lens) (mSv)	Equivalent dose (hands, feet, skin) (mSv)
Occupational exposure	20, averaged over five consecutive years, 50 in a single year[a]	20 mSv per year, averaged over a defined period of 5 years, with no single year exceeding 50 mSv	500
Exposure to apprentices 16–18 years of age	6	50	150
Public exposure	1, averaged over five consecutive years, 5 in a single year[b]	15	50

[a]Provided that the average effective dose over five consecutive years does not exceed 2 mSv/a.

[b]Provided that the average effective dose over five consecutive years does not exceed 1 mSv/a.

Blood Irradiation Chambers:

Gamma Irradiation Chambers (GIC), Gamma Chambers, Blood Irradiators (BI) or Gamma Cells are Self-contained Dry Source Storage Gamma Irradiators. A GIC unit mainly houses ^{60}Co or ^{137}Cs doubly encapsulated sources placed in a source cage assembly and is kept shielded at all times by lead encased in stainless steel material.

Within the GIC, the blood components are contained within a metal canister rotating turntable. Continuous rotation of the canister allows for the g rays from ^{137}Cs through pencil sources, which penetrate the entire portion of the blood component. The irradiation chamber is enclosed within a lead shield.

[60]Co containing Free standing irradiators as the source of g rays are comparable, except that the canister containing the blood component does not rotate.

In these chambers, tubes of 60 Co are placed in a circular array around the entire canister within the lead chamber. When freestanding irradiators are used, the rays are attenuated as they pass through air and blood at different rates. The magnitude of attenuation is more with ^{137}Cs than with ^{60} Co

Alternatively, Linear Accelerators have gained popularity for Blood irradiation.

Linear accelerators generate X-ray photon beams over a field of a given dimension and are projected on a tabletop structure. The blood component is then placed (flat) between biocompatible plastic sheets that can range several centimetres thick. The plastic sheet that wraps the top of the blood component, which is nearer to the gantry, generates an electronic equilibrium with secondary electrons at the point where they enter through the component container. The plastic sheet wrap on the bottom of the blood component provides for irradiation back-scattering. This helps to ensure the homogenous delivery of the x-ray photon beam.

The blood component is left stationary on the couch of the Linear Accelerator when the entire x-ray dose is delivered.

Alternatively, flipping over the blood component when one-half of the dose has been delivered can also be carried out; however, this process involves turning off and restarting the linear accelerator during the irradiation procedure.

Dose mapping with linear accelerators

Linear accelerators used for therapeutic radiation therapy are carefully monitored to ensure dose accuracy in the irradiation field. However, when blood components are treated with x-rays, the instrument settings vary compared to therapeutic settings. Hence, additional periodic quality control measures are necessary to assess the dose delivered to blood components.

An ideal dosimeter for this purpose is the tissue-compatible plastic phantom, which contains appropriate dosimeter material. An alternative approach involves using water-filled blood bags (simulating a blood unit) containing TLD chips. Besides, every year, dose mapping should be performed using a tissue compatible phantom.

The following should be measured when irradiating blood components in a linear accelerator:

i. distance between the x-ray source and the position where the blood components are placed;
ii. consistency in the strength of the x-ray beam used
iii. the intensity of the x-ray beam.

	Linear accelerators	Freestanding irradiators
Dose	2500 cGy to the centre of an irradiation field, minimum 1500 cGy elsewhere	2500 cGy to the central midplane of a canister minimum of 1500 cGy elsewhere.

Dose mapping	Yearly dose mapping with an ionisation chamber and a water phantom.	Routinely, once a year, Cs-137 or twice a year Co-60 and after significant repairs, the irradiation procedure should be tested using a fully filled canister with a dosimetry system to map the distribution.
Correction for radioisotopic decay	Not required	Cs-137; annually Co-60; every 3 month

Storage time (after irradiation) Red cells: 28 days; total storage time cannot exceed the maximum storage time for unirradiated red cells

Platelets: No change due to the irradiation.

Advantages of Cesium Irradiators:

- Fewer resources-both financial and human resources
- Low purchase, maintaining and operating cost
- Ease of use and lesser requirement for electricity

X-Ray Irradiators: Recently, the interest in X-ray-based irradiators has gained momentum because of the following drawbacks with Gamma Irradiators:

- use of radioactive source
- stringent health and safety regulations
- disasters like earthquakes, tsunamis or terrorism can cause health hazards due to leakage from these irradiators
- expensive for commissioning as well as decommissioning
- source amenable for decay and hence irradiation time may be increased as well a requirement for regular recalibration

Two forms:

1. A machine where a drawer holding blood bags is irradiated between two X-ray tubes
2. Blood bags are placed on a carousel which moves in a complete circle around a single X-ray tube

Comparison of X-ray irradiators against Gamma Irradiators

	X-ray irradiators	Irradiators Cesium based
Weight	2000 pounds	Up to 4000 pounds
Security and shielding	Lesser requirement	Very stringent
Turnaround time	Faster (<5 min)	Goes on increasing
Accommodation	Up to 6 RBCs at a time	Usually 3
Plasma haemoglobin	Slightly higher comparatively	
RBC Membrane permeability	Slightly higher	

Radiation Protection Protocol for Blood Irradiation:

Gamma Irradiation Chambers are extensively used in blood banks to irradiate blood and blood products/components for clinical and research purposes in various universities and academic and research institutes.

Therefore, regarding radiation protection, specific requirements must be met to ensure the safety of radiation workers and public members.

- **Certification and Documentation:**

Records relating to the sealed source(s) must provide the following information:

a. Make, model number and identification number of source and details of the contained radioisotope, activity and date of measurement of activity.
b. Physical and chemical form of the source
c. Sealed source classification certificate obtained from a national organisation (e.g. AERB/ ISO/ANSI)
d. Bend test certificate, as per the applicable standard
e. Leak test certificate, as per the applicable standard
f. Contamination test certificate, as per the applicable standard.
g. Special form test certificate by the transportation authorities if required
h. Documentation required by the Competent Authority.

The certificates listed above should be obtained from an accredited laboratory/ manufacturer

- **Leakage Radiation Levels for GIC:**

The exposure rates measured at 1 meter from the accessible surface of the GIC are calculated to the effective centre of the detector chamber and averaged over an area of 100 square centimetres (cm^2) with no linear dimension greater than 20 cm.

Measurements at a distance of 5 cm from the accessible surface of the GIC are measured as the effective centre of the detector chamber averaged over an area of 10 square centimetres (cm^2) having no linear dimension greater than 5 cm.

Mode of Operation	Location	Maximum Threshold
Irradiate/ Storage	5 cm from the accessible surface	200 micro Sv/hr
	1 m from the accessible surface	20 micro Sv/hr
Sample load/ Unload/ Transient	5 cm from the accessible surface	2 mSv/hr
	1 m from the accessible surface	100 micro Sv/hr

- **Radiation Protection Survey and Radiometry of GIC:**

The radiometry test report must include the following:

a. Make, model and serial number of the machine and the source used
b. Sealed source specifications must include the following:

     i.   Name of source manufacturer or supplier
    ii.   Identity of radionuclide source
   iii.   Source model, serial number and activity of each sealed source as of the date of manufacture
   iv.   Source geometry, total source activity as of the date of manufacture.

c. Date of radiation protection survey conducted

d. Measure the radiation levels with the GIC in different modes of operation with recordings of the positions where readings were taken.

e. Make, model, serial number and date of the recent calibration of the survey instrument.

f. Particulars of the individual responsible for radiometry and the dosimetric calculations for the survey.

- **Operational Safety Features:**

General radiation safety features should be provided to preclude the presence of radiation levels in excess.

a. The irradiator should not be operable until all shielding is in place and all other safety devices are actuated and activated.

b. The GIC mechanism and controls should be designed to protect against operational errors, such as should the irradiator be operated in an incorrect sequence. In case more than one control/command is actuated simultaneously, it shall not function.

c. Provision for manually returning the GIC to its 'not in use' mode in the event of power failure should be provided.

d. Termination of irradiation and return to its 'not in use' mode at any time must be provided.

e. Each irradiator must have a master control that should be used to prevent unauthorised operation. This control can be a key-operated switch.

f. For operational security, the GIC design should have safety features such as password protection, key-operated switch, mechanical lock and key etc.

- **Quality Assurance and Check:**

Aspects to be considered for developing an adequate QA & QC programme:

a. Quality assurance organisation and committee

b. Design control protocols

c. Manufacturing process controls and

d. Documentation and records of the programme

- **Radiological Safety Requirements:**

As part of the radiation protection programme, the employer should have the following safety infrastructure.

   o **Personnel Monitoring Service**

The appropriate personnel monitoring device has to be used to determine radiation doses received by each person who:

a. is involved in the routine operation and maintenance of the GIC unit, and

b. frequently uses the GIC unit for handling samples for irradiation.

When not in use, the TLD badges have to be kept in an isolated and specified location away

from GIC installation in a radiation-free area under the custody of the RSO.

- ○ **Radiation Monitoring**

  a. The employer/licensee should ensure that a suitable radiation measuring instrument is available in working condition to carry out the radiation protection survey of the GIC unit.
  b. The radiation survey meter must be periodically calibrated at least once in two years, and records maintained for the same.
  c. The calibration of a radiation survey meter must be traceable to the national/international standards laboratory.

- ○ **Radiation Protection Surveillance of GIC Unit**

  An initial radiation protection survey should be performed in the room and surroundings where the GIC unit is installed. The manufacturer/supplier should provide the radiation protection survey report and installation report to the user institution. These initial radiation levels are the baseline measurements at the site for future reference.

  The employer/licensee should ensure that the RSO carries out the routine radiation protection surveys of the GIC unit at least once in three months and maintain the records after each inspection.

  The radiation protection surveys of the GIC unit:

  To be undertaken in the event of any incident which may hamper the normal functioning of the GIC unit,

  e.g., stuck sample chamber,

  breakdown of wire rope/driving mechanism

  after every servicing/ repair of the GIC unit.

- • **Source Loading in a New GIC Unit**

To be carried out in a newly fabricated GIC unit manufactured as per the relevant Safety Standards and guidelines. The following measures are to be adopted:

a. The source of desired activity loaded in the source cage should not exceed the approved strength.

b. The radiation levels and contamination levels of the GIC unit loaded with a source should be measured, and records maintained with measurement time.

c. Tests/trials such as functionality, radiometry, dosimetry, proper markings and labelling should be carried out before dispatching the GIC unit to the concerned facility.

- **Source Replenishment**

In case of source replenishment, the manufacturer must perform checks on components, the systems such as source container assembly from a radiation safety point of view, critical weld joints (circumferential and longitudinal) of the outer shell of the container and for subsequent repair if required.

- **Procedure for Disposal**

The licensee should obtain prior approval from the Competent Authority for decommissioning, transporting and safely disposing of radioactive material. After this, the licensee should approach the manufacturer/supplier to decommission and transport disused sources in the GIC unit.

The room housing GIC can be released for any other use by the institution only after decommissioning the GIC installation.

- **Transport of GIC for Disposal**

The packaging and transport of the GIC unit should comply with the safe transport requirements of radioactive material as prescribed by the Competent Authority.

- **Emergency Response Plans and Preparedness**

The licensee should prepare emergency response plans, incorporating emergency scenarios and situations that may be encountered and action plan response to these emergencies to mitigate their consequences.

- **Reporting of Radiation Emergency**

Employer/licensee should report every unusual incident or emergency to the Competent Authority immediately or within 24 hours. The details should include the following:

    a. Date and time of its occurrence
    b. Brief description of the unusual incident or emergency
    c. Source activity at the time of the incident
    d. Action that was taken by the authority
    e. Probable cause of the incident
    f. Personnel radiation exposure due to the incident
    g. Lessons learned to prevent similar incidents and accidents in the future
    h. Improvement in emergency plans and preparedness.

Hyperkalemia as an effect of transfusion of irradiated blood: It has been estimated that the K+ concentration of CPDA-1 RBC at a haematocrit of 70 per cent at 35 days of storage (permitted shelf life) will be around 70-80 meq/litre. The transfusion dose in a neonate is 15 ml/kg; in a one kg neonate, only 0.3 to 0.4 meq K+ will be infused. This dose is smaller than the usual daily requirement of 2-3 meq/kg. However, this rationale will not apply to large-volume transfusions (>25 ml/kg), such as exchange transfusions

EQUIPMENT MAINTENANCE

Steps in equipment and materials management:

1. Selection
2. Procurement
3. Distribution
4. Maintenance

The goal of equipment and material management: provide the blood facility with all the resources needed to produce high-quality output as per the expectations of the end-users

Why maintenance?

- To make sure it works efficiently
- For longer life of the equipment
- Minimises chance of equipment failure

<table>
<tr><td>

Essential steps in establishing a planned maintenance programme:

- Create a register of all equipment that will require maintenance and calibration. Determine the interval
- Establish acceptable performance specifications for each type of equipment with acceptable fluctuation
- Have a Maintenance agreement in place
- Accurate record-keeping to provide a history of the equipment's performance and assist in making decisions

</td></tr>
</table>

Criteria for choosing a supplier

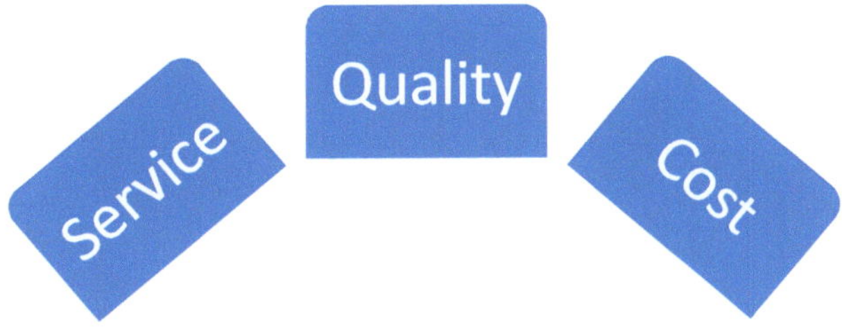

Factors to consider while choosing a supplier

Certification or accreditation by an accreditation agency

Assured continuity of supply and hold of stock.

Transparency to audit the facility.

Own quality audits, including customer feedback

Financial soundness

Their other installations

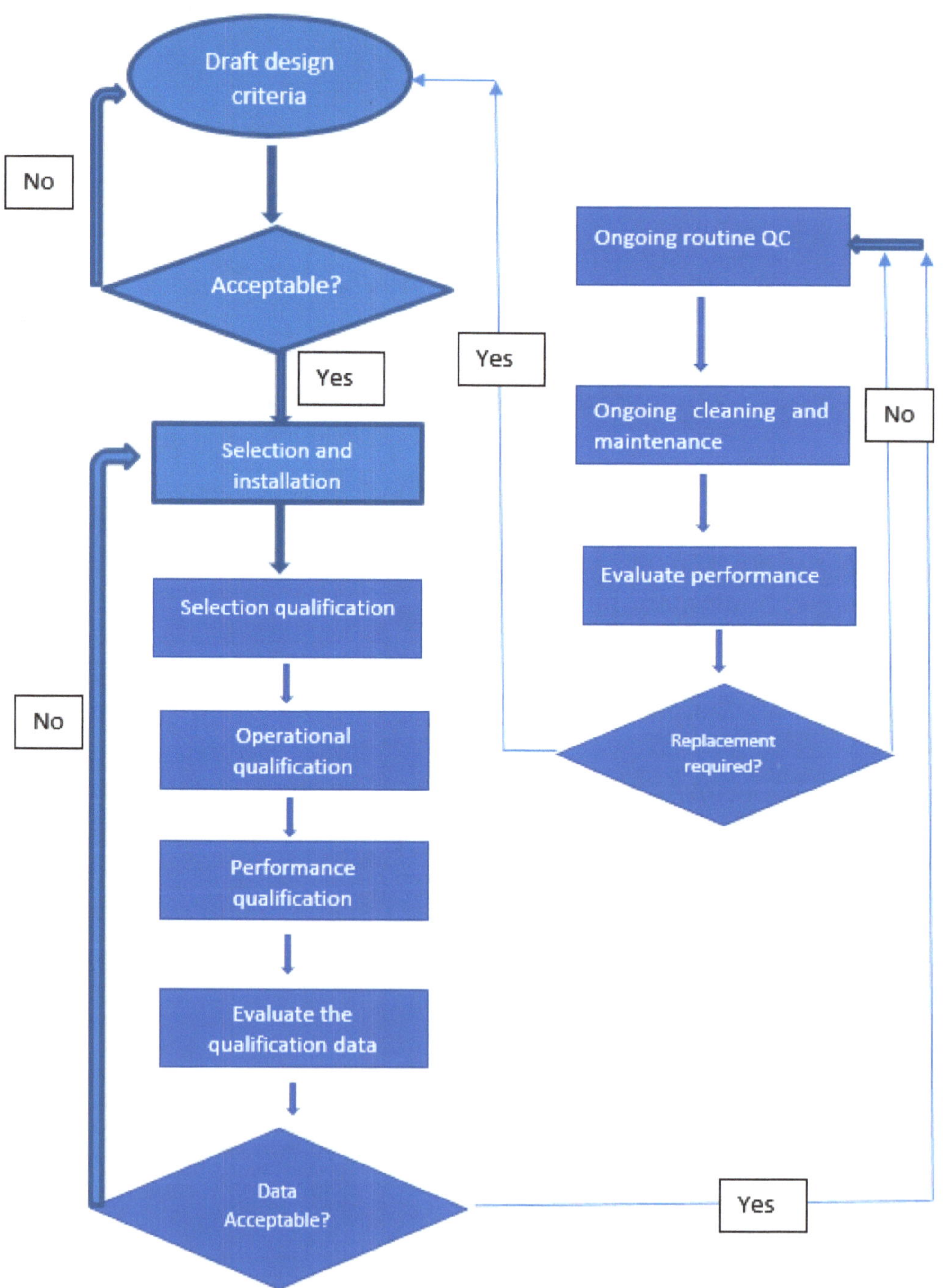

Figure 33. The Equipment cycle

Design Qualification: (DQ) process of documenting the functional requirements of an equipment. E.g. for a tabletop centrifuge, the Design qualifications would include the following:

- ✓ How many tubes must the centrifuge be able to hold at one time?
- ✓ What are the sizes of these tubes?
- ✓ What is the maximum gravitational force that will be required?
- ✓ What is the range of time that the automatic timer must cover?
- ✓ Is the user protected against aerosols? Is it possible to operate the centrifuge while the lid is open?

It would also include general elements like the Possible effect of temperature, humidity and lighting conditions in the working environment, the requirement for an uninterruptible power supply (UPS), the requirement of special supplies like distilled or deionised water, training requirements etc

Eliminating controllable environmental variables, such as temperature, humidity, light and extent of operator training, will reduce the variation in the overall process and make it more likely that the equipment will consistently deliver the expected performance.

Installation qualification: (IQ) involves establishing that the equipment's key aspects, including ancillary equipment such as power or purified water supplies, are installed strictly according to the manufacturer's specifications and that any additional recommendations have been addressed.

It will include steps to confirm that the equipment is received as specified, that it is undamaged and installed correctly, and that the environment into which it is installed meets the requirements of that equipment.

Operational qualification (OQ)

Calibrating, challenging, testing and evaluating the equipment after installation ensures that it functions as expected in the selected environment. It includes reviewing the standard operating procedures (SOPs) for the start-up, operation, maintenance, and equipment cleaning.

Performance qualification (PQ)

The process of ensuring that the instrument consistently and reliably performs according to the defined specifications on an ongoing basis in the environment in which it will be used routinely involves carrying out a series of tests using the equipment following the relevant SOPs. All test results must be evaluated to determine whether they meet the requirements of the organisation.

An example of a Refrigerated Centrifuge	
DQ	How many blood bags are to be centrifuged at one time? What is the size of the bags? What is the size of the centrifuge buckets? Will the centrifuge and the proposed rotor provide sufficient g to affect/ produce the separation required? What is the temperature range available/required? Does the centrifuge provide control over acceleration and braking? Is there a provision for customising centrifugation programmes to produce various components?
IQ	What variation in the temperature during a spin cycle is acceptable?
OQ	Required specifications for each blood component to be produced using the centrifuge enable the spinning speed, spinning time, and rate of acceleration and deceleration to be selected. Rewrite SOPs based on these
PQ	The SOP will produce acceptable components consistently. Acceptable fluctuation

At least three batches should be run to demonstrate that the SOP will produce acceptable components consistently

Management of Blood Component Inventory in the Blood Bank

– Dr. Shaiji PS

GOAL

The goal of a good blood component inventory management programme in a blood centre is to maintain enough stock of blood components to guarantee 100% availability and yet minimise expiry.

To ensure an adequate inventory without wastage, the following steps are necessary:

1. **Blood Need Assessment**

Blood centres should assess the need for blood components, which should be regularly reviewed. Methods for need assessment can be adapted depending on the location and previous experience.

Method 1. Based on the number of units of blood used in a specified period in a defined geographical area or population.

The calculation assumes that 1-2% of the population may require blood annually.

Method 1 can calculate the blood requirements of individual regions or districts within the country or if a particular blood bank is the only centre catering to a geographically distinct area.

Method 2: Based on acute hospital beds. Calculate seven units of blood per hospital bed(WHO, 1971) and 20.3 per acute care bed per year. Method 2 is helpful in the initial years of the blood bank, where no consistent prior data is available.

Method 3: Analyse previous blood usage and requests for blood to indicate whether the demand for blood is constant, increasing or decreasing and calculate the average demand daily/monthly.

An additional 10-20% of the calculated estimate should be collected for disasters/unexpected demands

Method 3 may be more centre specific and closer to the actual demand in an already established blood centre, directly calculated from the previous demand and issue.

2. Set Appropriate Inventory Levels

Once target inventory levels are determined, these levels should be maintained by a "stock up" policy. It is ideal to maintain a stock equivalent to approximately 4-6 days of average daily use of red blood cells and two days of average daily use of platelets (based on average annual use divided by the number of days when most blood is used). Inventory calculators/software can be used for this. When the stock falls below set levels, appropriate measures should be taken to replenish the same urgently.

Day's Cover/Issuable Stock Index

Day's Cover (Issuable stock index)is the number of days of available stock held in inventory for a particular product.

Issuable stock index (ISI) =Number of issuable(unreserved)units presently in inventory/Average daily use

Average daily use is the number of units ordered in a year/365(if blood is not issued on all 365 days of the year, this number can be changed accordingly)

E.g.:If 14,600 units of red cells are ordered over 12 months in a blood bank,

Average daily use is 14600 ÷ 365 = 40 units per day

 Number of available units in stock = 200

Days cover = 200 ÷ 40 = 5

The blood bank has RBCs adequate for five days' coverage. For each component, this should be calculated separately.

It is ideal to have a day's cover of 6 for RBCs and plasma. At least three days' coverage should be ensured in periods of shortage. For products like platelets, having a more extensive stock is not practical, yet a minimum of 2 days' cover is essential.

3. STOCK ENTRY

Manual

Many blood banks use a physical count of blood components daily and manually enter a register in India.

Daily Physical verification is cumbersome and time consuming, although it gives an additional opportunity to discard apparently poor quality(hemolysis/discolouration etc.)units and remove them from stock

Electronic

Automatic addition of collected units and deletion of issued units and TTD positives/discard makes it easier to manage inventory

Even in computerised stock maintenance systems, periodic physical verification is necessary. If coupled with an RFID system, convenience and traceability improve further.

Full transparency of stock levels, including remote refrigerators and storage centres, should be ensured on stock entry.

4. IMPLEMENTATION OF POLICIES TO CONSERVE INVENTORY

Target stock levels based on experience should be adjusted continuously. Profiling with lab software may be used to adjust based on daily demand patterns

When Blood utilisation practices change at the hospital(e.g., introducing new specialities), the target inventory levels should be revised. Adjust the inventory target levels if significant seasonal demand fluctuations occur, such as areas with seasonal residents or tourists/festivals/infections, etc

Store units sorted by age and use visual highlighting for units close to expiry; instruct staff

Keep large reserved stocks(assigned inventories for patient/patient groups) as low as possible. Question and challenge internal requests for blood to keep assigned inventories low and reduce just-in-case requests

Check Remote refrigerators(If any) regularly and return units to the primary storage

Careful handling of recurring orders and panic orders. Screening of orders, guidelines, audits and consultation with a transfusion medicine physician can help reduce unnecessary or inappropriate ordering of blood

For issuing, follow Strict First-In-First-Out (FIFO) principle

Split big orders into several small orders to get different shelf lives

Use standing orders to reduce workload and replenish using "top-up orders."

Use action levels and pre-defined order quantities for "out-of-hours" time to prevent panic orders

First In First Out policy(FIFO): Wherever appropriate, when products are received/manufactured, they should be sorted to be used on an oldest-product-first-out basis. Unless specific requirements for certain patient groups, ensure that a strict 'oldest unit first out' policy is adhered to.

Arrange inventory to ensure the oldest (the ones with the shortest remaining shelf life) are at the front of the storage shelf.

Alert staff to units that will be outdating soon. e.g., RBC (5 days), platelets (1 day), plasma protein products, and frozen products (three months). Ensure that they will be used first.

Use visual aids such as an expiring unit list on the storage unit or place distinctive tags on the units. Include reserved units (which may be kept in a separate area) in this process by moving them into useable inventory before they reach the end of their shelf life.

Identify units near expiry

If a product is getting close to expiry, pre-defined options might include transferring to another hospital or laboratory, rotating segregated inventories where possible, and highlighting that the product will soon expire. For example, BC can make up a sign/sticker for the fridge that clearly identifies stock with short expiry, enabling it to be the first selected for issue.

Return Policy

Indications for blood issues from the blood bank and return policy should be clearly defined to avoid wastage.

If blood is to be reintroduced into the inventory, ensure that temperature is maintained throughout the transit. Data loggers are ideal for this purpose. Also, ensure sterility was maintained.

Sending to storage centre/remote facility

It is better to choose fresher products but rotate them more regularly back into the general inventory

The product should have adequate shelf life left before expiry when moved from reserved or remote locations back to general inventory

Exceptions to FIFO

Some exceptional clinical circumstances where using the oldest blood first may not be appropriate includes Neonatal exchange transfusions. Hospitals should have a policy that describes the limited clinical situations where using the oldest blood first may not be appropriate.

Rare groups

O Rh(D) negative RBC for non-O Rh(D) negative recipients should be used only when indicated, i.e., lack of time/resources to find a donor. This practice should be monitored and reviewed regularly to ensure inventory levels are kept at optimum levels to avoid wastage and ensure a sufficient supply for patients who really need them.

Implement policies to address the management of group O Rh(D) negative RBCs to preserve these lower-incidence blood components. These policies should include reserving them for female patients of childbearing potential and children

Overstocking blood from very rare groups may result in RBCs not being readily available for patients with RBC antibodies in other hospitals. As far as possible, bleed such donors when the need is confirmed, especially when frozen storage facilities are unavailable.

Reserve

Limit crossmatch/reserve inventory.

Regular review and return to available inventory as soon as possible (within 24-48 hours) will reduce the number of units being held.

For surgical patients, a review of the patient's surgical blood use, the most recent postoperative haemoglobin result, and the presence of any clinically significant alloantibodies may assist with the decision

Avoid Wastage At Surgical Site

Increasing awareness of the value of blood components and products, timelines for availability, and the risks involved with transfusion can also improve practice and minimise wastage

MSBOS

Establish a maximum surgical blood order schedule (MSBOS). An MSBOS is based on a hospital's past RBC use and serves as a guideline for future surgical and other RBC transfusion requests. An MSBOS can guide ordering practice and avoid "just in case" ordering.

Endorsement by a hospital's transfusion committee, communication of the MSBOS guidelines to hospital physicians, surgeons, and nurse practitioners, and regular review of the MSBOS guidelines are critical to its success.

Crossmatch requests that exceed the MSBOS guidelines may require consultation. The use of preprinted order sets can also improve ordering practices.

DISCARDS AS A PERCENTAGE OF ISSUES (DAPI)

Discard as a Percentage of Issues (DAPI) is a good way to "discard data" of the blood centre comparable with other health providers. This will allow each BC to benchmark the discards against others. A certain level of discard, particularly fresh products with short expiry dates, is inevitable and appropriate to ensure that products are available where and when they are clinically necessary. However, a proportion of discards of blood and blood products is neither inevitable nor appropriate, which is termed wastage.

DAPI = Number of units discarded/ the total amount of blood and blood product units received X100

Example: If 100 RBC units are wasted over 12 months, and 10,000 RBC are issued in your facility over 12 months, DAPI is 1%

DAPI can also be referred to as WAPI (wastage as a percentage of issue). Generally, a discard that is neither inevitable nor appropriate is termed wastage.

5. **Clinician Awareness**

A. Alternate groups –Best Choices

For effective inventory management, knowledge about alternate blood groups used in shortage is essential for blood bank staff and ordering physicians. The choice of alternate components is listed below.

Alternative choices for the selection of RBC

RECIPIENT GROUP	O	A	B	AB
1st choice	O	A	B	AB
2nd choice	-	O	O	A
3rd choice	-	-	-	B
4th choice	-	-	-	O

Alternative choices for the selection of platelets

RECIPIENT GROUP	O	A	B	AB
1st choice	O	A	B	AB
2nd choice	A	AB	AB	A
3rd choice	B	B	A	B
4th choice	AB	O	O	O

Alternative choices for selection FFP AND CRYOPRECIPITATE

RECIPIENT GROUP	O	A	B	AB
1st choice	O	A	B	AB
2nd choice	A	AB	AB	-
3rd choice	B	-	-	-
4th choice	AB	-	-	-

NOTE:

- Individuals with blood group A can be transfused with group B FFP (and vice versa) only as a last option. If issued so, FFP is tested for high titre anti-B (or anti-A)
- ABO compatibility is not required for Cryoprecipitate except in the neonatal period.
- FFP and Cryoprecipitate can be transfused irrespective of RhD type.
- RhD-negative females of childbearing potential should receive RhD-negative platelets. If unavailable, RhD-positive platelets can be given with anti-D prophylaxis.
- All RhD-positive individuals can be transfused with RhD-negative packed red cells.
- RhD-negative individuals should always receive RhD-negative red cells. In dire emergency and lifesaving situations, if RhD negative units are unavailable, RhD positive red cells can be used, provided anti-D is absent.

6. Prioritisation

It is the responsibility of a blood centre to make sure that any patient who satisfies the criteria and indications for transfusion should be provided with blood. However, it becomes essential sometimes to prioritise the issue of blood between patients because blood is a limited resource, and inventories may not always be adequate. Factors that help us to prioritise are

a. Bleeding: A patient with bleeding/shock is given preference to the non-bleeding patient

b. Unstable /sick patients and neonates are given preference because of a chance of sudden deterioration

c. Primary disease: A disease in which the chance of bleeding is more is given preference(e.g. APML is given preference over aplastic anaemia for platelet transfusion)

d. Threshold laboratory value/trigger: In the absence of no risk factors in either patient, a patient with lower laboratory value is given preference, as well as Symptomatic patients

e. For Rh D negative groups, females of childbearing age should be given preference if indicated

f. in the absence of adequate inventory, elective procedures may be postponed to conserve blood for emergency

7. Collaboration

Bulk Transfer: Look for an opportunity to share blood components between two adjacent hospitals with different demands of the type of blood components.Implement redistribution to minimise outdated

Smaller hospitals can consider an arrangement to transfer "soon to outdate" blood components and products to a nearby larger hospital with a higher demand

Use internal service level agreements /MOUs to generate mutual understanding

Packing procedures must ensure that the blood components/products are maintained at the appropriate conditions during transport and that the appropriate documentation accompanies the transfer

8. Monitoring

Blood utilisation reviews

The hospital Transfusion Committee should monitor transfusion practices for all categories of blood and components, including monitoring of usage and discard and appropriateness of use in a combination of methods. All forms of review can be used to effect changes in transfusion practice. Utilisation reviews may be combined with other interventions such as education, practical usage of guidelines, and the attending physician's accountability.

Prospective (Real-Time) Review

Transfusion requests are reviewed in real-time using prespecified guidelines (i.e., review of individual transfusion requests before the issue of the components)so that it is possible to intervene or even stop or modify inappropriate transfusion requests

Concurrent Review

Review individual transfusion requests that occur in the 12–24 h following the transfusion episode. But the concurrent review can only alter the future blood transfusion practice

Retrospective Review

A retrospective review allows a review of aggregate transfusion data and trends in transfusion utilisation. The mean or the median number of component units transfused per hospitalised patient and procedure provides a more meaningful summary of component use. Results should be reviewed by the transfusion medicine/patient blood management committee.

Quality indicators of blood utilisation

1. Crossmatch to transfusion ratio (CT ratio)= number of units crossmatched/number of units transfused
2. Transfusion Probability (%T)=number of patients transfused/ number of patients crossmatchedx100
3. Transfusion index (TI)=number of units transfused/number of patients transfused

Lower these indicators, the better the transfusion utilisation. Hence each hospital can set its own benchmark compared to the previous experience and data.

Generally, A CT ratio of 2.5 or below, a Transfusion probability of ≥30%, and a TI of more than 0.5 indicate efficient blood utilisation.

9. Training

During regular training and refreshing courses make BC staff aware of the impact of wasting a unit. Motivate staff to keep wastage low

Ensure that experienced staff are placing orders and handling incoming deliveries Give intensive training to clinical staff who orders and handles blood regarding appropriate indications, handling, storage, the procedure of transfusion, conditions for return etc. Nonconformance may be reported to HTC.

Regular auditing of transfusion practices

Documentation of Results in Transfusion Medicine

– Dr. Shamee S

Introduction:

Documentation is an integral part of good laboratory practice. It allows us to track and review laboratory activities. Accurate documentation helps in problem-solving. Maintaining a detailed logbook of all the academic activities, tests, and procedures done during the postgraduate training period is very useful. It may provide you with the necessary data while drafting a scientific report or in the publication process.

Basics of Documentation in transfusion Medicine:

- Mention the condition of the specimen received
- Concurrent documentation: Record each reaction AS YOU READ IT
- Record POSITIVE reactions as + and NEGATIVE reactions as **0**
- Do NOT use a minus sign for negative results in serology
- Mention the units of measurement
- Do not use jargon/shortened forms of words (BG, Cxm, Tx)
- Mention the tests performed and essential steps
- Mention the reference (AABB method, Mollison's formula, etc.)
- Mention the interpretation of testing results

1. Immunohaematological Tests:

1.1 Blood grouping: The following pattern may be followed to document the results:

Table 1: The sample format to document the results of blood grouping

1.	Patient Details	Name, Hospital Number, Age, Gender
2.	Request form	ABO & Rh typing
3.	Sample identification	Match with the request form. Check for labelling errors or clerical errors
4.	Sample Appearance	Comment on the appearance. Mention the abnormal findings such as hemolysis or lipemia
5.	Method of testing	Tube method / Column agglutination technique /Microplate technique
6.	Reagent Used	QC; specificity - Passed Manufacturer; Lot No; Expiry

II Part:

Cell Grouping				Serum Grouping			
Anti A	Anti B	Anti D 1	Anti D 2	A cells	B Cells	O Cells	Auto Ctl.
4+	0	0	0	0	4+	0	0
Weak D typing	+/0 (if applicable weak D typing needs to be performed)						
Interpretation	"A" Rh-D negative; No discrepancy noted						
Resolution of discrepancy (if any)	Lectin study		Test	Positive Ctl.	Negative Ctl.	Remark	
	Antibody screening						
	Incubation at 4°C						
	Incubation at 37°C						
	Other relevant tests						

1.2 Direct Antiglobulin Testing (DAT):

Direct antiglobulin testing establishes the in-vivo sensitization of the red blood cells. It is performed as a part of a workup in patients with autoimmune hemolytic anaemia, transfusion reactions, delayed hemolytic reactions, and in a suspected case of hemolytic disease in newborns. If positive, further testing, such as elution testing or antibody subtyping, can be suggested. The systematic reporting method of DAT is shown in Table 2

Table 2: The sample format to report the results of DAT

1.	Patient Details	Name, Hospital Number, Age, Gender
2.	Request form	Direct Antiglobulin testing
3.	Clinical details	Diagnosis, Relevant clinical signs
4.	Relevant History	Autoimmune diseases, transfusion history Fever, URTI, Raynaud's phenomenon
5.	Laboratory Investigation	Haemoglobin, Reticulocyte count, total and direct bilirubin levels, LDH, findings on peripheral smear examination
6.	Sample identification	Match with the request form, Labeling error, if any?
7.	Sample Appearance	Auto-agglutination, Hemolysis, Lipemia
8.	Method of testing	Tube / Column agglutination technique
9.	Reagent Used	Manufacturer; Lot No; Expiry:

II Part

Poly-specific AHG	Test	Positive Control	Negative Control.	Auto Control	Check Cells	Interpretation
Grade of Reaction						
Monospecific AHG						
Anti IgG						
Anti C3d						

1.3 Red Cell Antibody Screening:

The initial part of the documentation is similar to that mentioned in table 2. Besides, a history related to pregnancy and blood transfusion can be mentioned. Table 3 shows the sample format for presenting the results of antibody screening. Following the interpretation of the results, the list of probable antibodies can be mentioned, and a workup for antibody identification can be suggested.

Table 3. Sample format for documenting the results of antibody screening

Test				Check cells	Pos Ctl.	Neg Ctl.	Auto Ctl.	Interpretation
	Saline, RT, ISP	At 37°C	At AHG	For tube tech				
Panel I								
Panel II								
Panel III								

Note: RT= Room temperature, ISP= Immediate Spin technique, AHG= Antihuman Globulin phase. Pos = Positive, Neg = Negative, Ctl = control

1.4 Pre-Transfusion Testing:

The initial part of reporting is the same as that of table 2. Pre-transfusion testing involves several major steps; the details are given in table 4.

Table 4. Steps of pre-transfusion testing

No	Steps	Details
1	Review of the request form	It must include the patient's full name, unique identification number, clinical indication, product details, date and time of request and dose of intended transfusion, any special requirement, relevant history, and lab parameters
2	Verification of patient identity, an inspection of the specimen	Patient identifiers need to be crosschecked with the request form and the labels on the blood samples
3	ABO and Rh typing	Report the blood group and check for the discrepancy (Table 1)
4	Antibody screening	Using 2 cell panel (table 3)
5	Selection of testing strategy – Type and screen or type and cross-match or IS technique	Depending on the product to be transfused and the clinical urgency, the appropriate method of compatibility testing needs to be selected.
6	Compatibility testing	The reporting format is shown in Table 5

Table 5. Compatibility testing report

Patient ID Details			Age Gender					
Ward/ Unit			Blood Group					
Sl No	Date and Time	Donor Unit No	Blood Group	Type of Component	Method of Crossmatching	Result of Crossmatching	Done by	Validated by

2. **Transfusion reactions:**

   Report the transfusion reaction workup under the following headings

   a. Patient Details
   b. Patient's History/ Examination
   c. Transfusion Details: This section includes details such as the indication for transfusion, the blood product transfused, unit number, volume, and the time of issue of the product taken for transfusion.
   d. Details of the transfusion reaction:

   - Signs and symptoms:
   - Vitals: Pre and post-transfusion
   - Classification: Immediate/delayed

   e. Reaction workup

   - Test performed by:
   - Samples received:
   - Check for the clerical error
   - Check the bag, the ports and the transfusion filter
   - Details of the blood product transfused: Unit number, Date of collection, date of expiry, bag lot number, manufacturers details
   - Serological testing: Given in Table 6

Table 6. The laboratory workup in a case with a suspected transfusion reaction

Tests	Pre-transfusion	Post-transfusion	Blood unit
ABO group			
Rh Blood group			
DAT			
Antibody screen			
Major Cross Match			
Minor Cross Match			
Plasma Hb			
Urine Hb			NA
Serum Bilirubin			NA
Additional Testing			
Gram stain	NA	NA	

- Interpretation: Probable diagnosis

  Imputability

  Corrective action; Preventive action

  Advice on the management of transfusion reaction and further transfusion support

  Reporting to the haemovigilance program

3. **Quality control:**

   3.1. Quality control of antisera: Perform the quality control testing of the given reagent and compare the results with the standard guidelines. The final comment is expected to state regarding the acceptance of the given reagent.

Table 7. Reporting the results of quality control testing of antisera

Type of Reagents	Result	Interpretation
Manufacturers details, lot number, expiry date		Acceptable/Not Acceptable
Physical appearance, temperature	Colour: Clarity: Volume:	Passed/failed
Titer (Potency)	Grading and scoring of the agglutination reaction	Passed/failed
Specificity	Using A1 cells, B cells, AB cells, and O cells (A2 if applicable)	Passed/failed
Avidity	In seconds	Passed/failed
Interpretation		

3.2 Quality control of Blood Components

When a blood component is given for quality control testing, the student shall check the overall quality of the product and comment if it is acceptable for transfusion. If it is not acceptable, the reason for rejection should be mentioned in such cases. Suggest possible causes for such deviation and the root cause analysis. Students are advised to prepare similar formats to report the results of the QC testing for all other blood components. (Table 8. 9.10)

It is essential to know the method of preparation of the blood component. For example, the WBC count in an RBC unit will vary depending on the preparation method.

Table 8. Reporting format for quality control testing of Red Cell Concentrates.

Parameter	Result	Quality Requirement
Unit Number		Mention DGHS standards for all the parameters
Type of Component		
Date of Collection		
Date of Expiry		
Appearance		
Volume		
Hct		
Hb g%		
WBC count		
Plasma Hb if the unit is near expiry		
Remark	Acceptable/ Reject	If rejected, give the justification

Table 9. Reporting of quality control testing of Platelet Concentrate

Parameter	Result	Quality Requirement
Unit Number		Mention the DGHS standards for all the parameters
Type of Component	RDP/SDP	
Date of Collection		
Date of Expiry		
Appearance		
Volume		
Swirling	Mention the score	
Platelet count /unit		
pH	Mention the method used to check the pH	
WBC count/unit	Mention the method used and express the count per bag	
RBC contamination	Express it mL	
Remark	Acceptable/Reject	If rejected, give the justification

Table 10. Reporting format for quality control testing of cryoprecipitate.

Parameter	Result	Quality Requirement
Unit Number		Mention the DGHS standards for all the parameters
Type of Component		
Date of Collection		
Date of Expiry		
Appearance		
Volume		
PT sec -FFP		
APTT sec		
Factor VIII		
Fibrinogen		
Remark	Acceptable/Reject	If rejected, give the justification

4. **Coagulation tests**

For all coagulation tests, it is crucial to consider the following checkpoints. And the reporting format is given in Table 11

Pre-analytical checkpoints	Analytical checkpoints	Post Analytical checkpoints
Sample identification	Patient test 1	Interpretation of results
Sample labelling	Patient test 2	Validating the results
Sample collection time	Control plasma	Clinical relevance
Sample transportation	Mean of tests 1 & 2	Further tests to be done
Reagents provided	INR calculation	
Cold chain maintenance	A normal lab reference range should follow the test results in brackets	
Water bath temperature		
Stopwatch calibration		
Control plasma identification		

Table 11. Reporting format for the basic coagulation tests

Patient sample ID	Name, Age, Gender, Hospital Number	Time of testing	
Sample collection time		Sample received time	
Control plasma Id	Lot number / serial number, Manufacturing date/expiry date		
Visual inspection of the samples	Appearance, Volume, Whole blood /PPP, Clots, Sample container type		
Reagents	Manufacturer, Lot, Expiry, Appearance		
Cold chain maintenance	Daily temp chart	Water bath temperature	
Pre-warming the reagents to 37 ^{0}C		Stopwatch & Pipette calibration	
QC of reagents	Ask for the Daily QC of the PT reagent and control plasma (PNP).		
Patient test	Test 1	Test 2	Mean
Control plasma test		INR	ISI of the reagent and use the formula
Result	Patient PT – seconds (range) Patient INR -		
Interpretation of PT results	1. Normal /2. Prolonged /3. Shortened		
Inference	Clinical relevance and any other test are suggested		

5. **Reporting of a peripheral smear:**

    The following steps may be followed while reporting a peripheral smear

    – The overall quality of the smear on inspection macroscopically
    – Microscopic screening of the smear: Assess the quality of the preparation. Mention red cell agglutination, rouleaux formation, or platelet aggregation if it is present; assess the number, distribution, and staining of the leucocytes.
    – RBC: Comment on size, shape, colour, distribution, inclusions
    – WBC: Total and differential count, abnormal cells
    – Platelets: count, abnormal cells
    – Parasites
    – Interpretation
    – Advice on further evaluation if required

6. **Incident reporting:**

The incident report shall provide the details of the incident or the near misses. The format for reporting the needle stick injury is given below.

Needlestick reporting format:

a. Demographics:

Name: Age   Gender.   Identification Number:

Circumstances in which injury occurred: Department/work area

b. Details of the injury:

Date and time

Time since injury

Wearing PPE: yes/no

c. The extent of exposure:

Mild/Moderate/severe

d. Source of exposure:

Known source: details....

Status of the source:

Unknown source

e. Status of the exposed person

Baseline details:

HBV Vaccination status, antibody titer

f. First aid details:
g. Counselling
h. Details of post-exposure prophylaxis
i. Root Cause Analysis:
j. Corrective action taken
k. Preventive action taken

Reported By   Date and Time:

DOCUMENTS AND STANDARD OPERATING PROCEDURES

Documentation provides traceability(details of processes- who, what, when, where, how) and trackability (logical sequence of steps)

Forms: templates for the capture of information

Labels: a piece of material attached to an object and containing information about that object

Record: information or data on a specific subject collected methodically, and the account kept in writing or other permanent forms.

Job aid: An excerpt (a piece of information) from an approved procedure or work instruction .e.g a table or flow chart/algorithm that needs to be referenced. They may be included as hyperlinks in computerised documents

Document: A piece of written, printed or electronic that provides information, especially of an official or legal nature

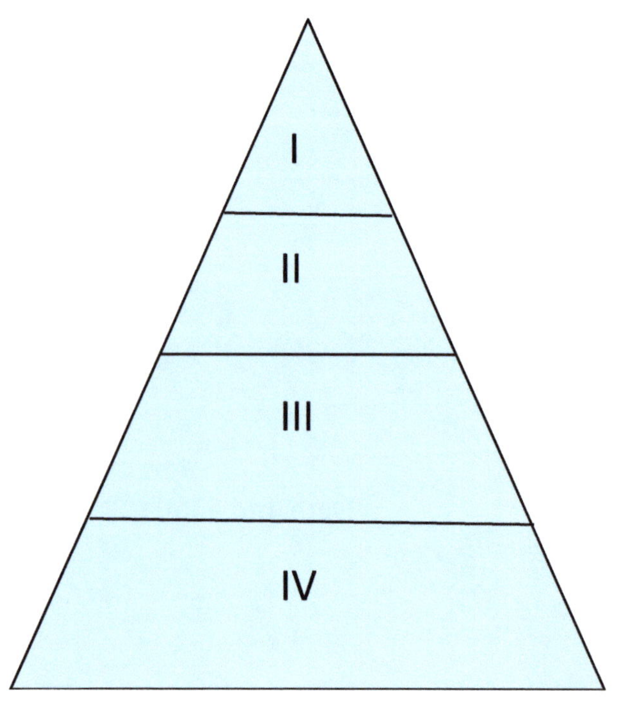

Hierarchy of QMS documents:

Level I - Quality Manual (mission, goals, objectives, and policy statements)

Level II - Responsibilities (training, quality control, validation, and process improvement)

Level III- SOPs

Level IV- Forms, documents, records

Policy: describes how an organisation operates, e.g. Dress code, smoking policy

Standard operating procedures: (SOP)s, also called work instructions, are documents that provide instructions on performing a task and describe who does what and when in sequence/order. They are key in achieving consistency and control in operations. The accreditation and licensing procedures also demand compulsory use of SOP. Individual blood banks must adapt and develop their blood bank-specific SOPs based on the infrastructure available, test procedures to be followed and availability of reagents. SOP needs to be developed for all critical procedures

A model SOP: Each SOP must be given a unique identification number along with the revision number if any

NAME OF THE BLOOD CENTRE

Number	Effective date	Pages	Author	Authorised by
				(quality manager)
Version	**Review period**	**Number of copies**	**Approved by**	**Date**
			(Blood bank Director)	

LOCATION	SUBJECT
FUNCTION	DISTRIBUTION

SCOPE & APPLICATION
What process is this SOP going to explain
What are its uses
RESPONSIBILITY
Who is responsible for implementing and performing the mentioned process/ procedure
REFERENCES
Relevant information/steps are borrowed or written as per...

MATERIAL REQUIRED
What all the things required to complete this process
PROCEDURE
Step-by-step instructions for performing this particular process
INTERPRETATION
How to interpret the results and what they mean
QUALITY ASSURANCE
How to ensure quality for this particular process
DOCUMENTATION
How to document the process and the findings

REGULATION BINDING TRANSFUSION SERVICES

	Licensing	Certification	Accreditation
Meaning	Grant formal authorization to do	To vouch for or confirm	To give credit
Definition	According to the state's policy powers, the state grants legal authority to practice/run within a designated scope.	recognition to an individual/ organization that has met predetermined qualifications	acknowledgement of an organization's responsibility for or achievement of something.
	Must have Punishable if no license	Better to have	Ideal to have
Coverage	Usually, the whole facility E.g., the Blood Centre	Usually, a procedure of the facility E.g., H.I.V. testing	Usually, a part/whole of the facility E.g., H.L.A. laboratory of a Blood centre
Requirement	Compulsory	Voluntary	Voluntary
Authority	By the Government/law	Usually, private/ autonomous bodies	Usually, private/ autonomous bodies

The Drug and Cosmetic Act has 5 chapters (I to V). Each chapter has various sections (1 to 38). Each section may have subsections a, b, c, etc.

A **bill** is a proposal for a new law or a proposal to change an existing law significantly. When the parliament approves a bill, it becomes **Act/law**.

A **Schedule** is a part of a Bill or part of an Act. Bills may have several Schedules that appear after the main Clauses in the text. They are often used to spell out in more detail how the provisions of the Bill are to work in practice. If a Bill becomes an Act of Parliament, its Schedules become the Schedules of that Act.

1945: Drugs and Cosmetic Rules: contains provisions for the classification of drugs under given schedules and guidelines for the storage, sale, display and prescription of each schedule

1967: Central Govt. (Ministry of Health) enacted a separate provision in Schedule F Part XII B of Drugs & Cosmetics Rules. For blood bank operations, various requirements were included, such as Accommodation, Technical staff, equipment, etc. State Drugs Controllers were authorized to issue the licences for blood banks. The standards for 'Whole Human Blood' was prescribed in Indian Pharmacopoeia.

1989: Made the test H.I.V. 1&2 antibodies of Whole Human Blood as a mandatory requirement before transfusion

1992-93: Drugs Controller General (India) was vested with the power of the Central Licence Approving Authority (C.L.A.A.) to approve the licence of Blood and Blood Products

1999: blood bank legislation has been extensively revised to include Good Manufacturing Practices, Standard Operating procedures, validation of equipment, etc.

2020-Mar-18: Amendment in Part X B & Part XII B pertaining to Blood centre and Blood components,

Section 3(b) of Chapter I of D&C	Blood is Drug
Part X-B Rules 122F to 122P	various procedures of – making applications by a blood bank, – fees to be paid for grant/renewal of licence by the applicant – conditions of the licence to be followed by the applicant after grant/renewal
Schedule F Part XII B	Requirements such as Accommodation, Technical staff, equipment, etc.
Schedule 'C' of the D & C Rules	Whole human blood is included in the Indian Pharmacopoeia

	Application (for Grant and Renewal under rule 122F)	Licence (under rule 122G)	Renewal (under rule 122G) H, I, P
Blood and Blood Components	Form 27-C	Form 28-C	Form 26-G
Blood products	Form 27-E	Form 28-E	Form 26-I
Umbilical Cord Blood stem cells	Form 27-F	Form 28-F	Form 26-J

License Fee (Rs/-)	6000/-
Inspection Fee (Rs/-)	1500/- (after that, 1500/- for every inspection)
License duplicate copy fee (Rs/-)	1000/-
Repeat application after rejection	250/- (if within 6 months)
For additional product	300/- for each product
For renewal (within 6 months after expiry)	1000/- for every month of delay

5 'S' of Blood Transfusion Service (The regulatory authority looks into):

Space: Building and accommodation

Staff: Doctors, technicians, nursing staff, social workers and counsellors, the housekeeping staff

Storage: Equipments for storage and space

System: Quality management, Hierarchy

Stability: The management and their credentials, support for camps, and hospitals for utilising the services of the blood centre

Steps in the blood bank licensing process
1. Application in form 27-C and fees by individual/Institution (called the Licensee)
2. Application scrutiny- State Drug Controller (DC) and S.B.T.C.
3. No Objection Certificate for grant of license by State Blood Transfusion Council S.B.T.C. after inspection
4. Joint inspection of the blood bank by the State and Central inspection team
5. Recommendation to Central Licensing Approving Authority (C.L.A.A.)
6. Grant of License

Section VI

Concluding Residency

THESIS SUBMISSION

37.1 HOW TO WRITE UP A THESIS?

Section	What to write...?
Introduction	Why did I pursue this study/topic?
Methodology	What did I do /How did I pursue the study?
Results	What did I find in the study?
Discussion	What do the findings of the study mean? What would be the implications of the results?
Conclusion	Decisions made after considering the inference and interpretation of the observations in the study
References	Enough details to identify and locate the citations

Introduction

Aims and objective:

This study aims to...

This study explores...

This study applies to...

Others: surveys, questions, highlights, outlines, features, investigate

Review of literature:

Objective - To make sure how well the student understands the research topic and writes up in his own words what is already known about the topic that he is planning his thesis on.

What to write?

A critical review of the literature available on the topic with their strengths and limitations.

How to write?

Let us take this example,

1. Write the title of your study.

   "Comparison of the effect of Irradiation on biochemical parameters of PRBCs stored in SAGM versus those stored in CPDA at the end of 4 weeks: A prospective experimental study."

2. Note down the keywords:

   Irradiation and its effects, Biochemical parameters, PRBC storage, SAGM, CPDA

3. So first, write about the irradiation:

   a. What it is,
   b. How is it done,
   c. Why is it done?

4. Then, write about the different effects of Irradiation specialities of how and whys of their effects.
5. Then write about various storage solutions for RBC preservation, how they are different, the methods available, and their effects.
6. Write about the various biochemical alterations during storage and their alteration by irradiation, factors, and mechanisms involved.
7. Then write about the studies, if similar ones are done in different parts, starting with the global studies, studies in the country, or similar locality.
8. Discuss the limitations or gaps in those studies. (bullet or points)

Elements to include in the Literature review					
Who	When	Where	How	What	Why
Authors	Year	Geographic area	Methodology	Results	Explanation (Discussion)

"Your review of the literature is ready." It usually would be **the most extended section** of your thesis, about **10-20 pages,** but more if it is imperative. Make sure you **do not copy verbatim**; read the articles, close them, and try to write about them on your own. If something is unavoidable and imperative to reproduce verbatim, **then include it in quotes and reference them appropriately.**

6 C's of a Good Literature Review
Concise: synthesis of a broad collection of literature
Clear: a rigorous collection of data
Critical: reflective and evaluative analysis
Convincing: appealing
Contributive: redundant/repetitive stuff to be removed
Comprehensive: include the recent most as well as those with diverse findings

How to do a literature search?

- ❖ Identify your sources: Journals (Primary), abstracting indices (Pubmed, Google Scholar, EMBASE, etc.), textbooks, and grey literature (unpublished resources like previous thesis, etc.)
- ❖ Search by keywords of the topic you are looking at. Try alternate words/acronyms, MeSH terms, singular/plurals

<table>
<tr><td>

How to avoid Plagiarism?

- Whenever you use another person's opinion, idea or theory- give a reference
- When you verbatim copy quotes or definitions, quote-unquote them
- Always read the article about the one you are writing, close it, try to write about it using your own words/paraphrase them, and take notes. [TRY TO READ THE WHOLE THING, DO NOT READ PIECEMEAL AND START WRTINIG]
- Use a plagiarism checker if you have access. Grammarly, iThenticate, Plagiarism checker, Urkund, etc
- Use relevant synonyms instead of phrases used by the original authors. ADD OR DELETE WORDS WHICH WOULD NOT GROSSLY ALTER THE MEANING

</td></tr>
</table>

Results:

- ❖ Present it in a logical sequence in the text, tables, and illustrations (But not the same thing in all the ways- avoid repetition)
- ❖ A minimal amount of data like a single number or very few categories like gender differentiation can just be mentioned in the text form
- ❖ Tables: Should have a title, column, and row headings. Units to be written for measures (gms, meters, %, etc.)—footnotes for details that cannot be included in the title. Write the summary statistics like p-values, CI, etc. Round up the numbers as much as possible and meaningful.

Discussion

- ❖ State the critical findings/results of your study
- ❖ Try to give a possible scientific and logical explanation for those findings and relate them to the research hypothesis
- ❖ Compare the results with other studies explaining as to why it was similar
- ❖ If they differ from other studies, try explaining why it could be so.
- ❖ Explain the strengths and weaknesses of your study
- ❖ State the conclusions
- ❖ Write about what implications the results could have and if they could be generalizable or not
- ❖ Write about the future directions for taking this study forward or doing it in a different way

References

A set of elements describing a document or a part of it that is sufficiently precise and detailed enough for a potential reader to identify and locate it.

What needs a reference?

> *"If you did not invent/create it and were not born knowing it- then you must reference it."*
>
> *-Faye Hicks*

Something which is common knowledge needs no reference. For example,

Irradiation is performed to prevent TA-GVHD. - **does not need a reference**

Irradiation leads to a series of biochemical changes, including .... -*needs a reference*

Generally, the **Vancouver style** is used for reference.

How to write references?

Articles from Journals:

Author1, Author2,.....up to 6 authors, et al. Title of the article. Journal name YYYY.Vol: Issue pages nn-nn.

Example: Bawazeer S, El-Telbany DFA, Al-Sawahli MM, Zayed G, Keed AAA, Abdelaziz AE, et al. Effect of nanostructured lipid carriers on transdermal delivery of tenoxicam in irradiated rats. Drug Deliv. 2020 Dec;27(1):1218-30

A section in a Book:

Chapter Author1, Author2,... et al. title of the chapter. In: Editor1, Editor 2... Title of the Book. Edition. Publisher; YYYY.pages (nn-nn)

Example: Eric AG, Edward LS, Alex BR. Transfusion-associated graft-versus-host disease.In: Toby LS. Rossi's Principles of Transfusion Medicine.5th ed: Wiley Blackwell, 1994. pg680-4

E-resources

Author1, Author2... Title of the article. Available from http://www............ Accessed on Month Date, YYYY.

Example: Cardigan R, New HV, Tinegate H, Thomas S. Washed red cells: theory and practice [published online ahead of print, 2020 Jul 7]. *Vox Sang.* 2020;10.1111/vox.12971. DOI:10.1111/vox.12971. Accessed on Aug 15, 2020

37.2 REFERENCE MANAGER

– Dr. Mohandoss M

A reference manager is a software package which helps researchers in performing three basic research steps:

1. Finding relevant literature
2. Allows to store papers and their bibliographic metadata in a personal database for later retrieval and writing
3. It allows researchers to insert citations and references in a chosen citation style when writing a text.

- Almost all the reference managers allow us to directly import from bibliographic databases through direct access from the reference manager and/or bookmarklets that import content from the web browser. References can also be imported from other reference managers or files in the BibTeX standard format with the help of import tools.
- Most reference managers provide tools for organizing the references into folders and subfolders. Few allow the inclusion of full-text papers in PDF format.
- They also offer tools for exporting citations and references into word processing programs by selecting relevant items from the database.

Digital Object Identifiers (DOIs) and Other Unique Identifiers

- Most journal articles are now uniquely identified by a digital object identifier (DOI).
- DOIs for journal articles are issued by CrossRef, a non-profit organization that has the most scholarly publishers as members. DOIs can also be used for other content like conference proceedings or book chapters.
- Other unique identifiers for scholarly content are the PubMed ID, PubMed Central ID, or the ArXiV ID. They make it much easier to handle bibliographic information

Citation styles and CSL (Citation Style Language)

- Citations can be formatted in different ways. The information to include (authors, title, journal, year, issue, pages), how to order and format this information, and reference these citations in the main text (e.g. by number or author/year).
- The publishers will look into unique identifiers that help them double-check the reference information against the database.
- Common styles are APA, MLA, Chicago, Vancouver
- As journals employ different reference styles, changing the citation style when a paper is resubmitted to another journal, the reference manager helps adjust to various citation styles, thereby reducing the time-consuming endeavour.

APA

Karafin, M. S., Blagg, L., Tobian, A. A. R., King, K. E., Ness, P. M., & Savage, W. J. (2012). ABO Antibody Titers are not Predictive of Hemolytic Reactions Due to Plasma Incompatible Platelet Transfusions. Transfusion, 52(10), 2087–2093. https://doi.org/10.1111/j.1537-2995.2012.03574.x

Vancouver

Karafin MS, Blagg L, Tobian AAR, King KE, Ness PM, Savage WJ. ABO Antibody Titers are not Predictive of Hemolytic Reactions Due to Plasma Incompatible Platelet Transfusions. Transfusion 2012;52:2087–93. doi:10.1111/j.1537-2995.2012.03574.x.

Nature

Karafin, M. S. *et al.* ABO Antibody Titers are not Predictive of Hemolytic Reactions Due to Plasma Incompatible Platelet Transfusions. *Transfusion* 52, 2087–2093 (2012).

Modern language association (MLA)

Karafin, Mathew S., et al. "ABO Antibody Titers Are Not Predictive of Hemolytic Reactions Due to Plasma Incompatible Platelet Transfusions." *Transfusion*, vol. 52, no. 10, 2012, pp. 2087–93, doi:10.1111/j.1537-2995.2012.03574.x.

Chicago manual of style

Karafin, Mathew S., Lorraine Blagg, Aaron A. R. Tobian, Karen E. King, Paul M. Ness, and William J. Savage. 2012. "ABO Antibody Titers Are Not Predictive of Hemolytic Reactions Due to Plasma Incompatible Platelet Transfusions." *Transfusion* 52 (10): 2087–93. https://doi.org/10.1111/j.1537-2995.2012.03574.x.

Reference Management Tools

Among the available reference managers, a few popular tools are described below.

EndNote

EndNote is a commercial reference management software that allows the import of bibliographic databases and full text. EndNote provides plugins for both Microsoft Word and OpenOffice. References can be exported to BibTeX. EndNote Web also provides the functionality for collaboration with other users. Users can even give group members read/write access to their references and import references from other people's libraries.

Mendeley

Mendeley, strength lies in its networking and collaborative features and provides facilities for efficiently managing PDF files. It offers both an offline and a web version with synchronized bibliographic information, allowing access from several systems and collaboration with other users. PDF files can be imported into Mendeley, and metadata such as authors, titles, and journals can be automatically extracted. It is possible to do a full-text search, highlight text in PDFs, and add sticky notes. Mendeley is free to use.

Zotero

Zotero, a popular open-source reference manager, offers Standalone functionality but runs as a separate program. Zotero also includes a hosted version to synchronize references across devices and share them in private or public groups. Zotero allows users to collect and organize various web sources such as citations, full-texts, web pages, images and audio files directly in the browser.

Papers

Papers is a commercial reference management software; its strength is that it is excellent in handling PDF documents (including metadata extraction) and has a polished user interface, whereas the collaborative features are less developed than in some other products. Papers use the Citation Style Language and provide a word processor plugin.

Others are JabRef, CiteULike, RefWorks, Citavi

LOGBOOK

A logbook is a verified record of the learner's progression, documenting the acquisition of the requisite knowledge, skills, attitude and/ or competencies.

A vital aspect of the new Competency-Based PG Curriculum is the emphasis on acquiring competencies as a requisite for progression in the course. The student's active learning process and his/her progression to the achievement of competencies / predetermined tasks need to be documented. A record of completed activities and competencies is necessary to ensure that the learner has acquired the key competencies. The logbook forms an integral part of the formative/ continuous assessment program. Generally, Institutions have their process and records based on local requirements incorporating the significant elements. This chapter will aid as a guide and provide tips to maintain a useful log.

Activity refers to a predefined task performed by learners that contributes to achieving objectives or competencies.

Remedial is a planned activity to correct deficiencies that prevent a learner from achieving an intended outcome.

Feedback is a formal active interaction performed after an observed activity (or activities) intended to facilitate positive change, growth and improvement of the learner through a guided reflection of the activity (ies) performed.

Whether logbooks are maintained in print or electronic format is left to the discretion of individual institutions.

General Components of a logbook:

The Faculty will determine the level of achievement or criteria that will determine satisfactory (meets expectations) completion of the activity

- Reflections can include how confident you were in performing a skill. Mention additional skills you need to gain, what actions you will take to learn new skills when completing them, what support and resources are required and how you will measure your progress. Furthermore, try to incorporate a learning plan.

- Narrative and creative writing experiences, participation, and presentations in group activities such as seminars, symposia etc., with moderator comments.
- Training conducted and interdepartmental activities
- Collected clinical or laboratory experiences, predetermined patient or community interactions such as field visits may also be included
- Competencies acquired in the postgraduate orientation classes, research methodology, computer skills, and other introductory courses etc., should be recorded
- All the competencies of the peripheral/allied specialities postings and external posting (outside the institute) should be captured
- Conferences/workshops attended, papers presented as posters or oral. Other achievements, if any.
- Publications that were made during the residency.
- Summary of the thesis.
- Records of periodic/internal assessments
- Psychomotor and Communication skills should be recorded year-wise.

Kirkpatrick's framework is often used in evaluating interventions in medical education. This framework suggests that a training program may be evaluated according to four levels. You can interpret or reflect based on the following stages as part of learning something new

1. Reaction: participants' opinions of the intervention.
2. Learning: learning outcomes.
3. Behaviour: behavioural change that happened as a result of acquiring the skill/competency
4. Results: the final result of the intervention

Let us take an example of, say, group counselling for donors. In the participants' opinion, you can write as to what would work or not, the barriers/facilitating factors etc. Behavioural changes that make you feel freer and more comfortable speaking to people. The final result of the intervention is that you can individually undertake counselling/motivation sessions for the donors.

The general schema of the logbook looks as follows: (As per MCI guidelines)

Sample template:

Sl No	Competency	Activity	Date completed	Rating	Decision	Signature	Feedback
1	Cognitive /Psychomotor /Counselling /Affective /Clinical /Organisational /diagnostic etc			Below expectations(B) Meets expectations(M) Exceeds expectations (E) OR Numerical Scores	Completed (C) To be Repeated (R) Remedial actions (Re)		

Sl No	Activity	The requisite number of Procedures (minimum)
Screening room		
1	Demonstrate proficiency in the selection of whole blood donors	500
2	Demonstrate proficiency in the selection of apheresis donors	25
Phlebotomy Room		
1	Demonstrate proficiency in the collection of whole blood collection	500
2	Demonstrate proficiency in evaluating and managing adverse reactions associated with blood donation/phlebotomy	25
3	Demonstrate knowledge and proficiency in therapeutic phlebotomy cases	5
Organisation skills and Quality Assurance		
1	Demonstrate proficiency in the organisation of outdoor blood donation camps and demonstrate skills to motivate blood donors/ organisers	10
2	Demonstrate proficiency in preparing SOP for the department.	5
3	Root cause analysis (RCA) and Corrective and Preventive Action (CAPA) as and when required	5
Component Laboratory		
1	Demonstrate proficiency in preparation of components as per department SOP – PRBCs, FFP, Platelet concentrate - Cryoprecipitate	500 each 25
2	Demonstrate proficiency in performing quality control tests on blood components such as PRBC, FFP, Platelets, Cryoprecipitate	25 each
Apheresis		
1	Demonstrate proficiency in the selection of apheresis machines and blood donors and be able to obtain apheresis product	25
TTI Laboratory		
1	Demonstrate proficiency in performing, interpreting, and documentation of blood donor screening tests for TTIs as per departmental SOP	500
2	Demonstrate proficiency in the preparation and interpretation of the LJ Chart	5
3	Demonstrate proficiency in Gram staining of biological fluids	10
Pretransfusion Laboratory		

1	Demonstrate proficiency in performing ABO/Rh grouping in donor/patient samples using department SOP	500
2	Demonstrate proficiency in performing crossmatches as per department SOP	50
3	Demonstrate proficiency in evaluating and recommending treatment plans for transfusion reactions	10
Immunohematology Laboratory		
1	DAT	50
2	IAT	50
3	Red cell antibody detection and identification	25
4	Titration of Anti D and Anti A, and Anti B	25
5	Elution	25
6	Demonstrate proficiency in the blood unit selection for a patient with AIHA.	5
7	Demonstrate proficiency in cryopreservation of reagent red cells	5

Peripheral postings

Department/ Centre	Duration (From ...to...)	Learning objectives	Signature	Feedback/ Remarks

Here are a few tips and points to remember:

- Generally, case studies on at least ten interesting cases (on component support, Immunohematology workup, biosafety issue, error management, emergency management etc.)
- Fill in the entries in the **logbook daily** and **not at the end** of the posting.
- Get the entries in the logbook verified by the Faculty in charge regularly and not keep it till the end of the course.
- Mention whether you observed or performed and the number of the activities.
- Ask your colleagues to observe and assist or correct you.
- Note that the logbook is evaluated/taken into consideration at the time of the Exit Exam.

Electronic Portfolios (E-Portfolios) in Postgraduate Medical Education

Chapter 39

– Dr. Zayapragassarazan

Documentation and assessment of self-directed learning, reflection and competency are a must in the current era of education and curriculum. With the adaptation of competency-based assessments and frameworks such as milestones and entrustable professional activities, portfolios have become a valuable tool in postgraduate medical education. In postgraduate medical education and training, portfolios are increasingly used as an assessment tool, documentation of competence, a database of procedure experience, and for revalidation purposes. With the advent of online learning, electronic portfolios (e-portfolios) have become popular in educational settings.

Portfolio – Meaning

A portfolio is a – "purposeful collection of student work that exhibits the student's efforts, progress and achievements in one or more areas." It is an assemblage of evidence demonstrating the continuing acquisition of skills, knowledge, attitudes, understanding and achievements. It is both retrospective and prospective and reflects the current stage of development and activity of the individual. Portfolios are used for multiple purposes, including assessment, providing students with feedback, career planning, and repository of student work and achievement. The main advantage of portfolios is that they host the fundamental elements needed to support the Competency-Based Medical Education assessment. These fundamental elements being flexibility, learner-centeredness, ease of communication between learners and teachers, learner engagement, assessment of progress over time and the platform to plan learning goals.

Conventional portfolio Vs e-portfolio

The portfolio encourages reflection and self-evaluation and collects evidence of learning and experiences as an educational tool. Portfolios can be either physical (paper-based) or electronic. Conventional portfolios are paper-based and are not much appreciated in the current scenario of digitalisation. Conventional portfolios are limited in their scope for collecting the learning evidence than electronic portfolios (e-portfolios). Electronic portfolios (e-portfolios) have become a popular alternative to paper-based portfolios because they offer the opportunity to review, communicate and provide feedback. An e-portfolio is a digitised collection of authentic and diverse evidence drawn from a more extensive archive constituting what a person has learned over time. It is an electronic format that students can use to record their goals, work, and achievements, reflect on their learning, share their learning and receive feedback and feedforward. An e-portfolio is also known as a digital, online, or web-based portfolio that collects electronic resources assembled and managed by a user on a digital platform or web. An e-portfolio can have content guidelines like a regular portfolio with the advantage that electronic files, multimedia, text, images, blog entries and hyperlinks can be attached. Another advantage of e-portfolios is that they can be seen from any computer or electronic device. Due to their easy access, the student and the teacher are more likely to use its content to achieve the expected reflective learning.

The primary use of conventional portfolios is for summative and formative assessment purposes. A summative portfolio can evaluate the student's final learning, and a formative portfolio can guide the student through the learning process and inform about their progress in learning or achievement of the levels of competencies. Furthermore, a wide range of credentials or learning evidence can be added to e-portfolios, and they are easily accessible and more acceptable to teachers and students. Given these merits, educators worldwide have recognised the e-portfolio as a tool that gathers evidence of knowledge, abilities, attitudes and values and have made recommendations on starting and maintaining an e-portfolio in medical residencies.

Salient features of the e-portfolio framework

A good ePortfolio is both about being a product and a process. Since it hosts a digital collection of artefacts, it is considered a product or a learning resource. The following attributes make any educational e-portfolio serve its purpose and achieve the stated goals.

The authenticity of the learning evidence: The learning evidence collected by the learners should be from an undisputed origin, not a copy of something. Students should show their responsibility for their learning by organising their e-portfolios and reflecting on their learning processes and findings.

Controllable and personalised: Students should organise their learning evidence collected by them, reflect on and assess their learning processes, and make necessary changes to their e-portfolios according to their reflections.

Communicative and interactive: e-portfolios should facilitate students' communication and interaction with their peers and teachers to improve their learning.

Dynamic in nature: The framework will facilitate the learners to update and organise their collection and selection of artefacts, the self-assessment and self-reflection of their learning process and improvement made according to self-assessment and self-reflection. All these will make an e-portfolio a dynamic one.

Reflect competency development: The portfolio reflects the students' competency development with reference to their curricular objectives and professional roles.

Integrative: e-portfolios facilitate creating connections between students' life and academic work.

Multipurpose in use, Multi-sourced: it provides students with feedback on their learning, teachers with the assessment of students' performances, and institutions with the opportunity to assess their programs, courses, or departments.

Motivational: it gives students ownership of their learning and improves their skills.

Reflective: e-portfolios require reflection on one's learning, so students can self-reflect and assess their learning processes via e-portfolios.

Evaluative in nature: it is objectively structured for assessment. Portfolios allow for authentic formative, structured and criterion-based evaluation and provide the opportunity for self-reflection by students.

e-portfolio tools

Many specialised and advanced programs for e-portfolios are available on the internet, and some of these programs need special training and come at a price in most cases. One of the disadvantages of free online programs is the low amount of storage. This can be overcome by uploading information as links from DropBox, YouTube, SlideShare, Google Drive, Blogs, etc. Some of the popular online platforms available for teachers and students to build their e-portfolios are listed below:

- *WordPress* is easy to use, popular, and versatile. WordPress is a free, open-source blogging tool and content management system that runs on a web hosting service that may be used as an e-Portfolio system. It is a great platform and a gateway for students to create their online portfolios.
- Blogging on blogger.com is the easiest to use, with excellent privacy control and comes with widgets. Blogger is free and available in 60 languages, including Indian regional languages, apart from English.
- *Mahara* is an online room with a pre-established portfolio design that can accommodate the contents and support the learning process. It requires training and is free to use. It supports translation into different languages using different packs.
- *Edublogs* is a student-centric learning platform that includes course blogs, e-portfolios, and managing student projects. Edublogs provides a stable, secure and hassle-free WordPress-based learning network for teachers and students. Education Blogging on edublogs.org is a free basic service, and other services require a fee.
- *Google sites* offer web pages with more control and organisation of information, privacy management, and ease of use.
- *Wikispaces* is another useful program for various learning activities, including the electronic portfolio.
- *Weebly* offers students a platform to create unique websites that will serve as effective digital portfolios. Students can build a professional website without technical knowledge with a simple drag-and-drop feature and responsive themes. It is free with limited features.
- *Evernote:* It is a cross-platform tool designed to take notes, organise content and archive it. It serves as an effective portfolio builder as it empowers students to write down notes, take photos, upload content, record audio, and tag items with specific keywords. The basic version of Evernote is free and limits to adding 60 MB of notes a month.

- *Foliospaces* is a free e-portfolio platform. It can be used as a personal space for learners to compile their academic works and evidence.
- *Pathbrite* helps to show your work digitally through an e-portfolio.

Section	Requirement	Paper-based Evidence	E-based Evidence
1	*Introduction:* Objectives and purpose of the portfolio and the scope and authenticity.	Printed series of pages.	Document attachment or hyperlink
2	*Learning outcomes:* List of learning outcomes that will be addressed and available for assessment. Learning outcomes based on Goals, Roles and Competencies by National Medical Commission.	Printed series of pages that highlights what was expected in the portfolio for each outcome.	Document attachment or hyperlink. A dashboard can also inform the user of what was submitted and what was expected.
3	*Learning plans and reflections on learning:* Each candidate is required to submit learning plans and reflections on their learning per month/posting in a section	Completed template and assessment from the supervisor, which could be handwritten or typed and inserted into the file.	Learning plans are revised through a series of electronic iterations. The supervisor approves the final version. Reflections on learning submitted via template and assessed by the supervisor
4	*Participation in educational sessions:* Includes a minimum prescribed hours/year and a variety of learning conversations such as: A: Clinical care B: Communication skills C: Team and leadership D: Teaching and training others E: Professionalism and Ethics F: Lifelong learning G: Others	Date, type of learning conversation, duration in hours and description filled in on a printed form and signed off by the supervisor.	Filled in online templates and approved by supervisor.

5	*Observations by the supervisor of consultations, procedures and teaching sessions:* A minimum of observations per year as decided by the institute	Multiple copies of the observation tools are included in the portfolio for use by the supervisor.	Filled in online templates and approved by supervisor. PDF copies can be made available for printing or sent via e-mail and filled out by hand if the supervisor does not have access to the portfolio.
6	*Written assignments:* A minimum of assignments per year. Completed assignments to be marked by the supervisor and added to the portfolio.	Assignments printed out and added to file.	Assignments are uploaded and validated by the supervisor.
7	*Logbook:* Consists of a list of core clinical skills and professional skills that needs to be acquired during the training programme and needs assessment at the end of each section postings A: Only theory B: Seen or have had demonstrated C: Apply/Perform under supervision D: Independent performance E: Taught others	Printed series of pages, each skill needs to be assigned an A, B, C or D, discussed/assessed by the supervisor, and signed with comments and date.	The online template of the logbook for each domain and each domain needs to be discussed and validated by the supervisor separately. A tally of individual procedures performed can also be added.
8	*Certification of essential skills:* A certificate of training in Bio-statistics, computers, medical ethics, leadership qualities, cost-effectiveness, preparation of reagents, handling equipments, educational technology etc., that are requirements to appear for the final examination.	Certificates can be added to the portfolio.	Certificates can be scanned and uploaded as a file.

9	*Self-directed learning:* MOOC courses, Distance Education Courses, Participation in Conferences, scientific presentations, publications, workshops, lectures, etc., paper and poster presentations.	Proof can be inserted in this section of the file.	Proof can be scanned and uploaded as a file.
10	*End of year assessment:* Portfolio Assessment Tool (PAT)	The assessor must examine the whole portfolio and extract the data needed to complete the assessment.	The assessor views the automatically collated scores in the template and adds a final score and any feedback.

THE ROAD AFTER POST-GRADUATION IN TRANSFUSION MEDICINE

– Dr. Puneeth Jain

MD/DNB in Immunohematology and Blood Transfusion or MD/DNB in Transfusion Medicine. All of us have been quite intrigued by the scope of this branch in the already vast field of medicine. Many times, a question is posed in front of the postgraduates to assess whether this branch intends to create just glorified blood bank specialists with an MD degree looking after a blood bank or if there is much more to it than just managing a blood bank.

It is a million-dollar question for people to make career choices and live with them. Many readers would have pondered this when choosing this branch or starting their specialist training. Some of us would still be pondering over it.

The history and birth of this broad speciality in India relate to a felt need experienced by the senior doctors/key opinion leaders (KOL) practising this field, wherein they envisaged a specialist qualification to train a cadre of doctors who can uplift the blood bank and bring in new ideas and technology in the existing domain to make it increasingly safe, affordable and quality rich for patients. Thus, grooming a blood bank into a department of Transfusion Medicine. While doing this would also help create and nurture a pool of specialist doctors who can take up important positions in policymaking with national and international bodies. However, time and again, we have seen that the scope of this field is far greater than the envisioned felt need. It depends on an individual to chart their path. It depends on how far one plans to look and take steps to fulfil it. It depends on what limits one has self-imposed on themselves.

The scope of transfusion medicine ranges from core clinical application to laboratory work and cutting-edge research. However, it is limited by the curriculum as it is a vast domain to cover in a three years training period. After a post-graduation in Transfusion medicine, people can chart their path depending on their liking. The idea of the training in this speciality is to impart the student with knowledge and experience, which can help them grow in the field and help the field grow with them. The knowledge gained can also help them decide on their prospects.

The path one chooses for the future will usually depend on the personal interest in the field, the passion for bench or bedside work, and the interest in trying new things (travelling uncharted territories). Some people would like to change the branch, as the case may be. They may choose to restart their journey into other clinical branches or move into core haematology, which encompasses transfusion medicine in most countries.

A few would like to gain additional qualifications and expertise to excel in the existing scope and domain of transfusion medicine permitted in our country. This can help them grow and bring more value to the institutes they decide to work for. A few specialists would want to get into pure research in the field of stem cells or immunology. An overwhelming majority would like to grow as faculty in teaching and training institutes and help more students realize their dream of becoming specialists in Transfusion Medicine.

Through this chapter, we would like to share a glimpse of what lies ahead after post-graduation in India and abroad for the PGs in Transfusion Medicine. Most of the description is based on my personal experiences

We have divided the avenues as follows:

India:

1.   Teaching faculty pathway
2.   Non-Teaching faculty pathway (Consultant)
3.   Fellowships
4.   Post-Doctoral Certificate Courses
5.   Super-speciality
6.   Core Hematology
7.   Civil Services: Medical/Non-Medical
8.   Research

Abroad:

1.   Clinical Pathway
2.   Research (PhD)
3.   Master's
4.   Fellowships/ Observership

Opportunities in India

1.   Teaching faculty pathway (Tenure track Assistant Professor-> Associate Professor-> Professor)

     Post-MD, one can work towards a career portfolio for becoming a teaching faculty in medical colleges/ autonomous institutes. Currently, various types of colleges offer teaching posts for Transfusion Medicine

     These are

     - Institutes of National Importance (AIIMS, PGI, JIPMER, SCTIMST......)
     - Autonomous Institutes (TMH, SGPGI, RML, RCCs........)
     - State Government-run medical colleges
     - Private Management based Medical Colleges

The primary requisite for joining any of these places as a teaching faculty is by gaining 3 years of teaching/training experience in a recognized department as a senior resident/tutor. Experience gained during a fellow/PDCC course may be counted depending on the institutional policy. The requirement for joining Private Management and state Government-run medical colleges ranges from 1 year to 3-year post-MD experience as a senior resident/Tutor, depending on the state and local rules.

2. Non-Teaching pathway (Tenure track Clinical assistant-> Associate-> Junior consultant->Consultant/Senior Consultant)

    Post MD, if a person identifies as the one for the private sector and does not want to go for teaching and training faculty, then they may join as clinical associate/clinical assistant in private hospitals which look up to postgraduates of transfusion medicine to manage their departments. This can be considered a parallel to the teaching pathway in the private sector. Even in this pathway, there is a chance to enter into teaching by joining institutes which offer DNB training in Transfusion Medicine. After sufficient experience post-MD and reaching a consultant position, one can venture into the DNB training program at their institute.

3. Fellowships (Transfusion Medicine specific)

    Fellowships in different subsections of transfusion medicine are designed to impart clinical and benchwork experience to postgraduates who want to further their career in a particular specialism, for example, Apheresis, Component therapy, Immunohematology etc. These may be university-recognized or institution recognized. The fellowship duration is limited to one year in most places.

4. Post-doctoral certificate courses

    Like fellowships, these courses are designed to impart additional knowledge and specialism to a candidate. The duration of PDCC can range from one to two years, depending on the institute. These are usually universities or institutions recognized.

5. Super-specialty

    Currently, MD/DNB in Transfusion Medicine is recognized as a feeder qualification for DM Medical genetics. Postgraduates interested in genetics can opt for this branch for super-speciality.

6. Core Hematology

    Currently, MD in Transfusion Medicine is not recognized as a feeder qualification for DM Clinical Hematology. However, graduates interested in learning about haematology practice can opt for fellowship courses in haematology, hemato-oncology and bone marrow transplant. These fellowships are offered by institutes like CMC Vellore, AIIMS Bhubaneshwar and Malabar Cancer Centre. MD in Immunohematology and Transfusion Medicine is an essential qualification to enter these fellowships.

7. Civil Services

If one is within the age limit and is interested, they can opt for the union public service commission (UPSC) examination and try their luck with civil services. One can also try for medical services UPSC examination if they intend to go into central medical services.

8. Research

Few institutes offer research courses exclusively curated to domains relevant to transfusion medicine. National Institute on Immunohematology, Mumbai, PGI Chandigarh, offer research PhD and Postdoc positions in the domain of transfusion medicine. AIIMS New Delhi offers PhD in transplant immunology for those interested in immunogenetics or HLA. One can even apply for a faculty position in NIIH suitable for a clinical scientist. One of the feeder qualifications for the post of clinical scientist is MD IHBT.

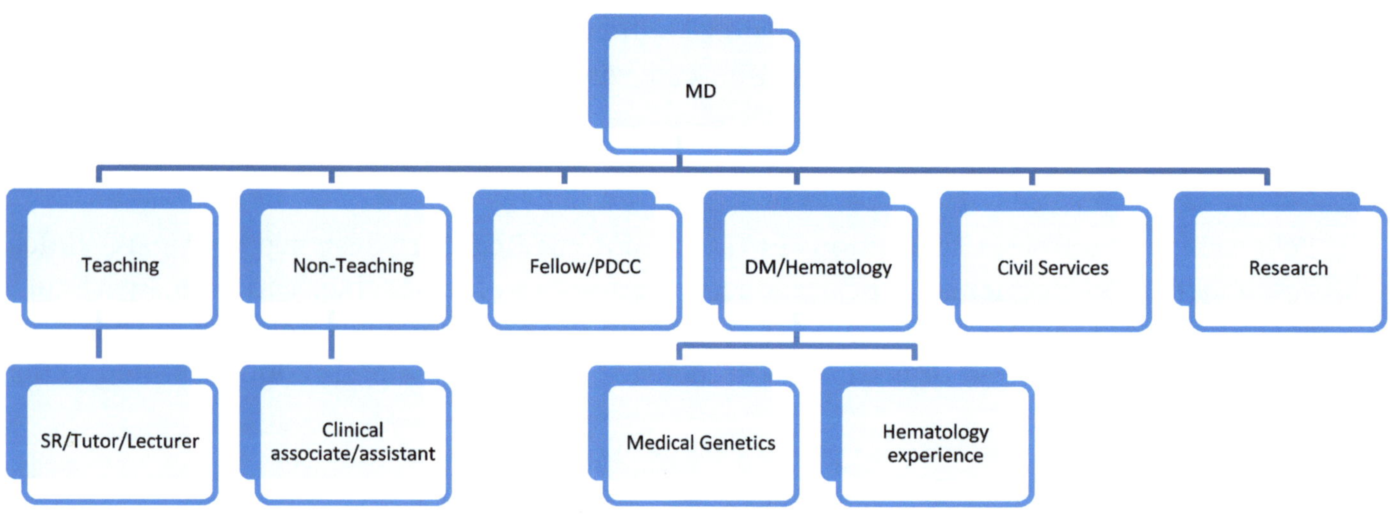

Opportunities for MD IHBT in India

Opportunities abroad

1. Clinical Pathway

MD/DNB IHBT is not recognized as a separate qualification in the US/UK/Ireland/Australia/ New Zealand/EU for the specialist registration pathway. Hence anyone intending to go to any of these countries will need to give a licensing exam as follows:

US: USMLE (Part 1 and 2)

UK: PLAB Part 1 and 2 OR MRCP Part 1, 2 and PACES

Australia/ New Zealand: Australian Medical Council (AMC) Part 1 and part 2

EU: It varies from country to country

Gulf countries: Apply for licensing exam/assessment. They recognize MD/DNB IHBT from India while giving specialist registration and full license to practice

For all the above, except in gulf countries, post-registration, one is considered an MBBS graduate with 3PGY (postgraduate years) experience. One can apply for the job based on this profile and even try to land a job in a country-specific training pathway.

E.g. In the UK, for practising Hematology, the following routes can be taken

a. PLAB 1 and 2 after/during MD IHBT→ GMC Registration with full license to practice →Foundation year 2 (competencies signed) →ACS/CC) (Acute care stem/ core training (2 years) → MRCP exam (part 1, part 2 and PACES) → Specialist training pathway (Hematology) for 5 years→ CCT completion→ Specialist registration (Hematology)→ Consultant in Hematology (and transfusion medicine)

   Total: 8-10 years

b. MRCP Part 1 and 2 and PACES (In India after or during MD final year)→ GMC Registration with full license to practice → FY/Trust grade/ HO posts (FY2 and CC competencies signed) for 1-2 years → Apply for specialist training pathway (no need to do ACS/CC posts)→ Specialist training pathway (Hematology) for 5 years→ CCT completion→ Specialist registration (Hematology)→ Consultant in Hematology (and transfusion medicine)

   Total: 7-8 years

A person can enter any other specialist training pathway after completing the MRCP (part 1, part 2 PACES) stage.

2. Research (PhD/ MD-PhD) pathway

   This pathway may seem to be interesting for those who are passionate about bench work and basic research. One can apply for a PhD post based on an MD IHBT degree and get into the research field in any country. The PhD course duration is 3-4 years in most countries, with a stipend paid in EU countries. In the UK, the PhD is paid. A tuition fee must be paid in the UK while pursuing a PhD. Funding for out-of-EU students is difficult, and there are not many options. Some scholarships (e.g. Commonwealth Scholarships) provide funding for pursuing a PhD in the UK. In the EU, there are no tuition fees for pursuing a PhD. There is a stipend available for PhD students in the UK and EU as per the norms fixed by the countries.

3. Master's (MSc or MRes) Courses

   These are one-year courses with a research project component which can be pursued post-PG to gain further knowledge in a particular specialism and may also serve as a baseline preparation for applying to a PhD. One year Master's course is offered in the UK. In the EU, the Master's duration is two years. Master's degree courses are paid courses with a tuition fee component. There is no stipend while pursuing a Master's course. However, many scholarships are available for pursuing a Master's course in the UK. These scholarships cover tuition fees and stipend to sustain living in these countries. The basic requirements for applying to these courses are graduation from the home country, an English language test and letters of recommendation.

4. Fellowships/ Observership

These can be paid/ funded fellowships for a duration ranging from a week to a couple of years. The fellow is attached to a hospital/ college with active involvement in learning and research. For clinical fellowships, the medical license of the host country is needed. Otherwise, the fellow will not be able to participate actively in clinical work. For research-based fellowships, many funding opportunities are available (e.g. Trialect.com)

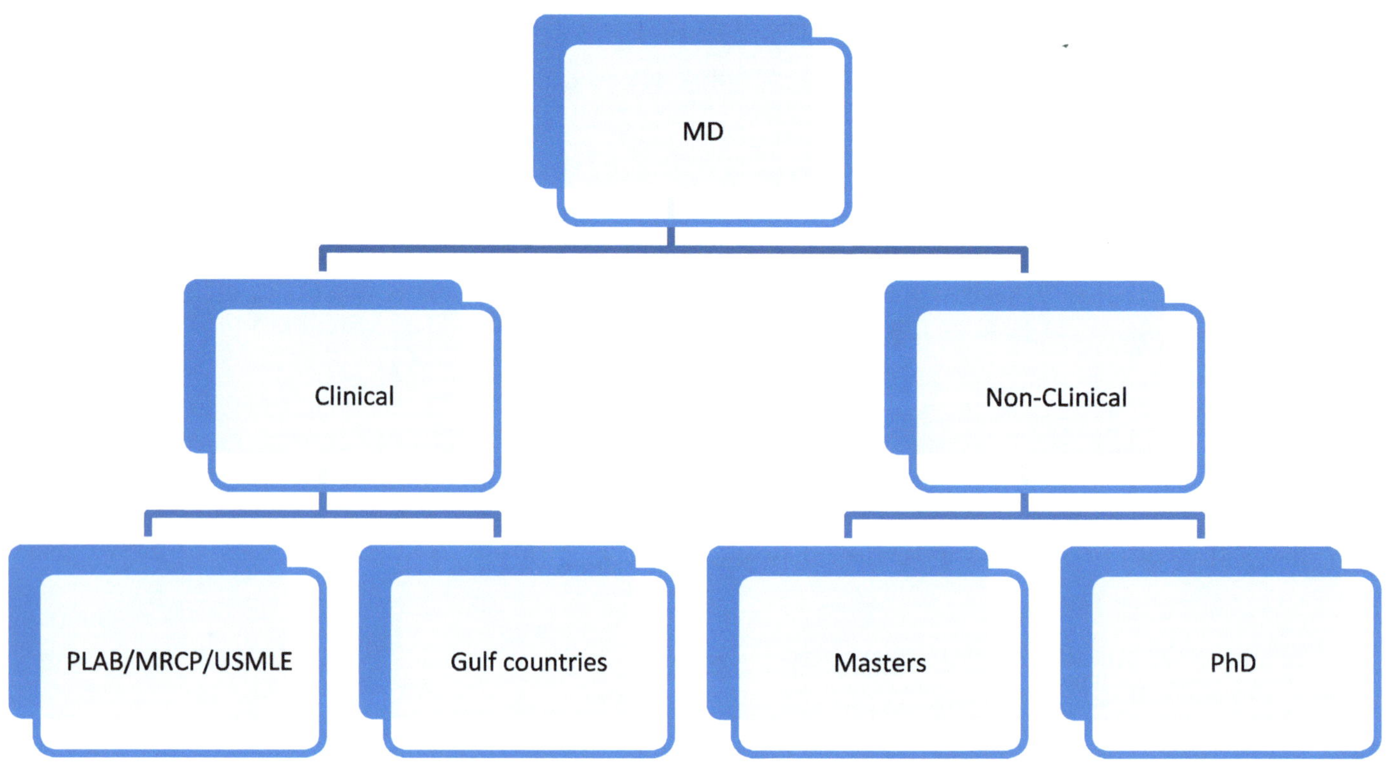

Opportunities for MD-IHBT outside India

Links for websites

1. https://www.chevening.org For Master's/Fellowship funding for UK courses
2. https://www.mhrd.gov.in For Commonwealth scholarship (for India chapter)
3. https://cscuk.fcdo.gov.uk/scholarships/commonwealth-shared-scholarships For commonwealth-shared scholarships across universities in the UK
4. https://www.daad.de/en/study-and-research-in-germany/scholarships For master's and PhD scholarships in Germany
5. https://www.gmc-uk.org General Medical Council Registration/ PLAB
6. https://www.mrcpuk.org For MRCP exam and registration
7. https://www.ielts.org For IELTS exam (English language)
8. https://www.ecfmg.org For ECFMG verification before PLAB and USMLE registration
9. https://www.usmle.org USMLE exams